Orthopaedics and Sports Medicine for Nurses

Common Problems in Management

Orthopaedics and Sports Medicine for Nurses

Common Problems in Management

EDITED BY

SHARON J. GATES, R.N., M.S.N., C.R.N.P., A.N.P.C.

Director, The Back Program
The Graduate Hospital
Clinical Instructor, Department of Nursing
College of Allied Health Sciences
Thomas Jefferson University
Philadelphia, Pennsylvania

PEKKA A. MOOAR, M.D.

Director, Delaware Valley Sports Medicine Center
Chief, Section of Sports Medicine
    and Orthopaedic Traumatology
Assistant Professor of Orthopaedic Surgery
The Medical College of Pennsylvania
Philadelphia, Pennsylvania

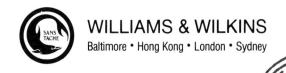

WILLIAMS & WILKINS
Baltimore • Hong Kong • London • Sydney

Editor: Susan M. Glover
Associate Editor: Marjorie Kidd Keating
Copy Editor: Mary E. Medland, Stephen Siegforth
Design: Saturn Graphics
Illustration Planning: Lorraine Wrzosek
Production: Raymond E. Reter

Accurate indications, adverse reactions, and dosage schedules for drugs are provided in this book, but it is possible that they may change. The reader is urged to review the package information data of the manufacturers of the medications mentioned.

The procedures in this book are based on the most current research and recommendations of responsible medical sources. The authors and publisher, however, disclaim responsibility for any adverse effects or consequences resulting from the misapplication or injudicious use of the material contained herein.

Printed in the United States of America

Library of Congress Cataloging-in-Publication Data

Orthopaedics and sports medicine for nurses.

  Includes bibliographies and index.
  1. Orthopedia.   2. Sports—Accidents and injuries.
3. Nursing.   I. Gates, Sharon J.   II. Mooar, Pekka A.
[DNLM: 1. Athletic Injuries—nursing.   2. Orthopedics—
nursing.   3. Sports Medicine.   WY 150 O77]
RD732.O775 1989   617'.3   88-33900
ISBN 0-683-03433-2

89 90 91 92 93
1 2 3 4 5 6 7 8 9 10

*To our families for their patience and understanding
during the preparation of this manuscript
Irving, Robert and Glenn
and
Sally, Ethan, Rebecca, and Sarah*

Foreword

Whether nurses care for adolescents, aging adults, or persons in their middle years, their encounters with problems of musculoskeletal injury and disease are likely to occur on a daily basis. People come to ambulatory care providers hoping for relief from pain or immobility; they seek sound information and useful advice. This manual is a response to a real need for cogent, focused guidelines to assist nurses in meeting such demands. Current trends toward more out-of-hospital care, the growing emphasis on self- and family management of chronic health problems at home, and the expanding field of sports medicine have all accelerated the need for such a text. Though orthopaedic problems are common across the life span, as this manual makes clear, the growing requirements of the elderly deserve special attention. Problems involving loss of mobility are among the three leading causes of nursing home admission. A clinical manual that focuses on ambulatory care needs will help nurses who practice in out-of-hospital settings to recognize, treat, and help prevent some of the most debilitating effects of aging and, perhaps, even avoid or postpone institutionalization.

The nurses and physicians who prepared this text are providing another service to clinicians and their patients. Their interdisciplinary approach to these complicated clinical problems speaks directly to the day-to-day concerns of practitioners. The different and complementary approaches of medicine and nursing are incorporated and merged. This innovative guide brings together relevant, significant orthopaedic content from both disciplines; it avoids the insularity of texts written solely for physicians or nurses. The clinician will find that information about relevant history, examination, laboratory diagnosis, and treatment of common orthopaedic problems is as easy to find and use as is content dealing with education of patients, adaptation to chronic illness, and prevention of sports injuries. Indeed, much of the manual emphasizes prevention and provides helpful aids to patient education and risk reduction. The juxtapositioning of this content with information on disease detection and treatment makes for a well-rounded, highly useful clinical work.

Joan E. Lynaugh, Ph.D., R.N.
Barbara Bates, M.D.
University of Pennsylvania
School of Nursing
Philadelphia, Pennsylvania

Preface

In 1983 we began to work together to develop a concept of collaborative practice in orthopaedics. We discovered that the collaboration between a nurse practitioner and an orthopaedic surgeon enhanced patient care through the merging of nursing and medical philosophies of care.

Our commitment to patient care through a collaborative practice model became the driving force behind the writing of this text. It is our hope that you, the reader, will find (as we have found) that practicing in a collaborative, complementary manner allows the patient to experience the uniqueness of both nursing and medicine. It is this collaboration that ultimately helps the patient to attain the best possible outcome.

In today's medical economic marketplace, the focus of patient care is shifting from the hospital to the community, and it is in this setting that nurses are being asked to manage efficiently and competently the care of patients. Each day nurses and nurse practitioners work in outpatient settings such as occupational health, primary care, secondary schools and colleges, and the emergency room, making clinical decisions that affect patient outcomes. These responsibilities speak to the necessity of the collaborative practice model.

This book utilizes the community health preventive model to direct patient care. The prevention concept has three levels in which nurses interact with patients: primary, secondary, and tertiary (Leavell et al., 1965). Primary prevention precedes dysfunction and has a twofold focus: (1) health promotion and (2) reduction of risks for illness. Primary intervention is aimed at educating a healthy population about adequate nutrition, exercise, and hygiene. Secondary prevention, which begins after dysfunction is recognized, includes the screening of individuals thought to be at high risk for illness, follow-up after early detection, and treatment for existing illness and disability. Tertiary prevention (rehabilitation) begins when the dysfunction has stabilized and interventions focus on restoration of function and the prevention and limitation of further disability.

This manual is written to guide nurses in the prevention and management of common orthopaedic and sports-related problems and to assist in the rehabilitation of patients with these problems. Where appropriate it contains a review of basic anatomy and function, techniques of physical examination, and specific health management guidelines, presented in a problem-oriented format. The early chapters focus on common age-related problems beginning with the adolescent and continuing through the older adult. The later chapters are oriented around specific regional problems. This book provides guidelines to answer the most frequently asked patient care questions regarding prevention, evaluation, treatment, and predicted outcome.

S.J.G.
P.A.M.

Acknowledgments

We gratefully acknowledge the assistance of many people without whom publication would not have been possible. We mention, in particular, Carol Hutelmyer, R.N., M.S.N., Vice-President of Patient Care, The Graduate Hospital, for providing an atmosphere conducive to the creation of the role of the nurse practitioner in collaborative practice, and for her support during formulation of this book; James E. Nixon, M.D., immediate past Chairman, Department of Orthopaedics, The Graduate Hospital, for his recognition and promotion of the role of the orthopaedic nurse practitioner; Suzanne Langner, R.N., Ph.D., G.N.P., Director of Nursing Research, The Graduate Hospital; and Amy Tuttle, R.D., B.S., Director of the Weight Management Program, The Health and Fitness Center of The Graduate Hospital, for their invaluable assistance in the critique of this book; The Graduate Hospital Administration for supporting The Back Program and for fostering an environment that permits creativity within nursing; to our manuscript typists, Regina Gibson, Susan Slavich, and Helen Schilinger for their commitment to this project; and lastly to Williams & Wilkins, especially Susan Glover, Nursing Editor, Linda Napora, Managing Editor, Marjorie Keating, Associate Editor, and Stephen Siegforth, Copyediting Supervisor.

Contributors

Jeffrey P. Bomze, M.D.
Sports Medicine Physician and
  Pediatrician
Human Performance Division
The Graduate Hospital
Human Performance and Sports
  Medicine Center
Wayne, Pennsylvania

**Tony Cook, R.N., M.S.N., F.N.P.C.,
G.N.P.C.**
Geriatric Nurse Practitioner
Carle Clinic Associates
Urbana, Illinois

Michael H. Cox, Ph.D.
Director, Human Performance Division
The Graduate Hospital
Human Performance and Sports
  Medicine Center
Wayne, Pennsylvania

**Sharon J. Gates, R.N., M.S.N.,
C.R.N.P., A.N.P.C.**
Director, The Back Program
The Graduate Hospital
Clinical Instructor, Department of
  Nursing, College of Allied Health
Thomas Jefferson University
Philadelphia, Pennsylvania

Harris Gellman, M.D.
Associate Professor of Orthopaedic
  Surgery
University of Southern California
Chief, Upper Extremity Clinic
Rancho Los Amigos Hospital
Los Angeles, California

**Joyce Lederman Lichtenstein, R.N.,
M.S.N.**
Program Coordinator, Department of
  Educational Services
Durham County General Hospital
Durham, North Carolina

Wendy W. McBrair, R.N., B.S.N.
Arthritis Clinical Nurse Specialist
Stretch Center for Arthritis Treatment
Arthritis Unit, West Jersey Hospital
Marlton Division
Marlton, New Jersey

**Lynn McCullough, R.N., M.S.N.,
P.N.P.C., O.N.C.**
Arkansas Spine Center
Little Rock, Arkansas

Daniel S. Miles, Ph.D.
Assistant Director, Human Performance
  Division
The Graduate Hospital
Human Performance and Sports
  Medicine Center
Wayne, Pennsylvania

Pekka A. Mooar, M.D.
Assistant Professor of Orthopaedic
  Surgery
Chief, Section of Sports Medicine and
  Orthopaedic Traumatology
Medical College of Pennsylvania
Director, Delaware Valley Sports
  Medicine Center
Philadelphia, Pennsylvania

James E. Nixon, M.D.
Clinical Professor of Orthopaedic Surgery
University of Pennsylvania School of
  Medicine
Immediate Past Chairman, Department
  of Orthopaedics
The Graduate Hospital
Philadelphia, Pennsylvania

Sally Pullman-Mooar, M.D.
Clinical Research Associate
University of Pennsylvania
Stretch Center for Arthritis Treatment
Arthritis Unit, West Jersey Hospital
Marlton Division
Marlton, New Jersey

Susan W. Salmond, R.N., Ed.D.
Assistant Professor of Nursing
Kean College
New Jersey

William H. Simon, M.D., F.A.C.S.
Clinical Associate Professor of
    Orthopaedic Surgery
University of Pennsylvania School of
    Medicine
Philadelphia, Pennsylvania

**Maryann Curran Tawa, R.N., M.S.N.,
    A.N.P.C.**
Department of Ambulatory Nursing,
    Emergency Services and Primary Care
Brigham and Women's Hospital
Boston, Massachusetts

Contents

chapter 1

Physical Fitness and Its Relation to Orthopaedics and Sports Medicine

MICHAEL H. COX, Ph.D.
DANIEL S. MILES, Ph.D.
JEFFREY P. BOMZE, M.D.

The human body is composed of a unique system of levers (bones) and pulleys (muscles). This anatomical arrangement allows for locomotion and exceptional mobility for human beings. Moreover, the good news is that the human body becomes more efficient with increased use of the musculoskeletal system. In fact, upon closer examination, it is apparent that the major organs of the body (e.g., the heart, lungs, etc.) have been designed to service the exercising body. The bad news is that with disuse, the body quickly becomes an inefficient organism.

Unfortunately, industrialization and technological advances in the Western world have decreased the individual physical demands once needed to sustain a day of work. Paralleling the industrial modernization have been associated increases in the diseases of disuse. In particular, a sedentary life-style has been shown to be related to certain musculoskeletal disorders, low back pain, osteoporosis, certain cancers, and coronary heart disease (CHD). Consequently, in societies dominated by inactivity, the prevalence of functional disabilities can become a serious public health issue in both economic and humanistic terms.

BODY FUNCTION AND EXERCISE TRAINING

Human physiology is such that the body adapts and improves with training. Furthermore, the beneficial effects of training can be realized at any age (Table 1.1). The physiological consequences of training include: (1) Improvements occur in the efficiency of the cardiovascular system. These cardiovascular responses are mediated by an increase in heart size, accompanied by larger stroke volumes at rest and during exercise, as well as an increase in maximal cardiac output. Blood volume also increases as an outcome of aerobic training, enhancing the oxygen delivery capacity of the cardiovascular system. Resting heart rate and exercise heart rate at submaximal workloads decrease as a result of cardiovascular endurance training. (2) Specific cellular changes take place in the muscle as a result of training. An increase in both the size and number of mitochondria, enabling muscle cells to extract and utilize oxygen more efficiently, is a well documented training response. Trained muscles also exhibit an improved ability to oxidize both fat and carbohydrate, which is of extreme importance in prolonged ex-

1

Table 1.1
Physiologic Adaptations as a Result of Endurance Training

	Rest	Submaximal Exercise	Maximal Exercise
Heart rate	Decrease	Decrease	Decrease
Stroke volume	Increase	Increase	Increase
Cardiac output	No change	No change	Increase
Aerobic power	No change	No change	Increase
a-$\bar{v}O_2$ difference	No change	Increase	Increase
Lactic acid	No change	Decrease	Increase
Muscle blood flow	No change	Decrease	Increase
Systolic blood pressure	Decrease	Decrease	No change
Diastolic blood pressure	Decrease	Decrease	No change
Ventilation	No change	Decrease	Increase

[a]Rest, submaximal, and maximal exercise are compared.

ercise. (3) Training increases maximal breathing volumes in exhaustive exercise. In submaximal exercise, however, trained individuals demonstrate a pronounced economy of breathing by ventilating less with any given workload. (4) Endurance training has been shown to decrease both systolic and diastolic blood pressure. These changes can occur in both normotensive and hypertensive individuals. (5) Body composition changes are often associated with regular training programs. Exercise often leads to an increase in lean body mass and a reduction in body fat. In the aging population proper exercise may retard a loss of lean mass and help maintain the integrity of the skeletal system.

The practical implications of exercise training should be obvious. The physically fit individual can do more work with less effort, has a larger cardiac reserve, can sustain intense efforts offsetting premature fatigue, and most likely has an improved quality of life. Moreover, it is unlikely that the fit individual will succumb to the modern diseases associated with an injudicious life-style.

GENERAL PRINCIPLES OF EXERCISE PRESCRIPTION

Evaluation of maximal aerobic power provides key information concerning the functional capabilities of the body. The magnitude of an individual's aerobic power reflects three coordinated mechanisms: (1) the ability of the lungs to bring oxygen into the body; (2) extraction and delivery of oxygen to the muscles; and (3) utilization of oxygen via aerobic metabolism. Changes in maximum aerobic power due to training have been reported to range anywhere from 5 to nearly 100%, although increases of greater than 25% have usually been associated with large body mass decreases and extremely low initial levels of cardiorespiratory fitness. Further, body composition changes seem to occur only if the intensity and duration of the activity elicit energy expenditures greater than 1200 kilojoules (approx. 300 kcal) per session and the activity is performed three or more times per week.

The American College of Sports Medicine has published a position statement entitled "The Recommended Quantity and Quality of Exercise for Developing and Maintaining Fitness in Healthy Adults." In brief, the extent of cardiorespiratory fitness and body composition changes is most influenced by an interaction of frequency, intensity, and duration of training. Recommended levels of activity include: (1) a training frequency of 3 to 5 days/week; (2) a training intensity of 60 to 90% of maximum heart rate reserve; and (3) a duration of activity greater than 15 minutes continuously. In general, these basic principles apply to all ages and both sexes.

ADOLESCENTS AND EXERCISE TRAINING

Physiologic responses to exercise training among adolescents are similar to those of adults. However, the basic difference that does exist is a quantitative one. Nevertheless, caution should be taken when generalizing about the aerobic and anaerobic characteristics of adolescents as, even among young people of the same age, there may be dramatic differences in physiological maturity.

Basically, both cross-sectional and longitudinal studies have shown physically active adolescents to have an aerobic advantage over their nonactive counterparts. However, the magnitude of this advantage is somewhat less than would be anticipated if a similar comparison were made between active and nonactive adults. In general, the maximal aerobic power is approximately 15 to 25% higher among active athletic youth, when compared to that of nonactive adolescents. Nevertheless, even these active youth have maximal aerobic values, expressed on a milliliter-per-kilogram body weight basis, anywhere from 3 to 15% lower than those of similarly active adults. These findings would suggest that adolescents are trainable and are certainly suitable for aerobic activities.

Activities requiring the use of large muscles groups such as swimming, cycling, and running are the exercises of choice to build aerobic fitness among adolescents as well as adults. On the other hand, it is questionable as to whether or not anaerobic activities are suitable for the young person. It has been demonstrated that adolescent boys can produce lactate levels that are only 60 to 70% of those reached by adults during exhaustive exercise. Thus it may be a frustrating endeavor for the young adolescent to attempt to train anaerobically.

Trainability of the young person is not an issue. Perhaps more important is helping young people develop a positive attitude towards physical activity. This may be the most important step towards young people participating in an active and health-conscious life-style.

ADULTS AND EXERCISE TRAINING

Most of the knowledge that has been accumulated relative to training has been gathered over the last 30 years, predomi-

nantly from studying adult males and females. General training responses and improvements are noticeable among most adults within 4 to 6 weeks after initiation of a properly designed fitness program. Where many adults get into trouble is with competitive sport activities. Overuse injuries involving the musculoskeletal system are common. Foot, knee, and hip problems associated with long distance running are typical. It is not unusual for the middle-aged racquetball or handball player to experience shoulder joint injuries or rotator cuff tears. Since most musculoskeletal injuries are avoidable, it is likely that the problem lies with the lack of training or preparation that is required to enable participation in competitive sports. Many times busy work schedules, family responsibilities, or other personal involvements preclude proper physical preparation for these activities, although the motivation to play is strong and at times may override common sense.

Besides the training principles stated earlier, there are at least two other principles of training that must be conscientiously adhered to in order to enable safe participation in competitive sports. The principle of overload is imperative in all quantitated exercise programs. This principle, simply stated, means that for improvement or adaptation to occur, a safe progressive exercise overload must be applied to those systems of the body being exercised. As the body adapts to each level of stimulation, corresponding physiologic improvements are noticeable. A second principle of training is the specificity principle. Training is specific to those metabolic and physiological systems overloaded. Thus, if a goal of a fitness program is to improve upper body strength, then the musculature of the upper body should be safely and progressively overloaded. Following these basic principles at any age can help prevent most common injuries of overuse.

THE MATURE ADULT (+60) AND EXERCISE TRAINING

Physiological adaptations to chronic exercise occur regardless of age. However, it is important to note that with aging there is a loss of function in all body systems. Although this is not well understood, it is probably this age-related functional loss that comparatively limits the amount of training improvements the elderly can realize. Nevertheless, older individuals who are habitually active show many physiological similarities to younger individuals. In this regard, it may be prudent to classify many individuals by physiological age, as opposed to chronological age.

Since most older adults are beyond their competitive years, a primary goal of an exercise program for this age group should be to improve the quality of life. This approach should lead to independence and an ability to handle the requirements of daily living. Precaution in prescribing exercise for older people should be adopted. Although the general principles of exercise training discussed earlier apply to the older adult, care should be taken in prescribing exercise to this population. Due to functional loss in most systems of the body, the elderly may be more susceptible to cardiovascular and musculoskeletal problems. For this reason, exercise requiring high-intensity levels is not recommended. Training programs should begin with a gentle progression of low-level intensity activities. Short-term reachable goals documenting gradual increases in activity are in order for this population.

Although the preceding has been a basic overview of exercise science and its relation to sports medicine, it should be recognized that habitual physical activity is an integral part of a healthy life-style. Obviously the health potential of exercise cannot be realized if a society remains inactive. The enforced exercise prescription of our hunting and food-gathering ancestors provided routine physical activity. Industrialization and modern technology have changed the direction of behavioral imperatives. In fact, it is estimated that 40% of Americans are completely sedentary while another 40% are active at levels well below a threshold that would produce gains in health. This fact exists, in spite of the edict by the U.S. Public Health Service that physical fitness and habitual physical activity are of prime importance in maintaining preventive health measures and population health status.

While intense exercise training may be an ambitious goal for many people, moderate levels of habitual daily physical activity improve health status and help provide protection against life-style-related diseases. Besides the physiological benefits of exercise there are many other personal benefits that are favorably affected. Some of these physiological, psychological, and behavioral benefits are summarized in Table 1.2.

SOME SPECIAL CONSIDERATIONS

In recent years a major health concern for women has been the risk of osteoporosis. Osteoporosis is characterized by bones that become increasingly porous and brittle. This condition leads to an increase in the risk of fractures.

In the United States it is estimated that 25% of the female population have a less-than-adequate calcium intake. Although this dietary imbalance is harmful at any age, after the age of 35, particularly in the postmenopausal years, the effects of inadequate calcium intake are extremely salient. For example, among elderly females osteoporosis accounts for nearly all hip fractures in the United States.

Obviously, adequate calcium intake is a prudent approach to offsetting premature bone loss. Nutritional scientists now believe that RDA requirements should be as high as 1000 mg/day for women and that this amount should increase another 500 mg/day after menopause. Bone mass loss may also be retarded through proper amounts of habitual physical activity. It is thought that exercise modifies bone metabolism. Several studies have documented greater bone mineral contents in active adults, when compared to those in age-matched sedentary controls. It would therefore appear that proper caloric intake with adequate amounts of calcium in the diet, combined with proper physical activity, may help maintain skeletal system integrity.

Table 1.2
Potential Benefits to Be Derived from an Exercise Program for Adolescents, Adults and Mature Adults

Adolescents	Adults	Mature Adults
Improve self-confidence and self-image	Reduce risk factors associated with CHD	Improve quality of life
Outlet for excess energy	Maintain weight control	Reduce anxiety and depression
Improve cardiorespiratory efficiency	Improve cardiorespiratory endurance	Improve sleeping habits
Improve muscular strength and endurance	Improve muscular strength and endurance	Improve self-confidence and maintain independence
Reduce risk factors associated with future CHD	Improve energy levels	
Development of motor coordination and flexibility	Improve sleeping habits	Maintain weight control
Social interaction through participation	Improve tolerance to stress	Improve flexibility and coordination
Development of prudent life-style habits	Improve self-confidence and self-image	Improve muscular strength and endurance
	Improve quality of relaxation time	Retard osteoporosis
	Improve job performance and job satisfaction	Sustain libido

Pregnancy and Exercise

Pregnancy can be considered a unique state of health that is associated with several physiological changes. These changes are mainly related to providing a stable and healthy environment for the fetus. The effect of exercise on a pregnant woman and her fetus is not clearly understood. The reader is advised to stay current in the literature in this area. For an overview, a recommended reading is *Exercise and Pregnancy*, edited by R. Raul and R.A. Wiswell (Williams & Wilkins, Baltimore, 1986).

Recent studies have suggested that properly prescribed exercise adds no additional risk to the mother. Weight-supported activity, such as cycling, may be a prudent approach since pregnancy is associated with weight gain and changes in the body's center of gravity. Nonetheless, current knowledge would suggest that moderate aerobic type exercise during uncomplicated pregnancies has no harmful effects on the mother.

Exercise effects on the fetus have not been well-studied. There has been concern that vigorous exercise during pregnancy could interrupt placental blood flow, although this has not been substantiated in humans. Thus far animal studies have shown no detrimental effects to fetal development or delivery due to exercise in pregnancy. Moreover, preliminary evidence in humans suggests that prudent moderate exercise during pregnancy in previously active women does not compromise fetal blood flow. Since data on this topic are still sparse, it is suggested that prudence and good judgment be used when recommending exercise for the pregnant mother (Fig. 1.1).

SUMMARY

The preceding is a brief overview of a complex topic. The main objective was to introduce the topic of physiology of exercise and make reference to this subject's application to sports medicine and life in general. For those readers so inclined, the authors suggest the general reference list for a more complete and detailed review of the topics covered.

ACKNOWLEDGMENTS

The authors wish to thank Ms. Harriet Leonard, Systems Analyst of The Graduate Hospital Human Performance and Sports Medicine Center, for timely editorial contributions and expert assistance in word processing.

These guidelines were issued by the American College of Obstetricians and Gynecologists to provide authoritative answers to numerous questions from patients and physicians. The guidelines have, however, been the subject of some debate.

Pregnancy and postpartum

1. Regular exercise (at least three times per week) is preferable to intermittent activity. Competitive activities should be discouraged.
2. Vigorous exercise should not be performed in hot, humid weather or during a period of febrile illness.
3. Ballistic movements (jerky, bouncy motions) should be avoided. Exercise should be done on a wooden floor or a tightly carpeted surface to reduce shock and provide a sure footing.
4. Deep flexion or extension of joints should be avoided because of connective tissue laxity. Activities that require jumping, jarring motions, or rapid changes in direction should be avoided because of the instability of the joints.
5. Vigorous exercise should be preceded by a five-minute period of muscle warm-up. This can be accomplished by slow walking or stationary cycling with low resistance.
6. Vigorous exercise should be followed by a period of gradually declining activity that includes gentle stationary stretching. Because connective tissue laxity increases the risk of joint injury, stretches should not be taken to the point of maximum resistance.

7. Heart rate should be measured at times of peak activity. Target heart rates and limits established in consultation with the physician should not be exceeded.
8. Care should be taken to rise from the floor gradually to avoid orthostatic hypotension. Some form of activity involving the legs should be continued for a brief period of time.
9. Liquids should be taken liberally before and after exercise to prevent dehydration. If necessary, activity should be interrupted to replenish fluids.
10. Women who have led sedentary life-styles should begin with physical activity of very low intensity and advance activity levels very gradually.
11. Activity should be stopped and the physician consulted if any unusual symptoms appear.

Pregnancy only

1. Maternal heart rate should not exceed 140 beats per minute.
2. Strenuous activities should not exceed 15 minutes in duration.
3. No exercise should be performed in the supine position after the fourth month of gestation has been completed.
4. Exercises that employ the Valsalva's maneuver should be avoided.
5. Calorie intake should be adequate to meet not only the extra energy needs of pregnancy but also of the exercise performed.
6. Maternal core temperature should not exceed 38°C (100.4°F).

Figure 1.1 ACOG guidelines for exercise during pregnancy and postpartum. Adapted with permission from the American College of Obstetricians and Gynecologists: *Exercise During Pregnancy and the Postnatal Period* (ACOG Home Exercise Programs). Washington, DC, ACOG, 1985, p. 4.

Suggested Readings

American College of Sports Medicine: *Resource Manual for Guidelines for Exercise Testing and Prescription.* Philadelphia, Lea & Febiger, 1988.

Dishman RK (ed): *Exercise Adherence: Its Impact on Public Health.* Champaign, IL, Human Kinetics Books, 1988.

Froelicher VF: *Exercise and the Heart: Clinical Concepts.* Chicago, Year Book Medical Publishers, 1987.

Klarreich SH (ed): *Health and Fitness in the Workplace: Health Education in Business Organizations.* New York, Praeger, 1987.

Lamb DR, Murray R (eds): *Perspectives in Exercise Science and Sports Medicine, Vol. 1: Prolonged Exercise.* Indianapolis, IN, Benchmark Press, 1988.

McArdle WD, Katch FI, Katch VL: *Exercise Physiology: Energy, Nutrition, and Human Performance.* Philadelphia, Lea & Febiger, 1986.

Patton RW, Corry JM, Gettman LR, Graf JS: *Implementing Health and Fitness Programs.* Champaign, IL, Human Kinetic Books, 1986.

Raul R, Wiswell RA (eds): *Exercise and Pregnancy.* Baltimore, Williams & Wilkins, 1986.

Shephard RJ: *Physical Activity and Growth.* Chicago, Year Book Medical Publishers, 1982.

Skinner JS (ed): *Exercise Testing and Exercise Prescription for Special Cases: Theoretical Basis and Clinical Application.* Philadelphia, Lea & Febiger, 1987.

GLOSSARY OF TERMS

Aerobic   Utilizing oxygen.

Aerobic endurance   The ability to sustain activities requiring a constant supply of oxygen.

Aerobic power   The maximal amount of oxygen consumed per unit of time. Also, maximal oxygen uptake or consumption = VO_{2max}.

Anaerobic   Without oxygen.

Anaerobic capacity   The ability to sustain strenuous activities of short duration (5 to 45 seconds) without utilizing aerobic metabolism.

Anaerobic power   The maximum rate at which energy can be produced in the absence of oxygen.

Body Composition   The proportion of fat and lean tissues in the body.

Fatigue   The inability to sustain a given level of effort over time.

Heart rate reserve   The capabilities above resting heart rate levels available to perform vigorous exercise.

Joule   A unit of energy measurement (a kilocalorie = 4.2 kilojoules).

Lean body mass   The mass of the body tissue exclusive of fat.

Oxygen uptake   The oxygen used by the cellular mitochondria.

Power   Work performed per unit of time.

Response   A physiological adjustment to either acute or chronic exercise.

Stroke volume   The amount of blood pumped out of the heart ventricle per beat.

Submaximal exercise   Exercise of less than maximal intensity.

chapter 2

The Adolescent

LYNN McCULLOUGH, R.N., M.S.N., P.N.P.C.
SUSAN W. SALMOND, R.N., Ed.D.

PHYSICAL CHANGES

The "adolescent growth spurt" is a phenomena well-known to both health care providers and parents of adolescents (ages 12 to 18). This growth occurs in both height and weight and is accompanied by the changes indicative of sexual and physical maturity. The increase in height may mean weight loss for some and weight gain for others. All adolescents should be assessed in all these parameters and assisted in dealing with these changes.

Previously athletic children may find they cannot continue to compete at their present level or become unsuited for a sport to which they have previously devoted a great deal of time and energy. An example of this would be a girl with much promise as a gymnast; however, at the onset of puberty she becomes too tall to perform maneuvers previously accomplished with ease. It is a well-known fact (usually due to delay in onset of menses) that successful female gymnasts usually are very small and petite. Another example is that of a boy who previously has been of average height and heavy build and excelled in football. At puberty, he may gain in height without gaining an equal amount of weight and, therefore, be unsuited for football and at greater risk for injury. These adolescents must be guided into sports for which they are physically suited in order to prevent injury, and just as importantly, assisted in dealing with their disappointment.

Conversely, formerly overweight, non-athletic children may also gain in height, and not in weight, and suddenly become interested in activities they previously would not participate in due to their weight. To minimize the risk of injury, they must be assessed fully and instructed in a program to improve their overall fitness.

Skeletal Development

During growth spurts (between the ages of 12 to 14 years), epiphyseal injuries occur more frequently in obese or in tall, thin boys (Fig. 2.1). Participation in contact sports during this time increases the youngster's risk for injury. At-risk adolescents should avoid contact sports until maturity of muscle and coordination has been achieved. The Tanner stages of sexual development aid assessment of skeletal maturity and development. Additionally, skeletal age can be determined by comparing an x-ray of the patient's hand with standards for different ages that appear in radiographic atlases (Greenspan, 1988). For those individuals who do participate in contact sports fewer injuries are known to occur if the teams are organized by height, weight, and general physical fitness.

DEVELOPMENTAL TASKS

According to Erikson (1963) the primary developmental task of adolescence is identity establishment versus role confusion. A part of identity establishment is developing a favorable self-concept and a sense of

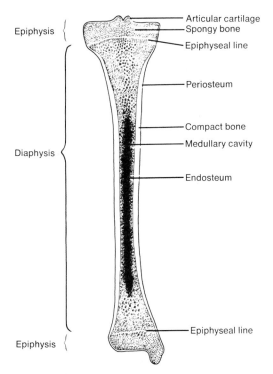

Epiphysis {

Articular cartilage
Spongy bone
Epiphyseal line

Periosteum

Compact bone
Medullary cavity

Diaphysis {

Endosteum

Epiphyseal line

Epiphysis {

Figure 2.1. Basic long bone structure. (From Hilt NE, Cogburn SB: *Manual of Orthopaedics*. St. Louis, CV Mosby, 1980.)

self-esteem. While the process of developing self-concept continues throughout life, during adolescence it is re-examined, questioned, revised, and solidified. Individuals with a favorable self-concept and high levels of self-esteem are usually successful, creative, independent, and well-equipped to handle the problems that arise in their lives. The physical condition of an individual is one of many factors that affects the development of self-esteem. Assisting adolescents in attaining their maximum health and physical conditioning will positively influence their self-esteem.

Maintenance of a positive body image is essential to the adolescent's developing self-esteem. The numerous changes that occur at this age can make this very difficult. Encouraging adolescents through this difficult period by reassuring them of the normalcy of these changes and their feelings about them will help in this development. Advising them of activities in which

they will probably be successful, based upon their individual strengths and weaknesses, will also aid in establishing a healthy, positive body image.

A key area to establishment of individuality is independence. It has often been said that the adolescent is one minute a child and the next minute an adult; consequently this time is confusing for both parents and adolescent. The adolescent is given increasing responsibility at home and at school and told that he/she is now old enough to take responsibility for his/her own actions. On the other hand, the adolescent is still responsible for following the parent's rules and frequently denied the right to make certain decisions, because he/she is still not ready to take total control. The adolescent does not see things in this same light; but feels that if he/she is responsible in one area, responsibility should be acknowledged in all areas. In order to develop skills in decision making, it is important to allow the adolescent to make as many decisions as independently as possible, even allowing the wrong decisions to be made on occasion. In the case of a decision that the adolescent may not make independently, allow him/her to participate in the decision-making process and take time to explain the rationale behind the final decision, whether or not it was the decision wanted.

It is of the utmost importance that adolescents be like their peers. Often it is very distressing to parents that peers have a great deal more influence over their child than parents. It is important for parents to realize that this is not a personal rejection of them by their child, but simply a step in the child's growth. Hopefully, the values and morals by which their child was brought up will favorably influence the choice of peers. On the other hand, adolescents will often test their parents by deliberately choosing friends of whom they know their parents will not approve. Often these are people they really do not want as friends, but they want to see the reaction of their parents (which may be viewed as evidence of their trust). It is important that the parents not overreact in these situations. Sitting down and discussing their concerns in a calm and reasonable manner, without spending too much time on the issue, will accomplish much more than simply forbidding them to see these particular friends.

In addition, adolescents are also influenced by a number of other individuals. Parents continue to be a source of influence as well as teachers, parents of their peers, older siblings (their own and those of their friends), and other adults with whom they have contact (church workers, coaches, and health care professionals). Other influencing factors are socioeconomic status, intellectual level of functioning, skills and abilities, and past experiences.

Adolescence is also a time of changes in cognitive development. The adolescent moves from the concrete and egocentric thinking of childhood to abstract conceptualization. With this comes the ability to view the world, and the self, from another's perspective (Mercer, 1979). Prior to this time, children can see only themselves and cannot see themselves as others do. They also begin to develop the ability to analyze problems and perceive the ramifications of a particular decision or choice.

The effect of illness or injury on this development is significant. Any illness or injury, even if of short duration or acute, makes them different from their peers for that period of time. Children with a chronic illness, or an injury that leaves them with a permanent disability, face different obstacles in establishing their identity and independence. They must be allowed to discuss their feelings in an open and honest manner. Contact should be maintained with their peers if at all possible. A significant loss of control occurs when adolescents are ill or injured, and this has a serious effect on their attitudes and reactions to others. They may become very uncooperative, belligerent, and even hostile. The adolescent who refuses to eat even though he knows inadequate nutrition will delay his recovery or the adolescent who refuses to cooperate with physical therapy exercises even if such noncompliance could leave a permanent disability are two examples. The issue of establishing independence and identity is so important that adolescents will find areas over which they can take control and make decisions. It is important to recognize this and find areas where they safely can make decisions and continue their development even while sick or injured. The adolescent with a chronic condition or permanent disability must be helped to identify with peers and to find alternative activities when he/she cannot participate in a conventional manner.

NONTRAUMATIC PROBLEMS

The discussion of common orthopaedic problems from nontraumatic causes will cover those problems affecting the upper extremity, the lower extremity, the spine, multiple areas of involvement, and chronic conditions.

Upper Extremity

There are few nontraumatic causes for problems in the upper extremity other than infection, congenital causes, or sequelae of injuries sustained at a younger age. An example of this would be an elbow deformity resulting from a fracture that did not heal properly.

Lower Extremity Sequelae

There are several categories of problems in the lower extremity. Numerous sequelae from earlier illnesses or injuries may be present. Some of these may only become evident at adolescence; it is important to know the patient's orthopaedic history, and whether follow-up care is being obtained, as well as the duration of any symptoms such as pain or limp. A septic joint or osteomyelitis at a young age may have resulted in permanent damage if joint cartilage was destroyed or growth plates were involved. Growth arrest may also occur from traumatic injuries (fractures, dislocations, crush injuries) suffered prior to adolescence, and could result in less than full range of motion of a joint, pain, or discrepancies in leg lengths. Legg-Calvé-Perthes disease, while usually diagnosed prior to adolescence, continues to have an effect throughout life. In adolescence, surgical procedures may be necessary to deal with the sequelae (i.e., trochanteric overgrowth or leg length discrepancy). In some cases, the diagnosis may not be made until adolescence. The child treated for congenital dysplasia of the hip may also need additional procedures for much the same sequelae. Appropriate intervention can make a tremendous difference in outcome in these children.

Leg Length Discrepancy

In addition to occurring as sequelae from other conditions, leg length discrepancies can also occur from hemihypertrophy/hemiatrophy and from unknown causes. There are a variety of interventions available for the treatment of discrepancies other than the traditional shoe lift (usually an unacceptable treatment modality to the adolescent). Procedures are available both to shorten a long extremity and to lengthen a short one. Determining which procedure is best in a given case is an individualized process. Regular, long-term follow-up is essential to decide the timing of procedures so that leg length equality will be achieved at the cessation of growth. It is important that leg length discrepancies (>2.0 cm) are treated as they may lead to knee, hip, and low back pain. Negative self-concept may develop due to the limp; participation in activities with peers promotes a positive self-concept and body image.

Slipped Capital Femoral Epiphysis (SCFE)

SCFE is one of the more common problems of the hip occurring in adolescence (see Chapter 8). This can occur as a chronic or acute condition or combination (i.e., a 2- to 3-month history of hip pain that is exacerbated after a fall or twisting injury to the hip). It is important that an accurate diagnosis be made as soon as possible to limit the amount of permanent disability. Any adolescent who presents with hip pain, limp, and external rotation of the leg should be assumed to have a slipped capital femoral epiphysis and referred for evaluation. Surgical intervention to prevent further

slippage is necessary to treat slipped capital femoral epiphysis.

Knee Problems

Chondromalacia patella (patellofemoral arthralgia) occurs frequently in adolescent girls. For a discussion see Chapter 9.

Foot Deformities

Complaints related to the foot are common in adolescence. Many of these problems can be treated with appropriate shoes. Pes planus (flat feet) rarely require more than a shoe with a good arch support or an insert with an arch. Calf or foot pain can initiate the need for treatment. Bunions, while not extremely common at this age, are common enough to warrant mention. In their desire to be like everyone else, adolescents may wear shoes which are not comfortable and lead to hallux valgus (bunions). Frequently, bunions, too, can be treated by wearing shoes which fit well and allow room for the toes. Occasionally there is the child with bunions resulting from metatarsus primus varus, which is severe enough to require surgical correction to realign the metatarsal bone.

Sever's disease is a common cause of heel pain. It frequently is most noticeable after running and is seen usually in boys. The pain can be localized to the insertion of the Achilles tendon into the calcaneous or the plantar fascial insertions into the calcaneous. The use of heel cups inside the shoe and modification of activities (activity restricted until painfree) are usually all that are required as treatment.

Persistent complaints of foot pain, which are worse with activity and unrelenting, require a thorough evaluation to determine if a coalition between bones of the foot is present. Often computerized tomography is necessary to make this determination. If a coalition is found, surgical resection may be necessary to prevent further pain or degenerative changes. For a discussion of bunions and Sever's disease see chapter 10.

Spine

The spine is an area that must receive special attention during the preadolescent and adolescent periods. The most common orthopaedic problem of adolescence is that of scoliosis. As scoliosis does not produce pain, regular back screening examinations are necessary whether or not there are complaints related to the back.

Scoliosis

Scoliosis is defined as a lateral curvature of the spine that is accompanied by vertebral rotation (Fig. 2.2). While scoliosis may occur from a variety of causes, including leg length discrepancies, spasticity, and structural anomalies, the most common cause is idiopathic, meaning the cause is not known. It is most common in the prepubescent and adolescent age groups. As scoliosis is not painful until a very large curve has developed, it is important to screen everyone in this age group; often the adolescent and the parents are unaware of the presence of the curve. Programs in the school for the screening of

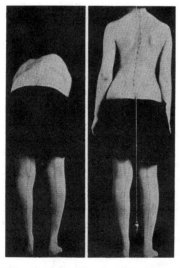

Figure 2.2. Scoliosis. In the upright position a scoliosis to the right is barely apparent. When the patient leans forward, however, the right hemithorax is thrown into relief, and the effect is much more obvious. (From Burnside JW, McGlynn TJ (eds): *Physical Diagnosis*, ed 17. Baltimore, Williams & Wilkins, 1987.)

scoliosis are now held in many states and are mandated by law in some. It is important that scoliosis be detected early, while the curve is small, so that treatment can be instituted. Untreated, large curves will continue to progress throughout life, and result in pulmonary and cardiac compromise, as well as back pain and a severe cosmetic deformity.

The first step in the evaluation for scoliosis, as with other conditions, is the history. As scoliosis is known to have a genetic component, it is important to ascertain if there is a known family history. Other important information needed includes any complaints related to the back and the presence of any neurological symptoms (numbness, tingling, loss of control of bowel or bladder, etc.). While idiopathic scoliosis does not ordinarily cause pain or neurologic compromise, this is information important to ascertain if the scoliosis may be a result of a cause other than an idiopathic one, or if there are other concurrent conditions. For females it is important to know the onset of menarche as this is a rough estimate of how soon the end of skeletal growth will occur. Generally 12 to 18 months of growth remain after the onset of menarche; this becomes an important factor in deciding treatment. The examination for screening of scoliosis is simple and takes very little time. The patient should be undressed except for underwear. It is helpful, but not absolutely necessary, for girls to remove their bras in order to afford the professional an unobstructed view of their backs. The first part of the exam consists of having the patient stand straight but relaxed with feet together and hands by the sides. The signs to look for at this time are:

1. Elevation of one shoulder;
2. Elevation or prominence of one scapula;
3. Elevation of the pelvis;
4. Difference in the space between the arm and the body;
5. Trunk shift with the head not aligned over the pelvis.

Any one of the signs listed above is probably not significant but the presence of two or more should raise a high index of suspicion for the presence of scoliosis and one should refer the patient to a physician. The next step in the exam is to examine the patient from the side while the patient is still standing as previously described. At this time the back is examined for the normal contours of thoracic kyphosis and lumbar lordosis. An exaggeration of these normal contours constitutes a reason for referral, particularly if accompanied by complaints of pain.

Next, have the patient place the hands together with the fingertips even and have him/her bend forward dropping the head to the chest and allowing the arms to dangle (but keeping the hands together). Examine for an unevenness of one side over the other. This unevenness is the result of a rib hump that occurs as a result of the scoliosis. As the vertebrae rotate and curve, the ribs are rotated as well, resulting in the rib hump. Have the patient bend slowly in order to watch as he/she bends and examine the thoracic, thoracolumbar, and lumbar regions. If he/she cannot bend far enough to obtain an adequate exam of the lumbar region due to hamstring tightness, have the patient bend the knees slightly. This will allow him/her to bend farther forward. As this is a somewhat subjective exam, a device called a scoliometer has been developed that allows a more accurate and specific exam. The scoliometer works on much the same principle as a carpenter's level and allows a numerical rating of the amount of rotation found. It is simple to use and relatively inexpensive. Any child with a noticeable rib hump on exam or with a scoliometer reading of five or more should be referred for further evaluation.

A very basic neurological exam should also be done. During the exam look for any dimples or hairy patches on the back indicative of spinal dysraphism or other skin signs such as café au lait spots indicative of neurofibromatosis. Scoliosis is more common in patients with spina bifida and neurofibromatosis. These patients may also have subtle neurologic findings.

Radiographs are vital for assessment of the curve. Progression is determined by serial films obtained on a regular basis. Films are obtained on a yearly basis if the curve is less than 20°. Films are obtained at more frequent intervals if the curve is greater than 20° and there is significant growth remaining. At the initial visit obtain a *standing scoliosis series* (anteroposterior and lateral views of the spine from the cervical area through the sacrum).

The treatment options for scoliosis include observation, bracing, electrical stimulation, and surgery. Treatment will be based on a number of factors including the degree of curvature, presence of structural abnormalities (hemivertebrae), the age of the child, skeletal maturity, location of the curvature, and psychosocial assessment of the child and family. Generally, curves 25 to 30° can be observed at 4- to 6-month intervals; curves between 30 and 40° will be braced or treated with electrical stimulation; and curves greater than 40 to 50° will be managed surgically. These are very broad guidelines, and it must be remembered that physicians will vary, and that the degree of curvature is not the only factor in determining treatment.

If bracing is to be instituted, it will be one of two types of braces. The most common is a low-profile brace that is covered entirely by clothing and is fairly nonrestrictive. The other type, which is still used in special circumstances, is the Milwaukee type of brace that has a pelvic portion and metal upper structure. This brace cannot be completely disguised by clothing and is much more restrictive. It is not as well tolerated as the low-profile type. Both braces are generally worn for 23 hours/day until skeletal growth is complete. On the average, a child will require full-time brace treatment for 2 to 2½ years. This is only a rough guideline; many circumstances affect both the hours for daily wear and the total time of treatment. Currently there is research being done on the efficacy of part-time wear, but the data are incomplete. A great deal of patient/family teaching is necessary for the patient who is being asked to wear a brace (Table 2.1). In addition to, and perhaps more important than, physical aspects of care are the emotional and psychological aspects. Patients will be followed at 4- to 6-month intervals while wearing their brace.

Electrical stimulation is an alternative to

Table 2.1
Instructions for Care of the Skin[a]

Skin Care: It is very important to prevent skin breakdown (that is, sore, red, raw skin). The skin under the brace needs to be toughened up, especially where the brace rubs hard.

To Protect the Skin:

1. Bathe daily (bath or shower)
2. Apply rubbing alcohol with your hands to all parts of the skin that the brace covers, especially the areas where the skin is pink and the areas where the brace presses a lot. The alcohol plus the friction between your hand and body toughens the skin.
3. Do not use creams, lotions, or powders under the brace. These will soften the skin.
4. Always wear a 100% cotton undershirt, tubular without side seams. The sleeveless men's (tank top) style is usually preferred by girls. Suggested brands include: Carter's (for younger children), Fruit of the Loom, Sears, or Hanes.
5. Wear your brace as tightly as possible! If you wear your brace loosely, it will move around and cause more skin problems by rubbing.
6. Observe your skin for pink or tender pressure areas. This is especially important when you first begin wearing your brace.

If there is skin breakdown (sore, red, raw skin) the brace must not be reapplied until the skin heals—one day or more. If this happens, call the Orthopaedic Nurse Specialist. The problem might be solved over the phone.

Sometimes the skin over the waist and hips get darker. This is common and is not a problem. When the brace treatment is over, this color will go away.

GOOD SKIN CARE REQUIRES
BRACE CARE EACH DAY!

---

[a]Reprinted with permission from McCullough L: *Scoliosis: Wearing a Brace.* Little Rock, AR, Dept. of Orthopedic Surgery, University of Arkansas for Medical Sciences, Arkansas Children's Hospital, 1980.

bracing in certain instances. This involves the use of surface electrodes placed on the back before bedtime. The electrodes are placed on the convex side of the curve and, with stimulation, correct the curve. The stimulation is provided cyclically throughout the night. Results from this treatment modality have been very mixed, and it is not used by all physicians. While (at least theoretically) avoiding the psychological problems associated with wearing a brace (as stimulation is only used at night), electrical stimulation is not without its problems. Most common is skin irritation, which can be severe enough that it cannot be overcome and the treatment must be discontinued. Other problems include inability to tolerate the stimulation, sleep disturbances that can result in nightmares and difficulties in school, and a lack of compliance (it is time consuming to get everything set at night and properly put away in the morning).

The goals of both bracing and electrical stimulation are the same, preventing progression of the curve. Neither will provide correction of a permanent nature. The curve present at the start of treatment will be the curve at the end of treatment. For this reason, bracing and stimulation are options for curves less than 40°. Curves of this magnitude have been shown to remain relatively stable throughout life with very little progression. People with curves of this size have no greater incidence of back pain than those without a curve.

Surgical correction is recommended for larger curves as these have been shown to be biomechanically unstable and will progress significantly, resulting in complications already discussed. Surgery is the only treatment that will provide permanent correction of the curve.

Surgery consists of a fusion of the spine in the corrected position through the use of various types of instrumentation and bone grafting. The type of instrumentation and surgical approach used is determined by the surgeon's evaluation of the patient, the nature and flexibility of the curve, and which technique he/she feels yields the best results. In most cases a postoperative cast can be avoided. If immobilization is needed a polypropylene brace, which can be removed on a daily basis for a shower, usually is used. In some cases, no immobilization is needed. The average hospital stay is 7 to 10 days with a 1- to 2-week period of recuperation at home. Essentially, all activities can be resumed after a 6-month period of restricted activities.

Back Pain

Most commonly back pain in adolescents results from overuse, a lack of conditioning, and/or poor body mechanics. These problems can usually be managed by a combination of rest, conditioning exercises, instruction in body mechanics, and the use of anti-inflammatories. Narcotics and muscle relaxants are rarely indicated. Although most back pain is not of a severe nature, there are a number of cases that are more serious. Every case of back pain severe enough to restrict activities and cause the patient to seek medical attention deserves a complete evaluation. Causes of back pain include spondylolisthesis, spondylolysis, and spinal tumors. The evaluation should include a thorough pain history, including social history, and should determine what stressors currently are present, as well as at the time the pain began. Other components of the workup include a complete neurological exam, complete x-rays, and often a bone scan. A MRI study can be helpful in some cases. After the cause of the pain is determined, treatment can be instituted (see Chapter 5).

Chronic Conditions

There are a number of chronic conditions that result in permanent disability with orthopaedic components. These include spina bifida, muscular dystrophy, and cerebral palsy. Surgical procedures to treat these diseases are ordinarily performed before adolescence, with the exception of spinal surgery, which is sometimes necessary in all of these diseases. Therefore, the focus of the nurse must be on helping these youngsters through the normal developmental tasks as well as helping them adjust to their limitations. As much independence as possible is a primary goal, and

the nurse must provide proper wheelchairs, accessories, and other assistive devices to ensure this. Outlets for physical activities such as competing in Special Olympics and other activities that give a sense of accomplishment must be provided. Assisting the patients in finding areas in which they can excel and discovering their personal strengths and weaknesses is extremely important.

Lesions of Bone

Lesions of bone usually present with a history of trauma and may present as pathological fractures. A pathological fracture should be considered in the child who presents with pain and swelling after minor trauma (which should not have been sufficient to produce a fracture), especially if the history of a lesion is elicited. Adolescence is also the time where certain malignant tumors of bone will appear. Any young person with signs of pain, swelling, or tumor must be immediately referred for complete evaluation. The use of limb salvage techniques, allografts, and prosthetic replacements has reduced the number of amputations that must be performed for malignant tumors, but the diagnosis must be made quickly for these to be treatment options.

TRAUMATIC PROBLEMS

Trauma is the primary cause of death in the adolescent age group, and motor vehicle accidents are the primary cause of this trauma. Adolescents are becoming drivers, both of cars and motorcycles. The trauma that results from motor vehicle accidents of any kind is frequently severe; in many cases the accidents could have been prevented or lessened in severity through the use of protective equipment, better driver education, and better judgment. As discussed previously, the adolescent is only beginning to develop more sophisticated abstract thinking that can be used to predict the outcomes of his/her decisions. There also is the feeling that he/she is invincible and accidents will always happen to someone else. Education is important in reducing these injuries but equally important is helping the injured adolescent to cope with the injuries and feelings.

There is almost always a feeling of guilt on the part of the adolescent, any friends who may have been involved, and the parents. Unless dealt with, this can be very destructive. Ideally this process should begin at the initial presentation for treatment. However, it is important that it does not end there. The adolescent who was driving while intoxicated and the adolescent who was the cause of an accident in which a friend or family member was injured or even killed must have help in dealing with the emotional and psychological impact of the accident. In many cases, a prolonged hospital stay is necessary due to the severity of the injuries. Multiple procedures may be necessary with more planned in the future. The adolescent has suffered a major unplanned interruption in life with a loss of control and the independence for which he/she has been striving. These patients will frequently exhibit the behavior discussed earlier and to a much more dramatic degree than the adolescent who has undergone a planned procedure for which he/she had time to prepare. After discharge, he/she will need assistance in reentering school and outside activities and dealing with any sequelae of the accident, such as casts, external fixators, scars, and restrictions in activities and abilities.

In addition to major trauma, adolescents frequently suffer from more minor trauma as they continue to "try their wings" and often become more active in competitive sports. These minor injuries usually take the form of sprains, strains, and fractures, frequently sports-related injuries. Upper extremity fractures can most often be treated on an outpatient basis. Fractures of the femur will almost always require hospitalization and surgical treatment. Fractures of the tibia and ankle may require hospitalization and surgical treatment, but in many cases can be handled on an outpatient basis. This is determined by the exact nature of the fracture. Follow-up care is imperative to insure that the fracture heals properly and that no changes in neurovascular status have occurred. The patient and family must be instructed in the care of the cast or fixator device, use of any assistive devices, and signs and symptoms that should be reported to the physician. Special arrangements for homebound schooling or early assistance with class changes will frequently be necessary. Communication with the school throughout the course of treatment is of great benefit in providing the student the opportunity to continue with education and to maintain contact with peers.

Sports

It is estimated that 20 million or more children (25% of girls and 50% of boys ages 8 to 16) are engaged in competitive sports in any given year. This fact, coupled with the lower overall level of fitness of youth and children, means greater numbers of children and adolescents will be seen with sports-related injuries. Therefore, although sports medicine has evolved as a specialty, it should not be limited to the orthopaedic sports medicine specialist. At some time almost all health care providers will be involved in the treatment of sports-related illnesses and injuries. This chapter will not discuss all possible sports-related injuries, but will discuss the most common, focusing on those most likely to present to the general health practitioner and those not requiring inpatient treatment.

Preparticipation Physical Exam

The purpose of the preparticipation physical exam is to detect any medical condition that could predispose the athlete to serious injury or death during sports participation. This includes identifying those medical conditions that could become worse by participation in sports activities. The current recommendation of the American Academy of Pediatrics is to screen all adolescents beginning a new sports program, and to obtain interval histories annually for those athletes continuing in the program. In adolescence, the most commonly encountered abnormalities are residual from previous sports-related injuries. The preparticipation physical serves as quality control for the treatment and the rehabilitation for that injury. The exam must be tailored to the sport with particular emphasis upon those areas of the body at risk for the particular sport.

The preparticipation physical exam (Fig. 2.3) should include a thorough history of previous illnesses and injuries, immunization record, general physical exam, maturational assessment, musculoskeletal examination, eye exam, and urinalysis. The general physical exam should include attention to the cardiovascular system to detect any abnormalities such as congenital or acquired heart disease, hypertension, arrhythmias, prolapsed mitral valves, and idiopathic hypertrophic subaortic stenosis. Particular attention should be paid to any individual with a history of fainting, chest pain during exercise, family history of heart disease, or findings of irregular heart rate or murmurs. Additional studies are often necessary to determine the fitness of such individuals for sports participation. Special attention should also be paid to any acute or chronic medical conditions (asthma, seizure disorders) that may require special management or may disqualify the adolescent from participation. Special precautions are also indicated for the athlete with a missing paired organ and the athlete recovering from an illness such as mononucleosis who may have an enlarged spleen and be in less than optimal physical condition. The evaluation of the maturation of the athlete is a very important component. The rapidly growing adolescent is at risk for injuries to ligaments and epiphyseal plates. The immature skeleton is subject to injuries that differ from those affecting the mature skeleton. Adolescents in early stages of development may benefit from being guided toward noncontact sports in order to protect them from injury. The musculoskeletal status also influences the risk of injury. Strength, flexibility, muscular development, and joint mobility can all be tested. At the very least, all joints should be put through a full range of motion.

In May 1988, the Committee on Sports Medicine of the American Academy of Pediatrics revised the 1976 American Medical Association list of recommendations for participation in competitive sports (Table 2.2).

The committee also issued a classification of sports based upon the amount of contact incurred. These guidelines can be used in determining whether participation in a sport may be detrimental to the health of the athlete (Table 2.3).

In working with handicapped children, other factors must also be considered in order to guide them into sports where they will have the least risk of injury and greatest chance of success. These factors include size, coordination, degree of physical fitness, physical health, stage of maturation, mental development, and emotional stability. Also to be considered are the physical and psychological benefits weighed against the potential frustration from repeated failure, the level of competition, and the need for special protective equipment. Careful physical assessment combined with consultation with family and the personnel who will be supervising the sports activity will allow most children to participate successfully in some form of sports activity.

Injuries

Injuries encountered can be divided into two main categories: those resulting from a sudden, violent application of stress (seen as fractures and ligament tears) and those resulting from recurring applications of stress (seen most commonly as stress fractures and overuse syndromes).

Acute Injuries

It must be reiterated that because the bones and ligaments of the immature skeleton have different biomechanical properties, they react differently to injuries and stresses. Fractures, which are for the most part unique to the growing skeleton, are plastic deformation, greenstick fractures, torus fractures, epiphyseal fractures, and apophyseal avulsions. Plastic deformation and greenstick fractures result from the ability of the immature bone to bend rather than break, and are treated as complete

Date of Exam_____ / _____ / _____

School Official _____

Exam Doctor _____

Cleveland Clinic Foundation

PREPARTICIPATION
SPORTS EXAM

	A	B	C
Contact: Coach			☐
School Nurse			☐
Family Doctor			☐
Family Dentist			☐

THIS IS NOT A SUBSTITUTE FOR A REGULAR PHYSICAL EXAM PERFORMED BY YOUR FAMILY DOCTOR

Name_____ Grade _____ Age _____ Birthdate _____ / _____ / _____

School _____ Sport _____ Sex _____

Parents _____ Address _____ Phone _____

Family Doctor _____ Address _____ Phone _____

HISTORY: Answer **No** or **Yes** with details and dates. Use reverse side if necessary.

I. Have you ever sustained **an injury** which prevented you from playing sports for **more than one day and** have you had any injuries **such as** (circle): skull fracture - **brain surgery concussion** - knocked out, **neck pain**/injury - arm/finger **numbness**, **back pain**/injury - leg/toe numbness, heatstroke/fainting - exhaustion, broken bone - **fracture**, joint **dislocation** - out of place, **deep bruise** - muscle pull, ligament **sprains**, tender kneecap/shin, **trick knee** - catching/locking,

_____

_____

II. Do you have a history of **and/or** take medicine (specify) for any medical problems **such as** (circle): **asthma** - allergy - wheezing - short of breath, heart **murmur/palpitation** - rheumatic fever - **high blood high blood pressure**, diabetes - high/low **sugar**, fainting - **seizure**, yellow jaundice - **hepatitis**, severe influenza/cold - **mononucleosis** - weakness, **anemia** - bruise easily - bleeding - sickle cell, loss of eyesight, hearing, testicle, kidney, etc., **hernia** - rupture - bulging, skin disease - boils - **rash**, or other?

_____

_____

III. Are you allergic to any medicine such as (circle) penicillin, iodine, novocaine or other?

_____

IV. Any family history of medically unexplained or cardiac caused sudden death under age 50?

_____

V. L.M.P. _____

BP___ / ___ P_____ Ht_____ Wt_____ Gross Vision: R_____ L_____, Pupils R_____ L_____ LAB: UA_____

EXAM:

1. Upper Extr: AC jts _____
   Symm _____
   ROM _____
2. Spine: Neck _____
   Fwd Bend_____
   Curve_____
3. Lower Extr: Gait _____
   1-Hop_____
   Duck _____
   Symm _____
   ROM _____

4. Heart:_____
5. Lungs: _____
6. Skin: _____
7. Abdo: Spleen _____
   Liver _____
8. GU: Hernia _____
   Testicles _____
9. Dental _____
10. Other _____
    _____
    _____

IMPRESSION:

☐ Satisfactory Exam

☐ Recommend further evaluation/rehabilitation regarding: _____

Contact your: School Nurse — Coach — Family Doctor — Family Dentist

CLEARANCE:

A — Cleared for: Collision — Contact — Noncontact sports

B — Cleared for: Collision — Contact — Noncontact sports after completing eval/rehab

C — NOT cleared for: Collision — Contact — Noncontact sports due to: _____

F 723 Rev. 5/87

Fig. 2.3. Preparticipation Sports Exam. (Permission to reprint granted by the Section of Sports Medicine, Department of Orthopaedic Surgery, Cleveland Clinic Foundation, Cleveland, Ohio.)

Table 2.2
Recommendations for Participation in Competitive Sports[a]

	Contact/ Collision	Limited Contact/Impact	Noncontact		
			Strenuous	Moderately Strenuous	Nonstrenuous
Atlantoaxial instability	No	No	Yes*	Yes	Yes
*Swimming: no butterfly, breast stroke, or diving starts					
Acute illnesses	*	*	*	*	*
*Needs individual assessment, eg, contagiousness to others, risk of worsening illness					
Cardiovascular					
Carditis	No	No	No	No	No
Hypertension					
Mild	Yes	Yes	Yes	Yes	Yes
Moderate	*	*	*	*	*
Severe	*	*	*	*	*
Congenital heart disease	†	†	†	†	†
*Needs individual assessment. †Patients with mild forms can be allowed a full range of physical activities; patients with moderate or severe forms, or who are postoperative, should be evaluated by a cardiologist before athletic participation.					
Eyes					
Absence or loss of function of one eye	*	*	*	*	*
Detached retina	†	†	†	†	†
*Availability of American Society for Testing and Materials (ASTM)-approved eye guards may allow competitor to participate in most sports, but this must be judged on an individual basis. †Consult ophthalmologist					
Inguinal hernia	Yes	Yes	Yes	Yes	Yes
Kidney: Absence of one	No	Yes	Yes	Yes	Yes
Liver: Enlarged	No	No	Yes	Yes	Yes
Musculoskeletal disorders	*	*	*	*	*
*Needs individual assessment					
Neurologic					
History of serious head or spine trauma, repeated concussions, or craniotomy	*	*	Yes	Yes	Yes
Convulsive disorder					
Well controlled	Yes	Yes	Yes	Yes	Yes
Poorly controlled	No	No	Yes†	Yes	Yes‡
*Needs individual assessment †No swimming or weight lifting ‡No archery or riflery					
Ovary: Absence of one	Yes	Yes	Yes	Yes	Yes
Respiratory					
Pulmonary insufficiency	*	*	*	*	Yes
Asthma	Yes	Yes	Yes	Yes	Yes
*May be allowed to compete if oxygenation remains satisfactory during a graded stress test					
Sickle cell trait	Yes	Yes	Yes	Yes	Yes
Skin: Boils, herpes, impetigo, scabies	*	*	Yes	Yes	Yes
*No gymnastics with mats, martial arts, wrestling, or contact sports until not contagious					
Spleen: Enlarged	No	No	No	Yes	Yes
Testicle: Absence or undescended	Yes*	Yes*	Yes	Yes	Yes
*Certain sports may require protective cup.					

[a](From Committee on Sports Medicine: Recommendations for participation in competitive sports. *Pediatrics* 81(5):737–739, 1988. Reproduced by permission of *Pediatrics*.)

Table 2.3
Classification of Sports[a]

| Contact/Collision | Limited Contact/Impact | Noncontact | | |
		Strenuous	Moderately Strenuous	Nonstrenuous
Boxing	Baseball	Aerobic dancing	Badminton	Archery
Field hockey	Basketball	Crew	Curling	Golf
Football	Bicycling	Fencing	Table tennis	Riflery
Ice Hockey	Diving	Field		
Lacrosse	Field	Discus		
Martial arts	High jump	Javelin		
Rodeo	Pole vault	Shot put		
Soccer	Gymnastics	Running		
Wrestling	Horseback riding	Swimming		
	Skating	Tennis		
	Ice	Track		
	Roller	Weight lifting		
	Skiing			
	Cross-country			
	Downhill			
	Water			
	Softball			
	Squash, handball			
	Volleyball			

[a](From Committee on Sports Medicine: Recommendations for participation in competitive sports. *Pediatrics* 81(5):737–739, 1988. Reproduced by permission of *Pediatrics*.)

fractures. Plastic deformation, if unrecognized and therefore untreated, can become a permanent deformity. Torus fractures result from the ability of the bone to react to both compression and tension forces. This results in an outward buckling of the thin cortex of the metaphysis. Epiphyseal fractures often occur in the immature skeleton while ligamentous injuries occur in the mature skeleton. This is due to the fact that the ligaments are stronger than the growth plate. Epiphyseal injuries require careful long-term follow-up as sequelae (leg length discrepancies) may not be immediately evident. Apophyseal fractures occur where major tendon units attach to bone at large prominences or tuberosities. Sudden, contractile forces of the attached muscle may result in separation of the plate rather than the attaching tendon. For example, in the adult a sudden extension of the knee with the hip flexed will create a pulled hamstring. In the immature skeleton, this same maneuver results in an avulsion of the ischial tuberosity, which may require surgical intervention. Other areas where this type of injury occurs are the lesser trochanter, where the iliopsoas muscle attaches; the anterior inferior iliac spine, where the rectus muscle attaches; and the iliac crest, where the lateral abdominal muscles attach. Ligament injuries occurring in isolation are rare in the immature skeleton because the adjacent epiphyseal plate will fail prior to failure of the ligament (as discussed earlier). These differences in injury patterns make it important to assess the skeletal maturity of the athlete to determine injuries for which he/she is most at risk. Instruction in injury prevention increases the understanding of associated risks (Table 2.4).

Stress Fractures

Stress fractures result from repetitive stresses that are concentrated on a specific area of bone. These occur most often in the tibia, fibula, metatarsals, and calcaneous. The symptoms are local pain that is increased by activity and relieved by rest. Initial radiographs will show no bony disruption, but 2 to 3 weeks after initial symptoms, periosteal new bone may be seen. If untreated, stress fractures can become complete fractures.

Table 2.4
Prevention of Overuse Injuries in Adolescents

1. Choose the right activity. Help the young athlete choose a sport that will be compatible with physical ability, skill level, and talent.
2. Evaluate equipment for proper working order. Teach the adolescent to change to new shoes as soon as wear is noticed (usually on the outside border first).
3. Obtain a preseason physical examination. Teach the adolescent that this will help to focus on both strengths and limitations allowing adequate time before the sport season begins to increase fitness with a proper exercise prescription.
4. Gradually build up body condition. Teach the importance of getting in shape 6 weeks before the season starts. Include strength, stretching, and cardiorespiratory conditioning in regimen. This will not only tone the body, but will also increase endurance. Fatigue is an important factor in injuries.
5. Warm-up before each practice or game.
6. Teach the importance of proper cool-down.
7. Help the young athlete understand not to play or practice when overtired.

Upper Extremity Injuries

The most common injuries of the shoulder girdle are acromioclavicular (AC) joint separations, fractures of the clavicle and proximal humerus, and problems associated with the rotator cuff. Shoulder dislocations are rare in skeletally immature individuals. It is more likely that injury to the shoulder will be seen as fractures to the proximal humeral epiphysis or metaphysis. There are some individuals who can voluntarily dislocate their shoulder; this should not be treated as an injury and can usually be ignored.

Fracture is a common injury of the elbow. This requires immediate medical attention as permanent damage can result when the swelling that accompanies these injuries compresses the neurovascular structures that are nearby. Dislocations of the elbow are not uncommon and may be accompanied by an avulsion of the medial epicondyle or a coronoid fracture. These should not be reduced except by trained medical personnel. "Little League elbow" is a phenomenon occurring from the repetitive activity of the acceleration phase of pitching that applies abnormal stresses on the growth centers of the elbow. Chronic overstress can lead to tendinitis, or osteochondral fractures of the capitellum or radial head, and to permanent disability. New regulations governing how much children can pitch within a given time hopefully will limit the number of individuals seen with this problem.

Wrist and finger fractures are also common. Baseball, or mallet finger, is a particular type of fracture occurring when the ball hits the tip of the extended finger. This is a hyperflexion injury. Failure to recognize this injury can result in permanent flexion deformity of the distal phalanx (see Chapter 7 for in-depth discussion).

Lower Extremities

Most injuries involving the hip are in the form of acute fracture or dislocation. These injuries are true medical emergencies. The blood supply to the femoral epiphysis is easily injured and can result in disruption of the flow to the femoral head, and ultimately avascular necrosis—a serious condition with permanent disability.

The knee is the site of frequent injury in the form of fractures, ligamentous injury, and various overuse syndromes. As mentioned previously, fractures will occur in the immature skeleton as the distal femoral epiphysis is weaker than the ligament. For this reason, fractures are seen rather than sprains.

Knee pain is a common complaint in adolescence. Increased stress on the patella is a frequent cause of knee pain in adolescents and if left untreated results in chondromalacia. Pain is increased in any activity that causes the knee to be flexed against pressure. This compresses the undersurface of the patella against the femoral condyles resulting in pain. On palpation of the undersurface of the patella tenderness is encountered. Having the athlete extend the knee and contract the quadriceps, while compressing the patella against the femoral condyles, will reproduce this pain. If there are no other associated conditions, this is usually a self-limiting condition and symptoms disappear with treatment. Treatment includes stretching exercises, and maintenance of muscle strength through isometric exercises of the quadriceps and hamstrings. Isotonic exercises that bring the knee from a beginning flexed position into extension should be avoided.

Subluxation or recurrent dislocation of the patella is not an uncommon problem. Subluxation (partial dislocation) of the patella occurs in patellar malalignment syndromes where the patella moves down the intercondylar area in an uneven manner. Subluxation of the patella often requires some form of treatment. Quadriceps strengthening exercises to improve patella femoral tracking are the mainstay of treatment. A patella stabilization sleeve is often beneficial. Surgery is indicated for persistent painful subluxation.

Dislocation of the patella occurs when the patella is completely displaced from the intercondylar joint. This is usually the result of a direct force that pushes the patella laterally and is usually accompanied by pain and swelling. The patella may spontaneously relocate or may require manipulation to relocate. Once a patella has dislocated, it is at risk to dislocate again. In the face of recurrent dislocations, the athlete may face the decision of surgery or the modification of athletic pursuits.

When the patellar tendon becomes inflamed and tender, patellar tendinitis results. This is usually due to an overuse syndrome. It is commonly known as "jumper's knee" because it is common in athletes participating in sports that involve jumping, such as basketball, modern dance, and high jumping. On examination, tenderness is found at the inferior pole of the patellar tendon. In chronic cases, the patellar tendon may atrophy, and in severe cases, rupture. Conservative treatment consisting of rest, heat, anti-inflammatory medication, and limitation of activity followed by progressive resistance exercises is usually all that is needed. A brace to restrain the patella should be worn when activity is resumed.

Apophysitis of the tibial tubercle is known as Osgood-Schlatter's disease and commonly affects adolescents. It develops during the period of most rapid growth (the prepubescent period in girls and early adolescence in boys). It is more common in boys and occurs bilaterally approximately 20 to 30% of the time. Symptoms include pain with activity, quadriceps atrophy, and a prominent, tender tibial tubercle. Treatment is symptomatic and consists of limitation of activities, bracing, progressive resistive exercises, ice massage, and anti-inflammatory medication if necessary. Complete immobilization should be avoided as this increases muscle atrophy and lengthens rehabilitation time (see Chapter 9).

Although uncommon, acute sprains and fractures of the spine are seen in children and adolescents. When they occur they should be treated as in the adult. Any injury to the spine, including the cervical spine, must be treated as a fracture and treated with immediate immobilization and transport to a medical facility. Improper handling of cervical spine fractures can increase neurologic deficit, or cause neurologic deficit where there previously had been none. Any athlete with a neck injury should be x-rayed. In addition, the presence of persistent, posttraumatic neck pain suggests the possibility of spinal fracture or instability.

Soft Tissue Injuries

Ninety-five percent of all injuries are soft tissue injuries. The most common of these are sprains, strains, and contusions. The likelihood of these injuries increases with the violence of the sport. Sprains are injuries affecting ligaments, while strains are injuries affecting the tendons. Both sprains and strains are graded on a scale of I, II, and III according to severity. The severity of sprains deals with the loss of joint stability. Grade I sprains are mild sprains with overstretching only and no loss of joint stability. Grade II sprains have some instability, while Grade III sprains have total loss of ligamentous continuity. The severity of strains relates to the extent of disruption. Grade I and II sprains and strains often can be treated symptomatically with rest and muscle rehabilitation. Grade III sprains and strains frequently require surgical repair. Contusions should be treated with ice and compression. Severe contusions may benefit from elevation and rest. Stretching and strengthening exercises are important in maintaining muscle flexibility and strength.

NUTRITIONAL AND METABOLIC CONCERNS IN THE ADOLESCENT CLIENT

Adolescence is a period of turmoil characterized by growth in five dimensions: physical, sexual, social, emotional, and cognitive. Changes in each dimension can affect the nutritional status of the adolescent. The practitioner must be aware of how each change affects specific nutritional needs and creates potential nutritional deficits. This awareness will lead to early identification of less than optimal nutritional patterns. Early intervention may facilitate adoption of lifelong healthy nutritional patterns which optimize well-being and performance.

Physical Dimension

The peak growth period during adolescence is only surpassed by the neonatal stage. Rapid growth rates, maturational changes, and intense sports/exercise involvement make the adolescent susceptible to nutritional deficiencies (Bailey et al., 1984; Paige, 1986; Manjarrez and Birrer, 1983). Nutritional needs during this peak growth period include energy needs, distribution of the basic four food groups, calcium, and iron requirements.

Energy

Energy needs are increased during adolescence. These escalating needs are a function of sex, biologic age, and maturation age, rather than simply chronologic age and, therefore, age-specific recommendations are difficult to define. Energy ranges are a more useful guide to establishing caloric needs of the adolescent (Paige, 1986). Table 2.5 presents energy and protein requirements for adolescent boys and girls. The peak growth period for girls is earlier and shorter than for boys, and energy and protein requirements are less for girls. Adolescent girls are therefore more prone to weight gain during this time.

Table 2.5
Energy and Protein Requirements for Adolescent Boys and Girls[a]

| Sex | Age | Energy Intake (kcal) | | Protein gm |
		Median	Range	
Males	11–14	2700	2000–3700	45
	15–18	2800	2100–3900	56
	19–22	2900	2200–3900	56
Females	11–14	2200	1500–3000	46
	15–22	2100	1200–3000	46

[a]Adapted from Food and Nutrition Board pamphlet.

Vitamins and Minerals

Research has shown that teenagers' diets are generally adequate in protein intake but likely to be deficient in vitamin C and calcium (Burtis et al., 1988; and Fahey et al., 1987). Calabrese (1985) concurred that nutritional density of adolescent diets was low, and also found marginal intake of vitamins A, D, folic acid, calcium, phosphorous, magnesium, and zinc. These deficits are not related to increased requirements of peak growth, but rather to nutritional patterns that include fad foods, fast-foods, and "junk" foods. Adherence to basic four guidelines can prevent these nutritional deficits, and generally does not require vitamin or mineral supplementation; however, supplementation is indicated if adequate nutritional patterns are not established.

Iron

Iron intake has been found to be deficient in adolescent girls, especially those actively involved in athletics. Vigorous physical activity causes an increased requirement for iron. When this requirement is combined with iron losses through menstruation, the female athlete is at risk for clinical or subclinical iron deficiency.

Although there is controversy over the effect of iron deficiency on performance, iron deficiency is believed to have an adverse effect on athletic endurance. The female athlete's diet history should be monitored for adequacy of iron intake (Elliot and Goldberg, 1985). Foods high in iron content include red meat, lamb, calf's liver, raisins, figs, and cooked peas and beans, grains and other vegetables contain lower quantities of iron. Subclinical or clinical iron deficiency requires oral iron supplementation, as iron-containing multivitamin preparations may not correct the deficiency. Cooking in iron skillets/pans and eating/drinking high vitamin C sources such as orange juice while ingesting iron-enriched foods increases absorption.

Calcium

Calcium requirements are increased during adolescence to meet the needs of rapid bone growth (Fahey et al., 1987). The NIH Consensus Conference (1987) adjusted the RDA of calcium upward, establishing a recommended level for adolescents at 1200 mg/day. The average American diet contains approximately 400 to 500 mg/day of calcium—a deficit of about 700 mg/day.

Calcium deficits can be further compounded by high-phosphorus or high-protein diets. Adolescents consume large quantities of processed foods, soda drinks, and junk foods. These foods are high in phosphorus content, and high levels of phosphate interfere with calcium absorption. Calcium requirements may be increased 400 mg/day in persons with a high-phosphate intake.

Dieting is another barrier to achieving calcium balance. High-protein diets are a common fad diet for adolescent boys. High-protein intakes cause hypercalciuria, which may lead to calcium deficiencies. If calcium intake is not adequate, the calcium is drawn from the bone.

Fasting diets and low-calorie diets also place the adolescent at risk for calcium deficits. Foods rich in calcium are often rich in calories and avoided by those counting calories. For the calorie conscious individual, it is best to recommend skim milk products, shellfish, and dark green vegetables (excluding spinach) for meeting calcium needs (see Appendix). Calcium requirements can easily be met by eating four or more daily servings of yogurt, cheese, or milk. This not only supplies the needed calcium but also the vitamin D necessary for calcium absorption. Calcium supplementation may be necessary to meet the recommended levels for the adolescent.

With the current emphasis on the relationship between calcium and bone health, many food products are now fortified with calcium. Fortified orange juice (providing elemental calcium of 300 mg/8 ounce) and fortified calcium-rich cereals are available. These products have the added advantage of supplying vitamin C and B vitamins that are frequently deficient in the adolescent diet. Calcium tablets are also available, generally inexpensive, and lack toxicity. Generic calcium carbonate is the least expensive form of calcium supplementation. Different brands contain varying amounts of elemental calcium; therefore, labels must be carefully read. Tums tablets contain elemental calcium of about 200 mg/tablet. Younger individuals should take calcium supplements on an empty stomach.

Nutrition and Sports

There are many myths and fads surrounding nutritional patterns that are supposed to produce optimal performance. The adolescent striving for athletic excellence falls prey to many of these performance diets marketed to help the athlete achieve the competitive edge. These diets are often expensive and may be lacking in essential nutritional components.

The nutritional recommendation for athletes is simple: eat a normal diet selected from the basic four foods (see Appendix M) with special attention to consuming sufficient calories to meet the demands of energy expenditure for a particular sport (Manjarrez and Birrer, 1983; Vitale, 1985; Elliot and Goldberg, 1985; and Dohm, 1984). Vigorous exercise does not cause an increased demand for specific nutrients but does increase caloric demands. As energy requirements are met from a variety of basic four foods, requirements for other essential nutrients will also be met.

Caloric Needs

Caloric requirements can best be met by complex carbohydrates such as bread, cereal, potatoes, rice, and pasta. Foods with a high-fat content should be avoided; they do not provide the level of energy supplied in high-carbohydrate foods and high-fat contents predispose the athlete to cardiovascular disease. The ideal caloric distribution pattern should maintain energy balance and provide 55% of energy as carbohydrate, 30% as fat, and 15% as protein.

Protein Needs

The consumption of high-protein diets is a prevalent practice among athletes. It is a dietary myth that a substantial amount of protein is needed to meet extra energy demands, improve athletic performance, and increase muscle mass (Manjarrez and Birrer, 1983). Muscle mass is not increased through a high-protein diet but through appropriate exercise.

In the early stages of training, protein requirements are slightly increased from the normal 1.5 gm/kg body weight for adolescents to approximately 1.6 to 2.0 gm/kg body weight, depending on the intensity of the exercise. After adaptation to training, protein intake returns to 1.0 to 1.5 gm/kg body weight. As most American diets provide about 15% of energy as protein, an athlete on an energy diet of 55 kcal/kg will have a protein intake of 2 gm/kg, still above the recommended dietary allowance.

Nutrient Need Variability

Energy and nutrient needs vary according to type of exercise and training. For purposes of discussion, training here is divided into three categories according to energy expenditure: strength exercise (weightlifting, wrestling), endurance exercise (long-distance running, soccer, cross-country skiing), and spurt-energy exercise (swimming, gymnastics, short-distance running, track-and-field events). Special considerations for each category will be presented.

Strength Exercise

Strength exercise includes activities such as weightlifting, wrestling, and certain football positions; this classification depends to a large degree on the muscle mass of the individual. Muscle enlargement or hypertrophy is the adaptation that occurs in response to consistent strength exercise. The stimulus for hypertrophy is not increased nutritional intake of protein; rather, the stimulus is within the muscle itself and involves stretch or force development (Dohm, 1984).

There is little scientific evidence that consumption of large protein supplements will have any beneficial effect on muscle hypertrophy, muscular strength, or physical performance. As long as the athlete consumes an adequate energy diet, protein needs are met by the normal diet that provides 15% of the energy as protein. During initial training phases, protein requirements are slightly increased, but still met by the 15% ratio.

Of concern in strength exercise sports, especially wrestling, is the practice of rapid weight loss to meet competition weight categories. This practice has negative effects on both the athlete's health and the athlete's competitive abilities. Rapid weight loss is accompanied by loss of lean body mass (strength, protein). This lean body mass is frequently replaced with adipose tissue rather than muscle protein. The rapid weight loss is also accompanied by dehydration that can threaten the athlete's well-being during competition.

The practice of carbohydrate loading is not recommended for this nonendurance activity. Carbohydrate loading only has an effect on performance when glycogen stores are depleted from exhaustive long-term exercise that occurs with the endurance sports. The effect of carbohydrate loading on the wrestler or weightlifter could be an impaired performance because of water accumulation in the muscle and a sensation of muscle stiffness (Elliot and Goldberg, 1985).

The pregame meal has been generally overrated. An athlete's performance is more dependent on long-term dietary practices than the last meal prior to an event. The pregame meal guidelines (Table 2.6) are not to assure supercompetition or superperformance but rather to minimize gastrointestinal problems during competition and maximize energy utilization. The guidelines for the pregame meal emphasize gastric emptying prior to competition and maintenance of low insulin levels to allow for free fatty acids to be used as an energy source (Elliot and Goldberg, 1985). Foods selected are a combination of foods from the basic four pattern, as well as additional simple carbohydrates to increase glycogen levels.

Endurance Exercises

Success in endurance exercise (cross-country skiing, long-distance running, soccer) depends on the ability to supply energy to the muscle for an extended period of time (Dohm, 1984). Increasing food intake (selected from basic four guidelines) to meet the increased caloric demand is the prime nutritional consideration. Estimates of sufficient caloric intake can be based on achievement of weight maintenance versus weight loss or gain.

Hepatic glycogen stores normally last about 12 hours. This level may be depleted in 4 hours when endurance exercise is ongoing, leading to a symptomatic hypoglycemia. Therefore, the goal in endurance exercise is to maximize precompetition glycogen levels and prevent hypoglycemia during the activity. This is generally accomplished by adequate nutritional intake on a permanent basis, a carbohydrate loading regimen 1 week precompetition, and glucose drinks during competition.

Glycogen stores in the muscle and liver play an important role in the athlete's ability to withstand prolonged activity (Manjarrez and Birrer, 1983). To augment glycogen stores, a carbohydrate loading plan (also called muscle glycogen supercompensation plan) was developed. Previously a three-phase process of carbohydrate loading, beginning 1 week precompetition, was advocated. However, because of the associated risks of fatigue, nausea, and the potential for chest pain, arrhythmias, angina, elevated triglycerides, and myoglobinuria with persistent loading, the practice has been abandoned.

The carbohydrate loading process currently recommended is nonexhausting. Athletes are advised to increase their carbohydrate consumption to 350 gm/day with their regular conditioning program. Three days prior to an event (as training tapers off) carbohydrates should gradually be increased until the athlete is consuming between 525 to 650 gm/day. The athlete should be advised that carbohydrate loading will not increase speed; rather the effect is that of performance with less fatigue (Fishman and Curhan, 1986).

Fluid intake is of primary concern during endurance sports. With prolonged exercise, the athlete may lose as much as 2 to 4 liters of sweat/hour or 6 to 8 lbs of body weight. For endurance events, 600 ml (21

Table 2.6
Nutritional Guidelines for the Pregame Meal

1. Avoid high fat or bulk content in the pregame meal; these foods delay gastric emptying.
2. Avoid simple carbohydrates (immediately prior to competition) as they increase insulin levels and cause a rebound hypoglycemia, and inhibit use of free fatty acids as an energy source (this is especially problematic in endurance exercise where there is a shift toward greater use of fat, thereby sparing glycogen and improving endurance). Simple carbohydrates are also hypertonic and cause fluid to move into the gut and cause cramping.
3. Avoid high protein meals precompetition as they slow digestive processes and cause increased urination.
4. Avoid solid food intake less than 3 to 4 hours prior to competition to assure gastric emptying.
5. Sample pregame meal may include:
   - 1 serving roasted or broiled meat or poultry[a]
   - 1 serving complex carbohydrate (potato, macaroni, rice, pasta)[a]
   - 1 serving vegetable[a]
   - 1 cup skim milk[a]
   - 1 teaspoon fat[a]
   - 1 serving fruit juice
   - 1 serving sugar cookies or plain cake
   - 2 cups additional beverages
   - Salt food well
6. Some athletes find it difficult to take solid foods because of pregame nerves. In these cases a liquid diet can be taken using products such as Sustacal, Ensure, and Nutriment.

[a]Foods selected directly from the basic four pattern.

ounces) of fluid should be drunk 2 hours prior to competition (the kidneys will process the fluid in 90 minutes, allowing the athlete time to urinate prior to the event) 400 to 500 ml (14 to 17 ounces) should be drunk 10 to 15 minutes prior to competition and small amounts (4 to 8 ounces) should be drunk every 20 to 30 minutes during the event. Although it is not recommended that glucose solutions be taken immediately prior to competition, once exercise has begun, the intake of glucose containing fluids does not have a deleterious effect on the regulation of blood glucose concentrations, and can be taken without an adverse influence on performance.

The postendurance meal should be high in carbohydrates (potatoes, pasta), and in those carbohydrates that replace lost electrolytes (oranges, fig newtons, bananas, etc.). The athlete should be advised to drink nonalcoholic beverages until the urine is clear.

Spurt-Energy or High-Intensity Exercise

Spurt-energy exercise such as swimming, gymnastics, and sprinting is characterized by brief periods of high-energy activity (a few seconds to a few minutes) with alternate rest periods. This activity is considered to be nonaerobic, with moderate caloric consumption. High-intensity exercise relies almost exclusively on muscle glycogen as an energy source. Increasing the percent of dietary carbohydrate allows the most efficient repletion of muscle glycogen and may improve performance during daily high-intensity workouts.

The most common problem in high-intensity exercise is weight control. Maintaining an ideal competitive weight is important for performance in all high-intensity exercise. The caloric intake required varies with the body size, age, nontraining activity level, and intensity of the training program. The swimmer will need significantly more calories than does the dancer or sprinter, as the energy cost of swimming is about four times greater than that of running (Grandjean, 1986). Maintenance of an ideal competitive weight throughout the

year is associated with the athlete having more power, more endurance, and more speed for competition. Starvation diets decrease performance by decreasing aerobic power and capacity, speed, coordination, strength and judgment.

This problem of weight control is especially true for female athletes striving for a painfully thin body image while simultaneously developing the motor skills necessary for performing. A higher incidence of anorexia nervosa is present in the female gymnast, dancer, and figure skater. In these sports there is a concern for appearance which is foreign to most other sporting activities. Calabrese (1985) found the diets of female gymnasts and dancers to be of low nutritional density and of low-calorie value. Ledoux (in Calabrese, 1985) had similar findings, but also found that this problem was more severe in the female athlete 15 years and older. These studies concluded that in order to achieve a low body weight, young women found it necessary to follow low-calorie regimens that ultimately resulted in nutritional deficits.

In addition to nutritional deficits, female athletes who consume low-calorie diets are at risk for delayed menarche, secondary amenorrhea, and irregular cycles. These abnormalities are likely to be caused by the combination of excessive dieting that limits the percentage of body fat and increased exercise patterns in relation to the caloric intake. The hypoestrogenemia caused by delayed menarche or irregular cycles affects the bone, causing osteopenia.

It is important to counsel teenage girls and their parents about the risks of nutritional deficits and the effect of delayed menarche on decreasing bone mass, predisposing the child to osteoporosis at an earlier age. Severe caloric restrictions can result in the loss of large quantities of electrolytes, minerals, glycogen stores, and muscle tissue. These result in symptoms of hypoglycemia, ketonuria, decreased urinary output, hypotension, weakness, and fainting. Guidelines for weight control should include modest caloric restriction (a decrease of 500 to 1000 kcal/day less than usual) along with an endurance exercise program (Calabrese, 1985). The difficulty in this regimen frequently is finding the time for endurance exercise when it is vital to practice the high-intensity exercise.

SEXUAL DEVELOPMENT: BODY IMAGE AND THE NEED TO BE THIN

The physical demands of puberty and the growth spurt have been discussed. In conjunction with the physical demands of puberty, it is important to take into account the developing body image of the adolescent. The ideal body image frequently presented to the adolescent through television and popular magazines is extremely thin, does not take into account body type variations. It is not surprising that a preoccupation exists in both sexes, but it is far more common in the adolescent girl than in the adolescent boy.

"Fear of fat" is being reported both in the medical literature as well as the consumer news as beginning as early as age 10. This is especially problematic, as dieting at this age will delay puberty and stunt growth.

Anorexia Nervosa

Anorexia nervosa is found most frequently in the vulnerable population of teenage girls and young women between the age of 10 and 20. Although this disorder is found in boys, it is only found one-tenth as often as in females. Anorexia can present with a broad variety of clinical signs, the foremost being severe weight loss in a person who is apparently otherwise healthy (Lucas, 1986). Hunger is present but suppressed. Self-inflicted weight loss, amenorrhea, decreased sexual interest, and a morbid fear of being unable to control eating characterize this syndrome. Assessment for these signs can lead to early intervention that could minimize the disorder or prevent complications of anorexia. Complications include: anemia, vitamin deficiencies, hypoproteinemia, bulimia, vomiting, dehydration, erosion of dental enamel, electrolyte disturbances, metabolic alkalosis, cardiac arrhythmias, and death.

Health care practitioners should be alert to this disorder. If identified in the early stages, it is frequently treatable with educational intervention, a gradual increase in food intake, and emotional support for the family and patient. More advanced forms require more intensive therapies.

SOCIAL/EMOTIONAL FACTORS IN ADOLESCENT NUTRITION

Eating is a way of socializing, and adolescence is characterized by a growing independence from the family and a tendency to follow the peer group. Fast-foods, fad diets, and fad foods become very popular during this time. The risk of fast-foods is primarily the high-caloric content that can lead to problems with weight control. Although the range of foods sold in fast-food restaurants is usually limited, the nutritional content of meals is generally adequate if proper selection is made (Yeung et al., 1983). It is best to help the adolescent select appropriate fast-foods rather than limit them, as limiting could interfere with socialization.

Fad diets are not recommended for the adolescent client. These diets are generally based on adult metabolism and should not be used in the teenage child. A study of adolescent girls (Storz and Greene, 1983) revealed that fad diets were most desired in the group requiring greater than 10% weight loss. These girls should be considered at high risk for fad diets and educated appropriately.

Obesity in the Adolescent

Coping patterns consisting of excessive food intake to handle stress may be established in the adolescent years. This is the ideal time for the practitioner to intervene to break this cycle before lifelong patterns are established. Many adolescents face threats to their self-esteem because of obesity or perceived fatness. The frightening reality is that many of these adolescents are not obese, but not the very slim image that has become the ideal.

There is much controversy about weight-control measures in the adolescent. Some professionals recommend minimizing weight control measures until after the growth spurt while others actively treat the weight problem prior to the growth spurt. During the growth spurt even mild dietary restrictions result in negative nitrogen balance. This does not occur when dietary restrictions are imposed after the growth spurt (Paige, 1986).

Because of the controversy concerning weight control measures, most nutritionists are recommending a behavioral modification approach that focuses on analyzing nutritional patterns. Identifying the cues that trigger overeating can lead to reshaping of behavior. Involvement of the parents is necessary so that buying patterns do not include high-calorie foods but include more low calorie foods. Eating environments should be monitored; watching television while eating, eating on the run, and stressful topics of conversation at the table should be avoided.

Cognitive Approach to Nutrition

The adolescent is not only emerging socially but is better able to take information and process it according to personal relevance. Educational approaches to nutrition counseling should include instruction on the basic four foods, with a special emphasis on the recommended ratio of protein, carbohydrates, and fats; include what these foods do and also why increasing intake is not necessarily beneficial.

In addition to instruction on the basic four foods, hazards of teenage dieting and anorexia should be discussed. Calcium balance and the multiple factors influencing bone growth and osteoporosis must be included, as it is during adolescence that peak bone mass is developing.

SUMMARY

Working with adolescents is a challenge that can be extremely rewarding if one understands the changes that occur at this time. An understanding of the physical, emotional, and psychological changes of adolescence increases the effectiveness of dealings with this age group. While generally a healthy time of life, there are a number of orthopaedic disorders specific to this age; it is important to know the effect the immature skeleton has on the injuries likely to be incurred by the adolescent.

The increasing number of adolescents participating in sports activities has also increased the number of athletes seen with sports-related injuries. As important as treating these injuries is the preparticipation physical exam to determine which adolescents are at increased risk for injury and even death. Appropriate choices of sports activities, as well as encouraging physical conditioning prior to participation, can decrease the number of injuries. Education regarding the importance of stretching exercises prior to events and exercises to condition muscles to prevent injuries, as well as appropriate treatment and rehabilitation, are responsibilities of all health care providers involved in the treatment of adolescents with sports-related injuries.

References

American Academy of Orthopaedic Surgeons: *Athletic Training Sports Medicine*. Chicago, Academy of Orthopaedic Surgeons, 1984.

Bradford D, Hensinger R (eds): *The Pediatric Spine*. New York, Georg Thieme Verlag, 1985.

Bunnell WP: An objective criterion for scoliosis screening. *J Bone Jt Surg* 66-A(9):1381–1387, 1984.

Burtis G, Davis J, Martin S: *Applied Nutrition and Diet Therapy*. Philadelphia, WB Saunders, 1988.

Calabrese L: Nutritional and medical aspects of gymnastics. *Clin Sports Med* 4(1):23–29, 1985.

Cleveland L, Peterkin B, Blum A, Becker S: Recommended dietary allowances as standards for family food plans. *J Nutr Educ* 15(1):8–14, 1983.

Committee on Sports Medicine, American Academy of Pediatrics, Smith NJ (ed): *Health Care for Young Athletes*. Evanston, IL, American Academy of Pediatrics, 1983.

Committee on Sports Medicine: Recommendations for participation in competitive sports. *Pediatrics* 81(5):737–739, 1988.

Dohm G: Protein nutrition for the athlete. *Clin Sports Med*, 3(3):595–602, 1984.

Elliot D, Goldberg M: Nutrition and exercise. *Med Clin North Am* 69(1):71–79, 1985.

Erikson E: *Childhood and Society*. New York, WW Norton, 1963.

Fahey P, Boltri J, Monk J: Key issues in nutrition during childhood and adolescence. *Postgrad Med* 81(4):301–305, 1987.

Fishman JA, Curhan HP: *Sports Nutrition: a Guide for the Professional Working with Active People.* Chicago, American Diet Association, 1986.

Gollnick P, Matoba H: Role of carbohydrate in exercise. *Clin Sports Med* 3(3):583–591,1984.

Gossett AT, Lincoln CE: The preparticipation physical exam: a first step toward injury prevention. *Surg Rounds Orthop* 2(7):53–55, 1988.

Grandjean A: Nutrition for swimmers. *Clin Sports Med* 5(1):65–75, 1986.

Greenspan A: *Orthopaedic Radiology.* Philadelphia, JB Lippincott, 1988.

Lovell WW, Winter RB (eds): *Pediatric Orthopaedics, ed 2.* Philadelphia, JB Lippincott, 1986.

Lucas A: Anorexia nervosa. *Hosp Med* March:127–149, 1986.

Manjarrez CK, Birrer R: Nutrition and athletic performance. *Am Family Phys* 28(5):105–115, 1983.

Marks A, Fisher M: Health assessment and screening during adolescence. *Pediatrics* 80(1)(Suppl):135–158, 1987.

McCarthy RE: Prevention of complications of scoliosis by early detection. *Clin Orthop Related Res* 222, 1987.

McCullough FL: *Self-Esteem of Diabetic Adolescents Compared with Non-Diabetic Adolescents.* Unpublished master's thesis, University of Arkansas for Medical Science, 1981.

Mercer R: *Perspective on Adolescent Health Care.* Philadelphia, JB Lippincott, 1979.

Moe JH, Winter RB, Bradford DS, Lonstein, JE: *Scoliosis Screening.* Philadelphia, WB Saunders, 1978.

Nachemson A: Adult scoliosis and back pain. *Spine* 4(6):513–517, 1979.

Ogden J: *Skeletal Injury in the Child.* Philadelphia, Lea and Febiger, 1982.

Paige D: Obesity in childhood and adolescence. *Postgrad Med* 79(1):233–245, 1986.

Rang M: *Children's Fractures,* ed 2. Philadelphia, JB Lippincott 1983.

Scott WN, Nisonson B, Nicholas JA: (ed): *Principles of Sports Medicine.* Baltimore, Williams & Wilkins, 1983.

Storz N, Green W: Body weight, body image, and perception of fad diets in adolescent girls. *J Nutr Educ* 15(1):15–17, 1983.

Tachdjian MO: *Pediatric Orthopaedics.* Philadelphia, WB Saunders, 1972.

Truswell A: ABC of nutrition. *Br Med J* 291:397–399, 1985.

Vitale J: Nutrition in sports medicine. *Clin Orthop Related Res* 1984.

Yeung D, Wyatt M, Habbick B, Wolfish M: Fast foods, food fads and the educational challenge. *Can Med Assoc J* 129:692–695, 1983.

chapter 3

The Adult

MARYANN CURRAN TAWA, R.N., M.S.N., A.N.P.C.
SUSAN W. SALMOND, R.N., Ed.D.

PSYCHOSOCIAL DEVELOPMENT

Adulthood has commonly been perceived as the time in which we abolish pre-existing anxieties and usher in an epoch of stability and freedom. By virtue of becoming a member of this elite classification (ages 18 to 60), one must assume responsibility for carrying the physiological and developmental baggage that the era dictates. When looking at the epidemiology of orthopedic risks and problems in the adult population, one must closely equate the developmental issues associated with this group.

Establishing ourselves as young adults will occur once we have given ourselves permission to gain closure on adolescent conflicts. Young adults are faced with challenges of both participation and completion of educational endeavors, of careers, and of entry into the labor force. Sufficient resources such as time, income, and accommodating location will permit young adults to participate in recreational sports in these years. Industries in the 1980s are committed to the concept of general health and fitness for their employees. On-site health assessment, institution of exercise facilities, and industry's partial sponsorship of work-related recreational trips, collectively contribute to the dual goal of promoting general fitness and supporting worker morale. Making the decision to marry, not to marry, or to defer marriage, feature prominently in the early adult years. The athletic arena has become a comfort-able place for socialization of many young adults. In fact, in some regions of the United States the upscale health club has superseded the night club for the successful introduction and networking of young people.

Defining the family is no easy task in the 1980s. The family takes many varied forms. Parenting may be actualized through the electively single parent, the divorced parent, the homosexual parent, the foster parent, and the "traditional" parent. Despite the different configurations of individuals who parent, the stress of balancing occupation, home, and family remains consistent. Personal fitness regimens are often neglected during the early child rearing years due to lack of time, income, and childcare facilities.

Traditionally, in the middle years the adult is cultivating and refining interpersonal relationships. Spouses may greatly modify their interaction with each other; the search for the "individual" behind the husband/wife role is a pressing task at this time. Married couples are permitted to refocus their attentions away from the children, and on renewed awareness of the initial relationship consituting the marriage (Kaluger and Kaluger, 1979). A mid-life crisis may ensue, and the potential for divorce is high. Intergenerational adjustments take much of the adults' time and energy. Becoming a grandparent and an in-law, as well as remaining a child and a parent provide many roles. Considering the extended period of the identity moratorium (Erikson, 1959) for youth and the medically elongated life span of many aged individuals, middle-aged adults can expect more family responsibilities rather than fewer. Intrapsychic flexibility is needed in the middle years, for it represents a period where children mature, parents die, and circles of friends may be broken by divorce, illness, and death.

The "empty nest," or the departure of the last child from home, has been identified as a hallmark event in the middle years. Most theorists concur that the anticipation of the empty nest is far worse than the actual experience. For many adults, the reorganization of the home and the re-establishment of the couple is beneficial. Many females, who have historically placed career pursuits on the back burner during their child rearing years, will now re-enter the work force. In 1965, Blenker described the stage of "filial maturity" in reference to the adult's adaptation to aging parents. Filial maturity implies the discovery of parents in terms of their individuality rather than in the role parents. The death of a parent has significant ramifications for the middle-aged individual who remains. This individual must now assume the position of maintaining the family tradition, legacy, and history, and giving advice to progeny (Hymovich and Barnard, 1979).

During middle-aged adulthood one begins to correlate small-scale civic responsibility with how one can fit into the broad scheme of civic and social improvement of the world. Contributing to the overall vision of community, national, and international development is permissible in these years. Jung (1971) described the last half of life as being less oriented to pragmatic tasks and more toward aesthetic concerns, spiritual development, and ego transcendence. Along with this altruism, middle-age is also the time when the adult can resume leisure activities and pursue self-satisfying hobbies. A balance of economic standards, demonstrated by spending money for personal gratification and putting it aside for future security, is another challenge of the middle years (Kaluger and Kaluger, 1979, p. 401).

PHYSIOLOGICAL CHANGES

The biological changes during the middle adult years occur gradually. This period represents a long "plateau" in the life span. The gradual and unrelenting physical displays of aging include graying of hair, wrinkling and sagging of flesh, and overall decrease in metabolic rate. Energy levels are no longer boundless; the adult now requires rest between strenuous activities. Skeletal muscle increases in bulk until age 50 and then begins its degenerative process by age 60. As gross motor coordination depends on skeletal muscle, this decline increases the risk of injury for the middle-aged recreational athlete. The concept of "physical fitness" often becomes a middle-aged obsession for both sexes. The thrust is on maintenance and improvement of cardiovascular function. A symbolic change in adulthood is that one *must prepare* for exercise through aerobic warm-up. This represents a contrast to adolescence and early adulthood when one would warm up only minimally, if at all.

Discussion of exercise recommendations for adults will follow in subsequent pages. There appears to be great uniformity among individuals with regard to physiological sense organ changes in adulthood. The individual's response to the sense organ changes is what remains diverse and puzzling. Eye changes often mark the middle-aged adult's realization that "loss of sense" is irreversibly connected with growing older. Presbyopia is the reduction in the elasticity of the crystalline lens of the eye that inhibits accommodation for near points of vision; middle-aged adults must now wear glasses to read. With middle-age, there is gradual deterioration and hardening of the auditory cells and nerves; presbycusis is compensated for by the use of hearing aids (Kaluger and Kaluger, 1979, p. 410). Collectively, these sense organ changes place the adult population groups at risk for domestic, recreational, and work-related orthopaedic injury.

The nurse provider is in an important position to participate in primary, secondary, and tertiary preventative measures with this group. Primary prevention includes periodic age-related health screening for the detection of eye and ear problems such as glaucoma and acuity loss, as well as patient education regarding anticipatory guidance on loss issues associated with aging. Secondary prevention includes performance of screening measures, such as tenometry readings to check for glaucoma and gross auditory acuity testing to evaluate hearing, and referrals to tertiary care centers for surgical and medical interventions as appropriate. Tertiary prevention focuses on patient education, such as instruction in home safety (elimination of scatter rugs, appropriate home lighting, etc.) and follow-up on newly implemented treatment programs.

Perception of self in the "adult role" in "middle-age" will influence anxiety; change of life becomes a common thematic anxiety for middle-aged adults. Climacteric in males and menopause in females evoke both biological and psychological states of change. Symptoms of menopause commence with hormonal shifts in females between the ages of 40 to 55 years. The shift is marked by reduction in ovarian and other gonadotropic organ activities. Physical symptoms include menstrual irregularities (with eventual cessation), changes in body contour (due to redistribution of fat), hot flashes, hair attenuation, and atrophy of splenic and lymphatic glandular tissue (Kaluger and Kaluger, 1979, p. 418). Psychologically, the cessation of menstruation, for some women, can be laden with much intrapersonal apprehension. It may represent absence of "female" potential; a new vacancy. In contrast, there are proportionally large numbers of women who adapt readily to the change.

There is no literal physical change in males comparable to the change in females. It is hypothesized that the emotional liability experienced by some males in climacteric is attributable to the progressive aging process and diminishing sexual drive. Unlike their female counterparts, male androgen levels decline slowly and reproductive function does not end until old age.

COMMON CONCERNS OF THE ADULT

Accidents of the Work Place

"An accident is an unplanned and uncontrolled event in which the action or reaction of an object, substances, person, or radiation results in personal injury or the probability thereof" (Petersen et al., 1980, p.33). In order to understand those factors that contribute to orthopaedic injury in the adult population, one must understand the ramifications of accidental occurrence. Accidents result from both direct and indirect causes. Direct causes can be conceptualized as those concrete, measurable culprits such as hazardous materials or poorly designed equipment. Indirect causes are analogous to "symptoms" of unsafe acts or unsafe conditions in a system. They may represent symptoms of poor management or policy, inadequate controls, lack of knowledge, improper assessment of existing hazards, or other personnel factors. Specific examples of unsafe acts include: improper use of equipment, improper lifting, use of illicit drugs or alcohol. Unsafe conditions include: defective equipment, poor housekeeping, improper illumination, or inadequate ventilation (Petersen et al., 1980, p.35).

A wide variety of allied health disciplines has proposed and tested theorems that indicate that accident liability is somewhat situational. Various tests have been devised to increase and quantify situational factors that may precipitate an accident. Often, an injurious event will ensue when one's coping mechanisms are taxed by life changes. Research indicates that accident liability, at this time, is greater than the susceptibility to illness. Health care providers employed in settings where they may encounter patients' emergencies should be cognizant of life changes when assessing causes of accidents.

The work place proves to be a familiar launching pad for orthopaedic injuries in the adult population. This is due to very practical considerations such as physical condition in the work environment, number of hours worked, and actual job functions. For example, the risk of developing low back pain is high in truck drivers, material handlers, nurses, and workers whose jobs require heavy physical demands, awkward postures, or postures that must be sustained for prolonged periods of time. Data submitted from insurance companies lead one to speculate that a worker is three times more susceptible to compensable low back injury if exposed to excessive manual handling tasks. The onset of low back pain in nurses takes place earlier in life and is largely precipitated by conditions at work, specifically, by activities involving repetitive lifting, such as lifting a patient in bed, helping a patient get out of bed, and moving beds.

About one-half of all workers' compensation cases involve musculoskeletal conditions. Although the vast majority of work-related orthopaedic injuries are minor in insult, they often result in some degree of permanent, partial disability for the worker. Seemingly "mild" strains and sprains can evolve into long-term residual disability resulting in lost work time and wages. Thus the prudent nurse provider will carefully weigh the multifactorial picture presentation when eliciting histories and strategizing treatment programs for the patient injured in the work place. It should be recognized by providers that a select subgroup of workers involved in occupational accidents does derive some secondary gain from the incident. The greater the time spent away from the work force, the more difficulty encountered with readaption to work routine. Some workers will pursue lengthy and perhaps unwarranted compensation periods post injury. Some workers may develop apprehensive attitudes relating to the safety of their work environment. Many injured workers receive unwelcome attention from colleagues when their "vacancy" is realized and work loads are intensified. Health care providers employed in occupational settings can intervene with counseling and directive activities to assist the worker with motivational issues. Sometimes merely addressing the hesitancy ob-

served by the provider will open the door for candid discussion. Workers permanently disabled, who may never resume their previously established occupation, may need referral to psychological or social service agencies for long-term intervention.

Workers' Compensation

Workers' compensation is a legal system designed to divert some of the costs of occupational injuries and illness from workers to employers. Nurses and physicians who provide direct care to patients who have sustained work-related injury must have a minimal working knowledge of workers' compensation laws in order to utilize the system efficiently. "Prior to the adoption of the first workers' compensation law in 1910, the worker was presumed to be a free agent, voluntarily taking a job and thereby assuming whatever risks were inherent in the job" (Rowe, 1985, p.7). The worker was expected to bear the burden of proof when negligence was suspected in the work environment. Hence, attorney and court fees poured in and future job security was held in abeyance. Workers' compensation legislation was aimed at redressing potential social injustice. In fact, the net result of the workers' compensation laws was to offer wider coverage than the pre-existing system. The compensation laws generally require employers, or their primary insurers, to reimburse part of injured workers' lost wages and all medical and rehabilitative expenses.

A worker can qualify for benefits if three conditions exist simultaneously. There must be injury or illness; the injury or illness must arise from the course of employment; and there must be medical/rehabilitative costs, lost wages, or disfigurement. In the United States, 50 states and three federal workers' compensation jurisdictions, each with its own statutes and regulations, exist today. Common features identified by all programs are summarized below:
1. Benefit formulas prescribed by law,
2. Medical and rehabilitative expenses covered in full,
3. Lost wages reimbursed partially (amount is state-regulated),

4. Employers equally responsible for paying benefit to injured worker,
5. Most claims are processed and paid by insurance companies derived from annual premiums,
6. Existence of a no-fault system of workers' compensation (Levy and Wegmen, 1983).

History and Physical Examination of the Injured Worker

Reconstructing a detailed and accurate scenario of events precipitating injury, and systematically describing the mechanism of insult, is crucial to industrial orthopaedics. The nurse provider is confronted with the task of developing an unbiased, factually corroborated database that is comprehensible for all participating members of the treatment team. Envisioning the client in the work environment is compulsory. On occasion, the provider may be called upon to translate psychosocial influences into the injurious response. Directed history taking, integrated with industrial orthopaedic themes, will provide the nurse provider with applicable treatment planning (Table 3.1).

The elements of the physical examination in the patient presenting with work-related orthopaedic injury require minor modification from standard technique. One variant the provider should be attuned to is that patients experiencing work related injury present for evaluation and treatment earlier than the general population. Subtle indications of trauma can be overlooked, if the examiner is not sensitive to the time sequence and mechanism of injury. For example, the patient with an eversion type 1st degree or 2nd degree ankle sprain may present to the industrial accident clinic (minutes after injury) prior to the onset of pain, swelling, ecchymosis, or deformity. Hours, or even days later, the physical manifestations of trauma may be easily identifiable to even the novice examiner. As more that one provider may interact with a client through the course of rehabilitation, descriptive physical examination communication is essential. Use of accepted physical assessment terminology and global abbreviations should be considered when documenting patient records. Tangible tools such as tape measures, goniometers, pinwheels, and reflex hammers assist precision in documentation.

Summarized below are six key points necessary for documentation of physical findings in the work-related injury patient. (Adapted from Rowe ML: *Orthopaedic Problems at Work*, New York, McGraw-Hill, 1985, pp. 10–12).

Negative Findings

Recording negative findings may be as important as recording the positive ones. The potential for full joint range of motion at initial encounter (before onset of swelling and spasm) precludes a diagnosis of tendon rupture. Documenting the untraumatized state of the associated structures involved in the injury may avert unwarranted claims in the future. If the early provider omits illustrating negative findings, subsequent concerns regarding the actual diagnosis may occur.

Point Tenderness

Recording the area or areas of point tenderness should be as routine to the objective assessment as are the gross changes of swelling, discoloration, deformity, and functional loss. Predictably, point tenderness may be evident only to the first examiner. With the passage of time, tender points may become diffusely distributed. Thus point tenderness may be a moot descriptive tool days or weeks after the initial insult.

Comparison with the Contralateral

Comparison of the injured or symptomatic extremity part with the opposite, unaffected part, is another helpful, descriptive assessment tool. Comparison between opposing joints sometimes informs the examiner that what is perceived as "deformed" may be a normal variant in this patient.

Range of Motion

Utilizing a meaningful method for recording limitations in range of motion is a crucial component in communicating mus-

Table 3.1.
Outline for Industrial Orthopaedic History[a]

I. Presenting complaint
  A. Complete and accurate description. Patient's words in quotes.
  B. If extremity, double check whether right or left and make sure all entries in the record are consistent.
  C. Mode of onset
    1. Sudden or gradual?
    2. Associated with single injury? Unaccustomed activity? Repetitive motion? Sudden pressure or temperature change?
    3. If associated with injury
      a. Detailed description (time, date, circumstances)
      b. Immediate effects? (deformity, swelling, discoloration, loss of function)
      c. If symptoms delayed, time and circumstances of onset
  D. Progress of condition since onset
  E. Effect of treatment, if any
    1. Local heat or cold application? Medication? Manipulation?
    2. Mobilization versus immobilization?
    3. Best position for comfort? Worst?

II. Past history
  A. Similar symptoms in past? When? Circumstances?
  B. Other musculo-skeletal symptoms? (contralateral area, arthritic, bursitic, rheumatic symptoms)

III. Family history (parents and siblings)
  A. Condition similar to patient's?
  B. Arthritis, bursitis, rheumatism, gout?
  C. Congenital musculo-skeletal defects?

IV. Socio-economic history
  A. Kind of work? Work record? Time on same job? Relationships in department? Job satisfaction?
  B. Evidence of adaptive resilience (medical record)
    1. Frequency of visits? Lost time? Frequency and duration appropriate to medical condition?
    2. Level of complaints versus objective findings in past?
    3. Home and family situation?
  C. Possible significance of present complaints in above areas?

[a]From Rowe ML: *Orthopaedic Problems at Work*. New York, Perinton Press, 1985.

culoskeletal injury response. Degree measurements of maximum angles of extension and of flexion of the unaffected joint should precede the analysis of the injured part. Contralateral comparison of range of motion will take into account the normal standard for each individual patient.

Circumference Measurements

Circumference measurements of the affected extremity can objectify the amount of soft tissue swelling sustained with injury, as well as assist with chronicling progress under designed treatment regimens. Passing the tape measure around the extremity perpendicular to its long axis and performing similar measurement con-tralaterally will assist with quantifying degree of disability.

Radiographs

X-rays are almost uniformly indicated in acute direct trauma situations. The health care provider should be familiar with the optimal views for visualizing the affected and associated parts (see Anatomical Regions for specific guidelines). Comparison of old films may be helpful when there is question of old fracture or joint space narrowing.

Prevention of Work-Related Injury

The responsibility for occurrence and prevention of orthopaedic accidents in the work place is shared by both industrial management and health care providers. Pre-existing state laws, Occupational and Safety Health Administration (OSHA) standards, and regional ordinances serve as readily identifiable reference guides for management teams (Petersen et al., 1980, p. 38). A combined moral and legal commitment to the worker and the work environment will enhance overall orthopaedic safety. This commitment may be demonstrated by strategies such as comprehensive job training, periodic on-site inspections, and expedient emergency care with accident occurrence. The nurse provider employed in industry is confronted with the task of individualizing preventative programs for "at risk" employees in the work milieu.

Patient screening programs, physical reeducation, and the redesign of manual jobs illustrate primary prevention efforts in the orthopaedic arena. Gross strength testing systems are a predictive screening tool for providers in the occupational setting. Several studies have suggested that a worker's likelihood of sustaining a back injury or other musculoskeletal disorder is three times greater when job lifting requirements approach or exceed strength capability as demonstrated on an isometric simulation of the job (Levy and Wegmen, 1983, p. 348). The nurse provider can facilitate the newly employed individuals' adaptation to their work duties by carefully correlating the screening data obtained with knowledge of the physical demands of the job.

Instructing workers on the proper methods for lifting is another area where nurses attuned to primary prevention can prevent orthopaedic injury in the work place. Reinforcing wise lifting measures includes keeping the object close to the body; lifting slowly, smoothly, and without twisting; and maintaining good physical health and muscle tone. Sometimes the energy required to lift correctly is greater than if performed incorrectly. Consequently the nurse may be challenged by patients to explain the rationales for avoiding short cuts with lifting. Redesigning manual handling jobs to reduce bending, twisting, and excessive weight is another practice concept of primary prevention for nurses in the work place. One-third of compensable low back injuries result from manual handling job design problems. Modification of physical space to suit the workers' anatomic individuality should be considered. For example, recommendations to raise counter spaces or add foot rests in the work environment may be a nursing intervention. In short- and long-term treatment planning, the occupational nurse provider should be attuned to the instructional elements of preventing worker fatigue and awkward posturing in the occupational setting. Some specific work place modifications adapted from the Liberty Mutual Insurance Company Loss Prevention Department follow.

1. Keep elbows down and shoulder abduction angle no larger than 30°.
2. Keep hands below shoulder level.
3. Avoid long reaches (not more than 16 inches).
4. Avoid using first 3 inches of work surface.
5. Avoid tilting head forward more than 30° and use head supports for greater angle.
6. Avoid tilting trunk forward.
7. Avoid sharp edges on work surface (a very common complaint easily solved by padding).
8. Allow for change in posture at worker's discretion.
9. Avoid hard floors for standing workers by supplying floor mats.
10. Provide proper seating which includes:
    (a) adjustable seat height,
    (b) adjustable back rest height.
11. Provide proper work surface height, adjustable if possible, for the sitting and standing operator.

Prevention of orthopaedic injuries often yields a two-fold task for those involved in the maintenance of the work environment. Controlling work place hazards is the rudimentary component that can be accomplished by skilled nonmedical personnel. Promoting safe behavior among employees must be the central long- and short-term goal of the occupational health care provider.

A brief discussion of the ergonomic concept here seems fitting. Coined "human factor engineering," ergonomics is an applied science dedicated to the design facilities, equipment, tools, and tasks that are most compatible with the anatomical, physiological, biomechanical, perceptual, and behavioral characteristics of humans (Levy and Wegmen, 1983, p. 112). This concept, in an orthopaedic mindset, is illustrated by the example of falls. Reducing falls in the work environment may be directly correlated with the mechanics of walking (forces and torques interfacing between floor and shoes) and the eventual design of nonslip surfaces. Quantitative analysis of the physical energy demands of a particular activity (i.e., lifting patients, mopping floors, or drilling oil) can assist in reducing unwarranted strain disorders. "As irony often dictates, this writer experienced a significant fall in the work place shortly after completing the reading and research for this chapter. The fast pace of the work environment and irregularly soled shoes, coupled with a steep stairwell, resulted in a loss of control and bilateral wrist and forearm fractures. Temporary disruption in professional endeavors, dependency induced in the home, and continued adaptation to the trauma, are just a few of the sequelae of work-related injury."

The costs of injuries in the work place extend beyond finance, liability claims, and medical and insurance premiums. There are hidden factors that intensify the overall perception of loss with each individual patient injury, and these factors must always be taken into consideration (Petersen et al., 1980).

The Recreational Athlete

Recreational athletes (both those seeking emotional benefits from sports as well as those seeking physiological rewards) are a contemporary concern in orthopaedic nursing. The nurse provider may encounter the recreational athlete prior to, during, or after exercise-induced injury. Treating the recreational athlete will require nursing intervention from the primary, secondary, and tertiary preventative perspectives. "Pop culture," with its myriad advertisements depicting finely toned torsos and intrigu-

ing exercise regimens within the confines of luxurious health spas, certainly contributes to the number of people engaging in recreational athletics. Therefore, a dilemma arises when the novice athlete is exposed to the disparity between the image of physical fitness and the reality of exercise in attaining fitness. The nurse provider can be a catalyst in both the assessment and instructional phases of the exercise prescription for the recreational athlete. Specific, primary, secondary, and tertiary framework recommendations for these nurse providers will be explained in more detail later in this chapter.

The noncardiac dangers of exercise can debilitate even the most enthusiastic of participants and can cause subsequent interruption in these programs. With a working knowledge of the potential noncardiac exercise dangers, the nurse provider can assist the patient's adaptation to the new regimen and prevent unwarranted sequelae. Exercise-induced asthma, heat-related illness, sprains, tendon ruptures, stress fractures, exacerbation of arthritis, hematuria and myoglobinuria, frost bite, and gout are a few such dangers.

As it relates to orthopaedics, the long-term effect of transient musculoskeletal injuries is not well known. It is believed that the musculoskeletal system can tolerate only a certain amount of trauma associated with cumulative exercising. At this time, there are no substantial data to confirm this, but it is estimated that the more aggressive the exerciser, the more evident the musculoskeletal system response (Fletcher, 1982). Musculoskeletal injuries can be minimized by directly educating the patient in exercise methodology, rate of progress, adequate warm-up and cool-down, and utilization of proper footwear and equipment. The shoe is the most essential accessory for every sport with the exception of aquatics. Shoewear is designed differently for various athletic pursuits and is sport specific. For example, aerobic footwear should not be worn for tennis or jogging. In general, the shoe should be constructed of materials that allow the feet to breathe, cushioned to absorb shock, and well padded around the laces.

The initial step towards fitness in the allegedly healthy group is the careful assessment of exercise limitations by the practitioner. This assessment represents a primary prevention measure. A working knowledge of patient risk factors (both intrinsic and extrinsic) will promote safety and enthusiasm in recreational sports, as well as decreased attrition from programs. The American College of Sports Medicine detailed guidelines on preexercise evaluation which include patient age, symptoms, usual physical activity, coronary heart disease risk factors, and disease (Gibson et al., 1983, p. 88).

The Exercise Prescription

Historically, health care providers have been great subscribers to general fitness regimens. Unfortunately, most have not been formally educated about how to translate proper exercise management to the patients. Instructions for exercise are often vague and lacking in technique. The exercise prescription has evolved into the therapeutic solution for both provider and patient. The exercise prescription should include written instruction for the type, intensity, duration, and frequency of exercise. Secondary and tertiary nursing prevention can be reinforced through adoption and support of exercise prescription principles and detection of patient divergence from safe exercise practices.

Type

Activity can be classified according to its conditioning effects and include cardiorespiratory, flexibility, and strength activity. The exercise prescription recommends a combination of all three types.

Aerobic activity, through swimming, cycling, dancing, or canoeing, will foster cardiorespiratory adaptation and activation of the endorphin system. Flexibility activities assist with extending and maintaining joint range of motion. Stretching should be performed to the point of tightness, but not pain. Flexibility is joint specific and sequentially geared toward every body part. To reduce the likelihood of soft tissue or muscle injury patients should be encouraged to perform flexibility exercises before and after strengthening and cardiovascular activities. Strength activities refer to effort against heavy resistance such as weight lifting, or isometric exercises that tense one set of muscles against a static object. These activities may deliver overall muscle hypertrophy, but do little for cardiovascular toning.

Pictorial displays often serve as a useful ambulatory care tool for patient education projects.

Intensity

There is an intensity in aerobic exercise that is sufficient to condition the musculature and cardiovascular apparatus without exceeding safe limits. Metabolic calculation of exercise duration is represented by a target zone. Cardiac output, oxygen consumption, and heart rate, collectively, will determine intensity of exercise. Exercise physiologists have selected target heart rate as the most realistic, objective measure for recreational exercise practice (Chapter 4 presents more details). A 6-second pulse checked at any pulse site, should be taken periodically throughout the session (Donn, 1987).

Duration

Duration of exercise refers to the time allocated per exercise session to the three basic components comprising time sequence.

Exercise regimens should include a 5- to 10-minute warm-up period, a stimulus period where the target heart rate is maintained, and a 5- to 10-minute cool-down period. As we age, both warm-up and cool-down periods need to be extended.

The warm-up period serves to prevent musculoskeletal strain and readies the cardiovascular system for the cumulative work. It consists of stretching, flexibility, and slow-paced activity. Heart rate should be below the target rate. The stimulus period immediately follows warm-up. It is the time of intense exercise when the target heart rate increases safely and is maintained. New exercise subscribers should aim for 15 to 20 minutes of stimulus with eventual increase to 40 to 50 minutes. For blood perfusion purposes, a cool-down period is mandatory for at least 5 to 10 minutes. If not performed, symptoms of vertigo, nausea, or even syncope may occur. Pulse should be monitored. The type of exercises performed is similar to those in the warm-up period (Gibson et al., 1983).

Frequency

Frequency of exercise refers to the number of exercise sessions per week that are included in the program. The usual average recommendation is to exercise at least 3 times weekly with no more than 2 days between workouts. Maintenance of this exercise prescription requires a lifetime of commitment, as fitness rapidly deteriorates with program fluctuations. The following is an example of an integrated exercise prescription (Fig. 3.1).

A regular exercise regimen can effectively combat both the physical and psychological stressors of aging.

Chronic Illness

As described previously in this chapter, the middle-aged adult years are considered to be quiescent and stable. The onset of chronic illness in adulthood becomes a disruptive diversion to quiet, untroubled days. Orthopaedic injury and degenerative changes impact greatly on life-style and relationships. The adult patients' initial introduction to the concept of "chronicity" on their wellness/illness continuance may influence their future behavior.

Arthritis

Arthritis is a major national health problem that affects people of varying demographic profiles. It has no preference for sex or race, but does have a proclivity for the middle-aged individual. Adaptation to chronic arthritis requires not only psychological and physiological compromises, but also financial and societal changes. The varying forms of arthritis place a significant burden on both individuals and the national economy. The costs can be divided into direct and indirect costs. The direct costs of arthritis include hospitalization, office visits, allied health professional services, medication, and convalescent care. The indirect costs of chronic arthritis include lost wages, lost homemaker services, and earnings lost due to death (Krishner, 1984).

Arthritis literally means "joint inflammation." It is thought to be a uniform manifestation of varying rheumatologic disorders. Rheumatologic diseases share some similar symptom patterns. The most prominent feature is that these disorders are chronic, last long periods of time, and recur intermittently throughout a person's lifetime. There are unpredictable periods of flare-ups and remissions. This chronicity factor dictates thoughtful treatment planning by providers. Despite their similarities, the various forms of arthritis have distinct points of difference. The major rheumatic diseases and their uniquely identifiable traits are found in Chapter 11 of this text.

Implementation of the nursing process can be approached from primary, secondary, and tertiary intervention modes with chronic arthritis and rheumatic disorders. The nurse provider may encounter patients prior to the onset of symptoms during acute stages of pain and inflammation, or in the rehabilitative/stabilizing arena.

With primary prevention, the nurse provider is in the optimal circumstantial condition to perform assessment strategies. Eliciting historical information on life-style practices, usual fitness regimens, personal health and family history is crucial to treatment planning. Assisting patients with the institution of proper diet, weight reduction, and exercise prescription will hopefully prove advantageous. Anticipatory guidance on the warning signs of potential arthritic changes should be reviewed with patients. They include the following:
1. Swelling of one or more joints;
2. Early morning stiffness;
3. Recurrent pain in any joint;
4. Limitation in range of motion of a joint;
5. Redness or warmth in a joint;
6. Unexplained weight loss, fever, or weakness combined with joint pain;

Exercise Prescription Form

Name	_____

Measurements	Height _____	Weight _____	
	Waist _____	Thighs _____	Skinfold _____
Stimulus exercise	Walking	Cycling	Other _____
(circle	Jogging	Rope skipping	_____
selections)	Swimming	Stationary running	_____

Frequency	Day	M	T	W	Th	F	Sa	Su
	Time	___	___	___	___	___	___	___

Duration	**Warm-up**	**Stimulus**	**Cool-down**
(Exercise routine)	5 to 10 minutes; stretching, bending, range of motion, slow-paced stimulus exercise	20 to 60 minutes	5 to 10 minutes; same as for warm-up

Intensity (Pulse monitoring) Count the pulse immediately upon stopping exercise. Find the beat within a second and count for six seconds. You must exercise at least 3 to 5 minutes before counting pulse.

Places to find pulse

Heart rate
Maximum _____
Target zone _____ beats·min⁻¹
_____ beats/six sec

Heart rate too slow? Increase speed
Heart rate too fast? Slow down

Alternative to using heart rate to measure intensity Perceived exertion

Remember
There is no such thing as instant fitness.
Go slowly at first.
There will be at least four to six weeks before results are evident.
If the training schedule is interrupted for a few days to weeks, resume program at a lower level.
Keep a record of weekly exercise accomplishments.
Walkers and joggers: wear identification.

Figure 3.1. Exercise prescription form. (From Gibson, Gerberich, Leon: Writing the exercise prescription. *The Physician and Sportsmedicine*. 11(7): 99, 1983. Reprinted by permission of THE PHYSICIAN AND SPORTSMEDICINE. Copyright McGraw-Hill, Inc.)

7. Duration of the above symptoms for greater than two weeks (Krishner, 1984).

Secondary prevention requires nursing action during the acute responses to arthritis. The nurse provider can prove instrumental in the provision of comfort measures and the prevention of deformity. Directed patient education on the subjects of pharmacologic and therapeutic intervention is beneficial at this time. Assisting both patient and family members with their exchanges with hospital systems is another nursing action for secondary prevention.

Tertiary prevention, or "seeing the patient through" rehabilitative measures of arthritis therapy, is the final area of nursing focus. At this point, the nurse provider strives to promote further adaptation to the elements of chronicity. Ongoing patient counseling and family interplay are fostered by prudent and thoughtful nursing action. Prevention of contractures through the use of splints may be implemented. The nurse assesses the patient for medication compliance and monitors the patient for potentially adverse side effects. Both provider and patient benefit from a good working knowledge of the home environment and modifications necessary to "make it work." Providing ongoing integrity and maintaining quality of life-style is an important mutual goal (for nurse and patient) during the tertiary prevention phase of arthritis care.

Osteoporosis

With 10 million American women having symptomatic disease, osteoporosis is the most common skeletal disease, and is the second most common cause of musculoskeletal disorders and morbidity in the elderly (Kaplan, 1983).

By definition, osteoporosis is a decrease in total bone calcium/ unit volume, which in turn leads to a more brittle bone. Plain radiographs may not show a decrease in the density until approximately 30 to 40% of the normal calcium is gone; often the first indication of underlying osteoporosis comes at the time of a fracture in the post-menopausal female. The most common fractures in women with osteoporosis are in the thoracic and lumbar spine, the distal radius, humerus, hips, and ribs.

The normal bone is constantly remodeling with osteoclastic and osteoblastic activity. The rate of remodeling depends on a balance between osteoclastic and osteoblastic activity and is regulated by many different factors, including; hormones, dietary calcium, phosphorus and vitamin D, exercise, gender, genetic predispositions, and environmental influences. At any given age, men have more body calcium than women.

After menopause, whether naturally or by oophorectomy, bone loss in women accelerates and may range from 0.5% to 2%/ year. This negative balance occurs because bone formation remains relatively constant, but resorption increases. The skeleton acts as the major calcium reservoir in the body; therefore, the blood levels of calcium will remain constant despite large changes in total body calcium.

Replacing the calcium content of osteoporotic bone is almost impossible; therefore, the two most important interventions for improvement in the condition are identifying premenopausal women who are at risk (bone densitometry of the spine and hips is frequently used for screening for the presence of osteoporosis) and working with postmenopausal women to lessen the rate at which calcium is lost.

Premenopausal women, especially those with a strong family history of osteoporosis, should be instructed in a preventive program to decelerate the rate at which calcium leaves the bones. Adequate dietary calcium is important; 1000 mg to 1500 mg/ day can be taken as a supplemental vitamin as long as there is no history of renal calculi. Daily weight bearing exercise has been found to be helpful in maintaining good bone stock. The elimination of environmental factors such as excessive alcohol consumption and cigarette smoking is also important. Women undergoing oophorectomy should discuss the risks of supplemental estrogens/progesterone compared with the risks of premature osteoporosis.

In the identified high-risk perimenopausal woman the nurse provider should consider the addition of estrogens, which have been found to decelerate bone loss. Hormone therapy should begin within three years following menopause (the time of most rapid bone loss). Referral and consultation with a gynecologist are recommended to determine the appropriate replacement therapy. In addition, as previously discussed, less controversial interventions should be undertaken.

The postmenopausal woman who sustains a fracture should have at least one evaluation for other causes of pathologic fractures. Radiographs should be obtained; they are often helpful for excluding a neoplastic process. A bone scan may need to be performed to identify a new fracture that may not be visible on x-ray. A complete blood count, sedimentation rate, alkaline phosphatase, and serum calcium test should be obtained and, if there is any evidence of an underlying pathologic process, a serum protein electrophoresis is needed to evaluate the patient for multiple myeloma. Osteoporotic fractures, as a rule, do not occur in men and if a male develops a nontraumatic fracture he should always be evaluated for an underlying malignancy, infection, or metabolic bone disease.

Treatment of osteoporosis should be aimed at prevention of calcium loss. Adequate dietary calcium of 1000 to 1500 mg/day is important as is vitamin D (400 IU). Exercise, such as walking or bike riding, may decrease the rate calcium is lost and elimination of toxic environmental agents should be encouraged. In patients at moderately high risk for fractures, or in whom fractures have occurred, discussion with a physician is indicated to determine the addition of estrogens, sodium fluoride, or calcitonin. Treatment of the vertebral fractures usually is conservative. The sharp pain subsides after 2 to 3 weeks, and most discomfort should be gone in 6 weeks. Neurologic complications rarely occur secondary to osteoporotic spinal fractures. Fractures in the limbs are managed by the orthopaedist, either through casting or appropriate surgical intervention. After the acute pain starts to subside, one should encourage the patient to increase gradually the number of minutes he/she can sit and then to resume normal activities when comfortable. The home environment should be screened for scatter rugs or slippery floors where falls may be likely (see Chapter 4). Spinal hyperextension exercises should be done and walking should be encouraged (see Chapter 5 for exercises).

Nursing interventions with osteoporotic patients should be directed toward minimizing loss of bone and prevention of fractures and related injuries. The nursing intervention model proves suitable for designing an inclusive patient care framework (Table 3.2).

NUTRITIONAL NEEDS OF THE ADULT

Good nutrition is vital both to maintain good health and to prevent disease. The following nutritional guidelines for the adult client give an age- and sex-appropriate perspective for optimal nutrition and disease prevention.

Nutritional Guidelines in the Adult

General nutritional guidelines presented by the United States Departments of Agriculture, and Health and Human Services, as well as contemporary dietary guidelines in Canada, Britain, and Scandinavia list seven suggestions:

1. Eat a variety of foods.
2. Maintain desirable weight.
3. Avoid too much fat, saturated fat, and cholesterol.
4. Eat foods with adequate starch and fiber.
5. Avoid too much sugar.
6. Avoid too much sodium.
7. If you drink alcoholic beverages, do so in moderation. (Sutnick, 1987, and Truswell, 1986).

These guidelines will be discussed and will be followed by a more in-depth look at nutrition in disease prevention and management.

The variety of foods selected should use the basic four food groups as a guide. The basic four model gives the individual an easy way to select food categories that will provide all of the needed nutrients. Many of the nutritional plans developed for weight control (Weight Watchers, Lean Cuisine, etc.) further categorize the basic four into six food categories or food exchanges. The expansion includes a group for fat and a separate group for fruits and vegetables. As the basic four is easier for the general public to recall, it will serve as the basis for this text.

The basic four food groups include: fruits and vegetables, grains and cereal, milk and dairy products, and proteins. Fruits and vegetables should be consumed liberally. Whole grains should be emphasized because refined products lack fiber and trace minerals. People must be reminded that the grain products are an excellent source of nutrients and that starchy foods are not high in calories unless extra fats or butter are added. From the protein group, legumes, fish, poultry, and very lean meats are preferred because they have lower fat content (Sutnick, 1987).

Maintenance of a desirable weight is achieved through a balance of activity and nutritional intake. General energy requirements for adults are based not only on chronologic age but on body size, sex, activity, and metabolic rate (Table 3.3). Generally, young adults require more calories;

Table 3.2
Nursing Interventions for Osteoporosis[a]

Primary prevention
(before the disease is present)
  Goal: Reducing risk factors

At-risk population
  Female sex
  Small frame
  Caucasian or Asian ethnicity
  Positive family history
  Lifelong low calcium intake
  Early menopause or oophorectomy
  Sedentary life-style
  Nulliparity
  Alcoholism
  High sodium intake
  Cigarette smoking
  High caffeine intake
  High phosphate intake
  High protein intake
  Steroids, heparin, anticonvulsants
  Hyperthyroidism, hyperparathyroidism

Health education
  Adequate calcium carbonate intake
    1000 mg qd before menopause
    1200 mg qd during menopause
    1500 mg qd after menopause
  Adequate vitamin D
    200 units qd before menopause
    400 units during and after menopause

  Exercise regimen
    Muscle building exercise (weightlifting)
    Weight bearing exercise (walking 30 minutes/
      day)

  Nutritional intake (48-hour diet recall)
    Referral to nutritionist when appropriate

Secondary prevention
  Goal: (1) To detect problem at an early stage
        (2) To prevent fractures and to limit dis-
            ability once the diagnosis is made

Screening
  CT or dual photon bone mass meas 1 to 2 years
  Thyroid functioning

Therapeutic regimen (health education)

Dietary

Ongoing nutritional support
  (1) Avoid bone meal as a calcium supplement, it
      may contain lead
  (2) Drink at least 8 ounces of water with each 1
      gm of calcium to decrease the risk of develop-
      ing renal stones

Dietary—continued
  (3) Increase calcium absorption by taking calcium
      supplement with the meal/snack that contains
      the least amount of fiber (fiber can reduce ab-
      sorption)
  (4) Take Lactaid as a supplement if there is a his-
      tory of lactose intolerance to aid absorption

Hormones
  Patient education regarding estrogen/progester-
    one replacement therapies
  Estrogen replacement in conjunction with physi-
    cian consultation
  Perimenopausal high-risk female
  Postmenopausal female with radiographic evi-
    dence of osteopenia

Exercise
  Walking, swimming, and social dancing
  Loading exercises for the upper extremities (lift-
    ing 1-lb weights to build the strength of the ra-
    dius for 15 min 3 times/week).
  Referral to a physical therapist for individualized
    exercise regimen

Tertiary prevention (symptomatic osteoporosis)
  Goal: (1) To promote patient adaptation to or-
            thopedic intervention
        (2) To restore the individual to optimal
            level of functioning

Expected Outcome

Fx	Healing time	Recovery
Wrist	6–12 weeks	3–6 months
Spine	4–8 weeks	1–2 years
Hip	6–12 weeks	1 year

Treatment regimen: may consist of
  Estrogen supplement
  Calcitonin
  Sodium fluoride
  Exercise i.e., walking (30 minutes 5 times/week),
  Loading exercises of the upper extremities (15
    minutes 3 times/week)

Health teaching regarding:
  Falls
  Back strain
    Keep commonly used items in reach
    Use proper body mechanics
    Maintain a safe home environment
    Proper usage of ortho support such as canes
      and crutches

---

[a]Primary Prevention segment only adapted from Lindsay R: Estrogens in prevention and treatment of osteoporosis. In *The Osteoporotic Syndrome: Detection, Prevention, and Treatment.* Orlando, FL, Grune & Stratton, 1987, p 101.

Table 3.3.
Recommended Energy Intakes[a]

Sex	Age	Energy Needs (with range)	
Male[b]			
	19–22	2900	(2500–3300)
	23–50	2700	(2300–3100)
	51–75	2400	(2000–2800)
	76+	2050	(1650–2450)
Female[c]			
	19–22	2100	(1700–2500)
	23–50	2000	(1600–2400)
	51–75	1800	(1400–2200)
	75+	1600	(1200–2000)

[a]From Food and Nutrition Board, National Academy of Sciences-National Research Council: *Recommended Dietary Allowances*, ed 9. Washington, DC, Food and Nutrition Board, National Academy of Sciences-National Research Council, 1980.
[b]based on 70 inches, 154 lbs.
[c]based on 64 inches, 120 lbs.

the caloric need gradually decreases with age. More regular exercise, less fat, alcohol, sugar, and salt, more cereals (preferably whole grain), vegetables, and fruit are the recurring themes for compliance with energy guidelines as well as with sound nutritional health.

The general recommendation to "avoid too much fat, saturated fat, and cholesterol" can be followed by reducing animal protein consumption, selecting lean meats only, broiling rather than frying foods, and using fats in limited amounts. Fats include butter, margarine, oils, salad dressings, cream, fried foods, potato chips, and pastries. Butter and margarine have the same fat and caloric content but margarine, a vegetable product, does not contain cholesterol. However, margarine made from cotton seed, palm, or coconut contains saturated fat (Sutnick, 1987).

Increasing dietary starch and fiber are easily accommodated into nutritional patterns. It is a myth that starchy foods are high in calories. It is the butter and sauces that are often applied to starchy foods that add the unnecessary calories. Starchy foods can be cooked and enjoyed by making some simple alterations: use nonstick coated pans to cook with or use the nonstick sprays; use wine or fruit or vegetable juices instead of butter and cream in sauces; and substitute yogurt for sour cream and mayonnaise in sauces, salads, and baked goods (Sut-

nick, 1987). Fresh fruits, vegetables, and whole grain consumption, based on the basic four guidelines, meets dietary starch and fiber needs.

Restriction of sodium and refined sugars intake is a key part in the balanced, healthful diet. Replace salt with herbs, spices, and other seasonings. Convenience foods should be avoided as they often contain more salt and sugar than products prepared at home (Sutnick, 1987). Refined sugars can be avoided by limiting the use of jellies, syrups, and candy.

Alcohol intake provides excessive calories with little or no nutrients. Alcohol consumption is associated with weight control problems and nutritional deficits; therefore, intake should be limited.

NUTRITION AND DISEASE PREVENTION

Heart Disease

Coronary heart disease has been linked to the intake of fat and cholesterol. The American Heart Association recommends a diet in which no more than 30 to 35% of calories comes from fat, with no more than 10% from saturated and 10% from polyunsaturated fats. Cholesterol intake should be restricted to 300 mg/day. Individuals who do not comply with these recommendations should have high-density lipoprotein (HDL) cholesterol levels screened to identify their risk for cardiovascular disease.

Advice to patients in the high-risk category should focus on controlling weight, lipid levels, hypertension, and cessation of cigarette smoking, and increasing exercise (Fahey et al., 1987). Weight reduction can lower cholesterol levels. The amount of fat in the diet for this high-risk category should be no greater than 20%, with one-third from polyunsaturated plant fats (safflower, sunflower, corn, cottonseed, soybean and sesame oils, and fish and shellfish), one-third from monosaturated fats (olive and peanut oils, fat found in chicken, turkey, and eggs), and one-third from saturated fats (found in beef, lamb, veal, pork, cheese, butter, coconut oil, and chocolate). Recent research has found that ingesting 2 tablespoons of pure olive oil daily reduces the risk for cardiac disease.

Cholesterol is found only in animal tissues, such as egg yolks, milk fats, and meats. The liver and intestines can synthesize all the cholesterol the body needs without intake but the average diet contains 479 mg/day. Cholesterol may be decreased by exchanging high-fat dairy products and egg yolks with low-fat milk and egg substitutes.

Omega-3 fatty acids are mainly found in fish and have, in some studies, been associated with decreasing the risk of cardiovascular disease. Intake of Omega-3 fatty acids can alter the synthesis of prostaglandins and appears to affect diseases such as atherosclerosis by inhibiting hepatic triglycerides (Burtis, 1988). Individuals must be cautioned not to attempt to purchase supplemental Omega-3 fatty acids as large dietary amounts of these fatty acids increase bleeding time.

Cancer

Many foods and nutrients have been linked to either a decreased or increased incidence of cancer. It must be emphasized that these are presently only links and are not fully supported through scientific research. Recommended guidelines integrate the nutrient-cancer link but are still within the basic four nutritional guidelines.

The classification of vitamins known as the antioxidants has been linked with lower cancer rates. According to the Committee on Diet, Nutrition, and Cancer (1982), beta carotene (the precursor to vitamin A in the body) has been associated with a reduced risk of cancer. As vitamin A toxicity is frequent and toxic, a vitamin A supplementation, beyond that contained in a multivitamin, is not recommended. Intake of vegetables that contain carotene and vitamin A (dark green vegetables and deep yellow fruits and vegetables) should be encouraged.

Vitamins E and C are also antioxidants, and some data indicate that they may inhibit cancer in humans. Dietary intake of vitamins E and C should be adequate if basic four guidelines are followed. Megavitamin therapy is not recommended because of the danger of hypervitaminosis. Fat-soluble vitamins A and D are more likely to cause bodily harm in megadose levels, but even the water-soluble vitamins at megadose level can cause serious adverse effects. Intake of vitamins and minerals above the recommended daily allowances (RDA) has not been shown to be more anticarcinogenic than normal levels.

Strong evidence indicates that dietary fat is associated not only with an increased incidence of heart disease but also with increased risks of cancer, especially of the breast, prostate, and large bowel (Fahey, 1987, and Sutnick, 1987). Dietary recommendations for cancer control recommend decreasing fat intake to less than 30% of total calories.

Dietary fiber has been associated with a decreased risk of colon cancer. Adequate fiber intake can be assured with an increased consumption of fruits, vegetables, and whole grain cereal products in the daily diet.

Other minerals associated with an anticarcinogenic tendency include zinc, selenium, manganese, and copper. These minerals are ingested in adequate quantities in the well-balanced diet.

Eating Disorders: Obesity

Obesity has become a national concern, especially in adult women. The causes for obesity are multifactoral and include excess food intake, decreased activity levels, depression with accompanying self-gratification through food, lack of knowledge, and lack of motivation. General nutrient guidelines include decreasing caloric intake, especially protein and fat intakes.

The RDA for energy for women age 23 to 50 years old is 2000 kcal (with a range from 1600 to 2400). A daily excess of 200 kcal will produce a gain of 20 lbs in 1 year; daily deficit of 500 kcal will produce a loss of about 1 lb/week. Reducing diets generally should not be less than 1200 kcal/day; if they are less it becomes difficult to provide adequate amounts of essential nutrients (Sutnick, 1987).

Exercising is an essential component of a weight loss regimen. Sedentary women may find that, despite a low-calorie intake, they have no weight loss (Sutnick, 1987). The simplest and safest exercise is brisk walking and bicycling and the aim is to build up to at least 30 minutes of aerobic exercise per day.

To successfully manage weight loss, one must pay attention to the behavioral cues that trigger eating. Strategies recommended to break common behavioral eating cues are to: (1) specify one room in the house where all food must be eaten and do not deviate from this rule; (2) change one's usual eating place at the table; (3) separate eating from other activities (such as watching T.V., reading, or talking on the phone), take the time to enjoy the food; (4) keep food out of sight; (5) keep fresh fruits and vegetables for snacks in attractive containers; (6) do not serve "family style" (i.e., do not leave food containers on the table); and (7) assess one's emotional status and determine which feelings or events may trigger unnecessary eating (Snetselaar, 1983).

Eating Disorders: Bulimia

Bulimia is most common among young adult women. This eating disorder is characterized by episodes of binge eating, when large quantities of food are consumed in a relatively short time, followed by self-induced evacuation efforts of vomiting, and/or use of laxatives and diuretics or periods of starvation (Kelley et al., 1985). Bulimia is not always associated with significant weight loss; the bulimic individual might even be somewhat overweight.

Bulimics have strong appetites and may binge several times a day with intakes ranging from 1200 to 11,500 kcal per episode. Binge food is usually high in calories, and binging is ordinarily related to stress.

This disorder is characterized by a preoccupation with weight and body size, an exaggerated fear of becoming obese, and depression. Complications of bulimia include hypokalemia resulting from body fluid and electrolyte losses, sore throat, swollen parotid glands, and frequently include dental hygiene problems such as destruction of dental enamel (Kelley et al., 1985). Prolonged bulimia will be accompanied by decreased calcium intake and possible hypoestrogenemia that will result in loss of bone mineralization and increased incidence of osteoporosis.

Therapeutic treatment strategies must focus not only on the issue of eating behavior but also on the self-esteem and mood of the patient. Psychological care is the most important aspect of the eating disorder; however the patient must be able to control adequately his/her eating behavior before psychological treatment can be beneficial. Nutritional goals are for normalization of eating habits. A gradual return to a normal caloric intake with a balance of nutrients is desired. Regular meals should be encouraged to minimize the likelihood of eating binges or long periods of fasting.

Osteoporosis

Osteoporosis affects as many as 50% of women over age 45. Estrogen deficiency is a known cause of osteoporosis. There is growing evidence of calcium deficiency as a causal factor and the NIH consensus conference (1986) recommended preventative therapy as early as adolescence.

Osteoporosis is not a disease limited to the elderly; development of clinical osteoporosis is seen shortly after menopause. Data from the Mayo Clinic (1982) suggest that bone loss leading to osteoporotic hip fractures may start as early as age 25 for some men and women. The development of osteoporosis is influenced by the dietary and activity patterns of the adult. The time to intervene is not when the individual is a senior citizen but earlier in adulthood when the individual's nutrient intake can be adapted to influence the eventual outcome. High dietary calcium intake may suppress age-related bone loss and reduce the fracture rate in patients with osteoporosis.

Factors that negatively influence the relationship between calcium absorption and metabolism must be identified and eliminated. The link between cigarette smoking and osteoporosis has not been clearly established, but documentation shows that cigarette smokers have less bone mass. Excessive alcohol intake is associated with a decreased bone mass as is chronic use of corticosteroids, heparin, dilantin, methotrexate, isoniazid, and aluminum containing antacids. High intakes of caffeine, protein and phosphorous also interfere with calcium absorption, and these intakes should be monitored.

Calcium intake requirements are based on sex and, in women, on menopause status. Premenopausal women, estrogen treated women, and men should have a daily intake of 1000 mg of elemental calcium. Postmenopausal women not on estrogen treatment should have a daily intake of 1500 mg of calcium. Pregnant or nursing women should increase their requirements by 400 mg/day.

The average American has a daily calcium intake of 450 to 550 mg/day, less than one-half of the requirement to maintain calcium homeostasis. To increase the dietary calcium intake significantly, people must consume more milk or more foods such as cheese and yogurt. Tofu and dark green vegetables are also good sources of calcium. Calcium-fortified orange juice, bread, and breakfast cereals are also available (see Appendix M, p. 288).

The difficulty associated with adequate intakes of dietary calcium is the associated caloric value of the foods. Skim milk and low fat yogurts and cheese should be recommended not only for the reduced caloric value but also for the lower fat content. The reality is that most Americans, especially women, will not adequately increase their dietary consumption of calcium. This is somewhat understandable when achieving a 1500-mg intake level using high-calcium content dairy products would account for approximately one-third of a woman's caloric intake. Supplementation with a calcium carbonate product is a feasible adjunct to nutrient intake.

Vitamin D is essential for calcium absorption and utilization. Vitamin D can be synthesized in the skin when the skin is exposed to ultraviolet light. The RDA for vitamin D is approximately 200 IU/day. For high-risk osteoporotic individuals this RDA is increased to 400 IU. This RDA can be obtained in milk (fortified with 400 IU/quart) and fortified breakfast cereals. Naturally occurring sources of vitamin D include fish oils, egg yolks, butter, and liver.

Calcium intake is not the complete answer to the problem of osteoporosis. Patient education must also include explanations of the role of exercise, cigarette smoking, vitamin D, caffeine, and alcohol.

Arthritis

Nutritional deficits occur in approximately 25% of patients with rheumatoid arthritis. Helliwell et al. (1984) reported an increased incidence of malnutrition in patients with rheumatoid arthritis, as compared to that in the normal population. Malnutrition is accompanied by loss of lean body mass and muscular strength that would impact severely on the already limited mobility of the arthritic patient. In addition, malnutrition interferes with the body's ability to fight stress and infection and predisposes the patient to additional medical complications. It is imperative, therefore, to understand the factors that contribute to the nutritional deficit and to intervene as quickly as possible, if necessary.

The symptomatic arthritic client will have a decreased appetite (secondary to pain and general malaise). In addition, oral dryness, a frequent complaint among patients with arthritis, can cause periodontal problems that complicate mastication. Oral lubricants (saliva substitutes) should be used by these patients before meals for symptomatic relief and to facilitate mechanical removal of food particles (Arthritis Facts, 1985). When the patient is acutely symptomatic, a change to a soft diet may be necessary. Sugar-free hard candies and chewing gum may also minimize the dry mouth symptoms.

Temporomandibular joint problems are common in the arthritis patient. Inflammatory arthritis can affect this joint, particularly in patients with rheumatoid arthritis. This inflammation causes stiffness and limitation of joint motion that can interfere with mastication.

Oral complications in the patient with arthritis may also be manifestations of drug toxicity. Gold compounds, penicillamine, and methotrexate may cause oral lesions or a severe oral stomatitis. The goal in all cases of oral distress is to provide a diet that does not cause increased discomfort with chewing and that still provides optimum nutrition. This can generally be achieved with a soft diet, but liquid supplementation may be necessary.

Obesity may be a problem in patients with arthritis, especially in those with mobility deficits. Nutritional counseling combined with a planned exercise and activity program to meet the specific individual requirements are necessary for these patients. The health care provider should caution patients against adopting poor eating habits to promote a "cure"; there are no magic foods.

Trauma and Fracture Healing

Although good nutrition may not prevent the trauma resulting from a car accident, it is an integral part of the healing process. Major injury such as trauma and long bone fracture initiates a hypermetabolic and catabolic response. The hypermetabolic response corresponds to the severity of the injury and necessitates an increased caloric intake to meet the energy demand. Without a sufficient increase in the caloric content, the body will meet these increased metabolic demands by breaking down its own endogenous protein stores—a process known as gluconeogenesis (Salmond, 1984).

In the early phase of trauma, large amounts of endogenous protein are lost to a general catabolic reaction as well as to gluconeogenesis that supplies the needed glucose for energy demands. This accelerated loss of protein is decreased as the body adapts by using fat as an energy source. Adaptation slows protein loss from a high of 75 gm/day to about 25 gm/day. Adequate protein and energy are essential

to prevent further loss of endogenous protein.

Loss of endogenous protein will appear as symptoms and complications of protein-calorie malnutrition. The effects of protein-calorie malnutrition lead to problems with wound healing (delayed healing, infection), mobility (weakness, apathy, diminished muscular strength), and diminished resistance (higher incidence of sepsis, pneumonia, and mortality). These complications greatly interfere with the fracture healing process.

Loss of protein is further aggravated by the immobility that often accompanies trauma and multiple fractures. The modalities used to stabilize a fracture frequently impose a regimen of immobility on the patient; therefore, additional protein is catabolized from disuse (Salmond, 1984). Jensen (1982) identified a 43% incidence of nutritional deficits in a group of 129 orthopaedic surgery patients. It is clear that the fracture patient suffering from the catabolism of trauma and immobility is at risk for developing problems associated with protein caloric malnutrition. These patients must be assessed for nutritional deficits and provided adequate nutritional meals or substitutes.

Nutritional requirements for healing depend upon the severity of the trauma and the stage of fracture healing. Adequate calories and protein intake must be provided to optimize the anabolism necessary for repair and growth (Table 3.4). Protein and vitamin C are key nutrients for stages I and II of fracture healing. For successful completion of stages III, IV, and V, the essential nutrients required include protein, calcium, phosphorous, magnesium, and vitamin C (a needed nutrient for soft tissue healing). Lack of adequate nutrition during the fracture healing process is hypothesized to result in an increased incidence of delayed and nonunion (Salmond, 1984, and Griffith, 1982).

A balanced diet rich in protein, vitamin C, calcium, and phosphorous is the key to supplying adequate nutrients. In the early stages of trauma the increased caloric and protein demands can be met by increases in both the carbohydrate and protein con-

Table 3.4.
Nutrient Requirements for Bone Healing

Stage	Healing Process	Nutrient Need
I	Hematoma formation Semisolid clot begins to fasten broken ends together	Protein[a]
II	Organization of the hematoma vascularization of hematoma fibroblastic proliferation phagocytosis Granulation tissue formation precursor to scar tissue Fibrous union at end of stage II	Protein[a] Vitamin C[b]
III	Chondroblastic and osteoblastic activity granulation tissue infiltrated by chondroblasts and osteoblasts Cartilage replaces granulation (chondroblastic) Nonossified bone replaces granulation (osteoblastic)	Protein[a] Calcium Phosphorus Vitamin D
IV	Ossification inorganic bone salts deposited External callus formation immature bone provides structural rigidity	Protein[a] Calcium Phosphorus Vitamin D
V	Remodeling and reshaping mature bone replaces immature bone bone of maximum structural strength	Protein[a] Calcium Phosphorus Vitamin D

[a]If adequate carbohydrate is not supplied, protein will not be spared and used for bone repair but will be used for energy.
[b]Vitamin C remains a needed nutrient, not for fracture healing but for soft tissue healing.

tent of the diet. In severe trauma energy demands may approach 5000 cal/day. Adequate carbohydrate as an energy source must be provided to enhance the body's protein-sparing capacity. Caloric supplementation may be provided by milkshakes (meeting carbohydrate and protein demands) or canned meal replacement formulas and puddings. These foods supply not only carbohydrate but also additional essential nutrients such as calcium, vitamin D, and phosphorous. A multivitamin preparation and supplemental calcium are also indicated.

References

Alvioli LV: *The Osteoporotic Syndrome: Detection, Prevention and Treatment.* Orlando, Fl, Grune & Stratton, 1987.

American Heart Association: *Diet and Coronary Heart Disease.* Dallas, American Heart Association, 1978.

Arthritis Facts: Arthritis complications. *Postgrad Med* 78(3):92–97, 1985.

Blenker M: Social structure and the family genera-

tional relationships. In Shanas E (ed): *Social work in family relationships with some thoughts on filial maturity.* New York, Prentice Hall, 1965.

Burtis G, Davis J, Martin S: *Applied Nutrition and Diet Therapy.* Philadelphia, WB Saunders, 1988.

Committee on Diet, Nutrition, and Cancer, National Research Council: *Diet, Nutrition, and Cancer. Directions for Research.* Washington, DC, National Academy Press, 1982.

Dickelmann N: *Primary Health Care of the Well Adult.* New York, McGraw-Hill, 1977.

Donn M: Guidelines for an effective personal fitness prescription. *Nurse Pract* 12(9):14–16, 1987.

Erikson E: Identity and the life cycle. *Psychol Issues,* Vol. I. New York, International Universities Press, 1959.

Fahey P, Boltri J, Monk J: Key issues in nutrition: disease prevention through adulthood and old age. *Postgrad Med* 82(1):135–141, 1987.

Fletcher G: *Exercise in the Practice of Medicine.* Mt. Kisco, NY, Futura, 1982.

Gibson S, Gerberich S, Leon A: Writing the exercise prescription: an individualized approach *Phys Sportsmed* 11 (7):87–99, 1983.

Goroll AMI, Mulley A: *Primary Care Medicine.* Philadelphia, JB Lippincott, 1981.

Griffith B: The positive impact of nutritional support on fracture healing. *A.S.P.E.N. Update* 2(3):6, 1982.

Helliwell M, Coombes E, Moody B, Batstone G, Robertson J: Nutritional status in patients with rheumatoid arthritis. *Ann Rheum Dis* 43:386–390, 1984.

Hymovich D, Barnard M (ed) *Family Health Care.* New York, McGraw Hill, 1980, p 144.

Jensen J: Nutrition in orthopaedic surgery. *J Bone Joint Surg* 64(9):1263–1272, 1982.

Jung C: The Stages of Life. In Campbell J (ed): *The Portable Jung,* New York, Viking Press, 1971.

Kaluger G, Kaluger M: *Human Development.* St. Louis, CV Mosby, 1979, p 399.

Kaplan FS: Osteoporosis. *Clin Symposia* (CIBA) 35 (5):1–32, 1983. In Kelley WN., Harris E, Ruddy S, Sledge CB (eds): *Textbook of Rheumatology.* Philadelphia, WB Saunders 1985.

Krishner I: *Understanding Arthritis.* New York, Arthritis Foundation, Scribner & Sons, 1984.

Levy B, Wegmen D: *Occupational Health.* Boston, Little, Brown, 1983.

Mayo Clinic. *J Clin Invest* Clin Abstr 70:716–725, 1982.

National Institute of Health Consensus Conference: *Osteoporosis, Cause, Treatment, Prevention.* U.S. Department of Health and Human Services. NIH Publication No. 86-2226, 1986.

Petersen D, Heinrich HW, Ruos N: *Industrial Accident Prevention.* New York, McGraw-Hill, 1980, p 35.

Rowe ML: *Orthopaedic Problems at Work.* New York, Perinton Press, 1985, p 7.

Salmond S: The role of nutrition in fracture healing. *Orthopaedic Nurs* 3(4):27–33, 1984.

Snetselaar L: *Nutrition Counseling Skills.* Rockville, MD, Aspen Systems, 1983.

Sutnick M: Nutrition: calcium, cholesterol, and calories. *Med Clin North Am* 71(1):123–133, 1987.

Truswell A: ABC of nutrition. *Br Med J* 291:466–469, 1986.

chapter 4

The Mature Adult

TONY COOK, R.N., M.S.N., F.N.P.C., G.N.P.C.
JOYCE LEDERMAN LICHTENSTEIN, R.N., M.S.N.
SUSAN W. SALMOND, R.N., Ed.D.

Much attention has been focused recently on the "graying of America" and the consequences of the growing numbers of people age 60 years and older. But the mature adult population is a diverse and heterogeneous one that, contemporary stereotypes and misconceptions notwithstanding, defies easy characterization. The physical health characteristics, self-care abilities, and social and psychological assets of the working 62-year-old woman will differ markedly from those of her 87-year-old mother for whom she is the primary care giver. Yet as nurses we provide care for both. Implementation of a preventative model to care effectively for this population requires a broad and unique knowledge base. This chapter provides the nurse with a baseline working knowledge of contemporary geriatrics as it applies to the care of the mature adult in general, and to specific age-related mobility and orthopaedic problems in particular.

DEMOGRAPHICS OF AGING

The mature adult population is commonly divided into subgroups based on age. Thus the "older population" denotes those individuals ages 55 to 60 years, the "elderly" those age 65 years and older, the "aged" those ages 75 to 84 years, and the "extreme aged" or "old old" those age 85 years and older. These differentiations are often useful in comparing certain characteristics between groups such as morbidity

and mortality or functional characteristics. More commonly, though, population statistics are reported for the "elderly" in general.

In 1985 the United States population numbered approximately 238.7 million people, and about 12% (28.5 million) of Americans were ages 65 years or older (National Center for Health Statistics, et al., 1987). The absolute and proportional numbers of the elderly have been growing steadily since the turn of the century with the groups ages 75 to 84 and age 85 and older experiencing the greatest growth. From 1970 to 1980 the growth of the elderly population (28%) was more than twice that of the United States population in general (11%). This trend will continue until about 2030, when the effect of the post-World War II "baby boom" will taper off. Using "middle population series" estimates, the United States Census Bureau has predicted that by 2020 (1) the number of elderly will increase to over 50 million, and (2) about 30% of the population will be over age 55 years.

There is no typical mature adult, but certain demographic characteristics are well documented and are useful in identifying potential problems and related areas of prevention. These characteristics include (1) gender differences, (2) racial differences, (3) socioeconomic status, and (4) physical health and functional abilities.

There are more older women than older men, and the ratio of men to women decreases with age. In 1980 there were 68 men for every 100 women age 65 and older, but only 55 men for every 100 women age 75 and older (National Center for Health Statistics et al., 1987). The older man is much more likely to be married and living with a spouse than is the older woman. In 1981 75% of men, but only 33% of women, age 65 and older were living with a spouse, while 51% of women were widowed and 40% lived alone.

Almost 12% of the United States white population is 65 years or older, compared to 7.8% (a significantly smaller percentage) of the black population (National Center for Health Statistics et al., 1987). This is due in part to the greater mortality for blacks than whites at most ages, resulting in fewer numbers of blacks surviving to old age. Certainly other factors are involved such as different patterns of health care utilization and socioeconomic status.

The economics of aging in the United States are an issue that has generated much debate for decades. While most of us look forward to our retirement and the subsequent years of freedom and independence, for many older Americans the retirement years portend a gradual or precipitous attrition in financial resources. For some retirement means simply an exacerbation or acceleration of an on-going cycle of poverty.

The majority of American elderly are not poor, but only a small minority can be considered affluent. In 1985 less than 6% of households headed by an elderly American had an annual income exceeding $50,000 (U.S. Department of Commerce, Bureau of the Census, 1986). Conversely, 12.6% of elderly Americans lived below the poverty level. Moreover, for certain subgroups poverty is pervasive. In 1986 39% of elderly blacks, 26% of elderly Hispanics, and 32% of elderly women living alone were impoverished (Storey, 1983). By 1985 more than one-half (54.5%) of elderly black women living alone had incomes at or below the poverty level (Villers Foundation, 1987).

Certainly the economic status of most elderly Americans falls somewhere between affluence and poverty. Their incomes meet or, to varying degrees, exceed their cost of living. But such factors as the rising cost of health care, heavy reliance on government sources of income (e.g., Social Security), and increasing out of pocket medical expenses threaten their economic viability. It has been suggested that, "if poverty among the elderly were measured in the same way as for the non-elderly . . . at least 45% of the elderly . . . are either poor or economically vulnerable" (Villers Foundation, 1987).

Perhaps no characteristics of the mature adult population are more stereotyped and misconstrued than general physical health and functional abilities. The visual media tends to portray older adults dichotomously as either loving, retired, bespectacled grandparents, or as dependent, disfigured, incapacitated octogenarians. While the former may be closer to reality than the latter, such generalizations belie the diversity of this population, and perpetuate myths of aging.

When asked to assess their own health during household surveys in 1983 and 1984, almost one-half of respondents ages 55 to 64 years (44.8%) and more than one-third of those age 65 years and older (35.9%) described it as "excellent or very good" (National Center for Health Statistics et al., 1987). Of particular significance are the self-reported data concerning activities of daily living.

Activities of daily living (ADLS) are commonly used descriptions of everyday functional self-care abilities and are commonly divided into two categories: basic ADLS and instrumental ADLS. Basic ADLS include mobility (walking), bathing, dressing, eating, and toileting. Instrumental ADLS include shopping, meal preparation, housework, and use of transportation. During the 1984 National Health Interview Survey noninstitutionalized civilian residents of the United States were queried about both basic ADLS and instrumental ADLS. With regard to basic ADLS the most common limitation was in walking, a limitation reported by 15% of those age 65 years and older. In descending order of prevalence were limitations in bathing (10%), dressing (approximately 7.5%), toileting (approximately 5%), and eating (less than

3%). Heavy housework was the instrumental ADLS most likely to be limited (more than 20%), followed by shopping (more than 10%) and meal preparation (approximately 7%).

Most mature adults are in good health and have few limitations in their activities or functional abilities. The vast majority live independently and require little or no outside help. Nevertheless, advanced age is associated with declining function and increased dependence on others. For a small, but growing, minority of elders, institutionalized care becomes necessary. In 1985 slightly less than 5% of those age 65 and older, 10% of those age 75 and older, and 22% of those age 85 years and older resided in institutions (National Center for Health Statistics et al., 1987). However, 5 to 10% of the noninstitutionalized elderly population receive some type of in-home care, and it has been estimated that more than 75% of such care is provided by family and friends (Stoller et al., 1983). Such caregivers are generally spouses or adult daughters of the dependent elder. The physical, psychological, emotional, and economic burdens of caregiving are great and the social ramifications complicated.

PSYCHOSOCIAL DEVELOPMENT

Mature adults are survivors. Sixty or more years ago, when they were born and growing up, death by the fifth or sixth decade was not unusual. Over several decades their lives have been influenced by unprecedented global political, economic, and social changes. Through maturation and adaptation they gained the psychosocial skills needed to endure and thrive in the face of those changes. "Normal" human growth and maturation explain only part of this developmental process; changing social norms and attitudes have further influenced their lives. Knowledge of the developmental process of aging and its associated hazards (such as suicide and alcohol abuse) are prerequisites for successful interaction and collaboration with the mature adult.

The mature adult must make many adjustments throughout the advancing years.

The mature adult is faced with a myriad of maturational events that predispose him/her to psychological decline and to despair. Old age is characterized by many types of losses, often permanent and often irreplacable. The death of a spouse, family, and friends often force the survivor party to learn new, seemingly impossible skills, to adjust to the loss of significant support systems, and sometimes to find a new place to call home. Once considered a highly productive member of a fast-moving society, the mature adult must now face retirement. Coupled with retirement is a decrease in annual income, and often a decrease in perceived self-worth. Days which were never long enough may now be too long and inadequately filled with meaningful activities.

Erikson reminds us that people do not cease developing once adulthood has been reached. Psychosocial development is a lifelong process. The psychosocial development task for mature adults is to confront the ends of their lives. Erikson termed this his final stage of psychosocial development, as one of Integrity versus Despair (Erikson, 1963). The elderly review their life experiences in an effort to find congruence between the experiences and the values they adopted throughout their lives (Lappe, 1987). If the previous stages of life have been satisfactory, then old age is colored with a sense of integrity, a sense of a life well-lived, a sense of tranquility, wholeness, and quiet confidence. Ego integrity is attained when the elderly are able to adapt positively to the constant changes throughout their lives. If, however, reflection brings disappointment and regret, and life is viewed as a series of lost opportunities and failures, then the final years will be years of despair.

Aging brings role devaluation, in the United States there is a stigma to growing old. Mature adults must adjust to physiological and psychological decline. Poor health, chronic illnesses, loss of bodily functions, and lack of autonomy contribute to feelings of grief, loss, helplessness, and increased isolation (Ryan and Patterson, 1987). Loneliness appears to be associated more with loss than with isolation; the recently widowed have been found to be the most lonely. This feeling of loneliness is more significant if the widowed individuals are childless or rarely interact with their children (Townsend, 1968). A significant direct relationship between physical incapacity and self-reported loneliness in the elderly has also been demonstrated (Tunstall, 1966; Townsend, 1968; Berg et al., 1981).

It is important to know the psychosocial developmental needs of mature adults in order to develop a plan of care. Mature adult orthopaedic clients need to be supported in order to develop feelings of self-esteem, self-acceptance, and inner tranquillity. They require assistance in developing latent abilities (Fitzsimons, 1985) and making adjustments to the many losses confronting them.

An intact social support network is necessary to help mature adults maintain well-being. This is especially true in times of crises when information is needed to provide a sense of security and self-worth (Preston and Grimes, 1987). The nurse provider must assist mature adults in identifying social support systems. It is helpful to determine who is involved in these support systems, how their assistance is assessed, and when assessed, if the assistance is satisfying. If barriers or breakdowns in the system are perceived, the nurse provider must identify the source. This network can be expanded by involving family and friends and, when necessary, can help mature adults to replace losses. The number and lengths of visits by existing support systems is not as important as the regularity of the visit (Preston and Grimes, 1987). Mature adults require support systems that are reliable and dependable, as well as available and effective.

Clients age 60 years and older want to make their own decisions regarding their lives but often do not have the resources to make informed decisions. It is important for them to know that the mechanisms are in place and support systems are available. It is equally important that clients are knowledgeable regarding the problem-solving techniques available for their use. The client should be provided information about opportunities and affiliations that are available. With advancing age, there is less

need for competition among peers; companionship and a sense of belonging become increasingly important. The mature adult's decision to be involved in activities that are meaningful should be supported, and these clients should be encouraged to utilize their experiences to enrich the lives of others.

Not all mature adults successfully adapt to, or cope with, the physical and emotional challenges of aging. Inadequate coping can be manifested behaviorally in many ways, such as preoccupation with physical changes and discomforts, social withdrawal and isolation, and overt depression. These manifestations usually are recognized without difficulty and are likely to be resolved with appropriate interventions such as counseling. For some mature adults inadequate coping is manifested in hazardous maladaptive behaviors (i.e., alcohol abuse and suicide). Each of these problems, while not unique to mature adults, has important implications and repercussions about which all health care providers must be knowledgeable.

PHYSIOLOGIC CHANGES OF AGING THAT IMPACT ON MOBILITY

Aging is a biologic process that begins at birth and continues unremittingly until death. Physiologically aging is characterized by a decline in the functional and reserve capacities of all body systems, and a pansystemic deterioration of homeostatic mechanisms. Concurrent with the physiologic changes are changes in body composition and anatomic structures. While aging per se is not pathologic, advancing age is clearly correlated with increases in acute and chronic disease.

Skin

Perhaps the most visible changes of aging are those that affect the skin and supporting structures. A gradual thinning of the dermis accompanies aging (Walther and Harber, 1984). There is a decrease in subcutaneous adipose tissue, an increase in the density of connective tissue, and a decrease in total water content. Collagen and elastin components degenerate, and there is a gradual atrophy of epidermal secretory glands and hair follicles (Berman et al., 1988). The result is skin that is wrinkled, prone to dryness, increasingly fragile, and less effective as a defense barrier.

Cardiovascular Changes

As with most other organs, heart functions start declining by the fourth decade. After age 30 cardiac output decreases by 1% and stroke volume by 0.7% per year, respectively (Berman et al., 1988). Thus, a 70-year-old adult has approximately one-half the cardiac reserve of a young adult. With increasing age comes a linear decrease in the maximal heart rate, a greater increase in systolic blood pressure with exercise, and a prolonged period of time needed to return to the resting heart rate and blood pressure after exercise (Beard, 1983). Although healthy older adults can maintain cardiac output during exercise, they can not generate as great an increase in cardiac output as young adults. Both arterial blood pressure and total peripheral resistance increase with age. The net effect of normal cardiovascular decline is a decrease in organ perfusion, resulting in a 50% reduction in renal blood flow and a 20% reduction in cerebral blood flow by age 80 (Berman et al., 1988). In addition, aging baroreceptors in the carotid sinus are less sensitive to decreased blood pressure that results from postural changes. Orthostatic hypotension (defined as a drop in systolic blood pressure of 20 or more mm Hg from lying to standing) becomes increasingly prevalent with age and affects between 20 and 33% of those age 75 years and older (Beard, 1983). These changes increase the risk of falls.

Respiratory Changes

With aging, there is a gradual increase in the anteroposterior diameter of the chest and a progressive kyphosis, that results in decreased compliance of the chest wall (Goldman, 1979). The alveoli are reduced in number, but increased in size. Lung volume decreases and lung weight is decreased by about 21% (Berman et al., 1988). After age 30, there are significant changes in important functional parameters: (1) vital capacity decreases by approximately 30 cc/year; (2) functional residual capacity increases by 50%; (3) residual volume can increase up to 100%; and (4) forced expiratory flow rate decreases regardless of lung volume. However, resting tidal volume and total lung capacity do not change significantly. Arterial oxygen tension (PaO_2) decreases by 10 to 20% with aging, but the arterial pressure of carbon dioxide ($PaCO_2$) remains the same and any change indicates pathology.

While maximum breathing capacity decreases linearly with age, in the absence of disease or respiratory risk factors (e.g., smoking), these normal changes will be largely unnoticed in terms of everyday functioning. When there is concern about possible significant functional impairment, the match test can provide a reliable assessment of forced expiratory volume. If the patient is unable to blow out a burning match held 6 inches from the wide open mouth, further pulmonary function screening is indicated.

Muscular and Skeletal Changes

There is a gradual but progressive decrease in both muscle mass and strength with aging, most prominently in the lower extremities. (Whipple et al., 1987). Aging joints show deterioration of articular cartilage by age 30, and joint spaces slowly but progressively narrow due to loss of water from cartilage (Goldman, 1979). More than 35% of adults ages 55 to 64 years and nearly one-half of those age 65 years and older have some type of chronic arthritic condition (National Center for Health Statistics et al., 1987). Independent of these arthritic changes, the older adults' limbs and joints are more stiff, less flexible, and more easily strained or stressed.

Loss of bone mass, or osteoporosis, affects all adults and is influenced by many factors such as sex, race, and coexisting conditions. Primary osteoporosis occurs in two pathophysiologic types: type I, or postmenopausal, affects only women, and type II, or age-related, affects both men and women (Bellantoni and Blackman, 1988). Women affected by both types can lose 50% of their trabecular bone mass and 35% of their cortical bone mass, while men can lose 6 to 8% of their trabecular and 3 to 5% of their cortical bone mass.

Osteoporotic bone is brittle, less dense than normal bone, and contributes significantly to fractures primarily of the hip, shoulder, wrist, and vertebral bodies. Loss of vertebral bone mass results in varying degrees of spinal kyphosis (the "dowagers hump" common in many older women) and ultimately impacts on stature, posture, gait, and balance.

Neurologic and Sensory Changes

Loss of neurons begins in young adulthood at the rate of approximately 50,000 to 100,000 neurons/day; lost neurons are not regenerated. There is a gradual decrease in brain size and, concurrent increase in the size of the ventricles. But cortical function remains normal and, with the exception of mild short-term memory loss, any cognitive impairment indicates pathology and warrants investigation. "Senility" is not part of normal aging.

Peripheral nerve conduction gradually slows down, and deep tendon reflexes are frequently diminished somewhat, especially in the lower extremities. Certain superficial reflexes may disappear (e.g., cremasteric and abdominal). Vibratory and tactile sensations decline, especially in the lower extremities, and may be accompanied by peripheral neuropathy resulting from chronic disease such as diabetes and peripheral vascular disease. Sensitivity and responsiveness to extremes of temperature decline significantly and place the mature adult at increased risk of hypo- and hyperthermia. Mobility is affected by a gradual but variable impairment of balance, diminished body-orienting reflexes and posture control, and decreased ability in

the height the adult can step. Intermittent rapid, low-amplitude muscle tremors and fasciculations in the lower extremities may occur normally, but muscle fibrillation is an abnormal finding.

The ability to see, hear, taste, and smell decline with age as the result of specific anatomic changes. Presbyopia, or loss of accommodation and near vision, Typically occurs by age 50 and results from loss of elasticity of lens and ciliary muscle. There is a decrease in the number of retinal receptors, gradual corneal degeneration, and decreased tear production. Aging pupils are smaller and less reactive to light. Visual acuity, the ability to properly adapt to the dark, and the range of visual field decline. Color vision is impaired; this affects discrimination between greens and blues more than between yellows and reds. Typical eye disorders include cataracts, macular degeneration, glaucoma, and retinopathy. Visual changes that are abnormal and require investigation include blurred vision, diplopia, and perception of halos or rainbows around lights and may result in frequent eyeglass prescription changes.

More than 50% of people age 65 years and older are affected by presbycusis, the degenerative bilateral sensorineural hearing loss that accompanies normal aging. Loss of high-frequency (high-pitched) sounds may occur first, and certain sounds may be particularly difficult to differentiate (e.g., the consonants D,B,X,Z,T,F, and G). A sudden or acute change in hearing is abnormal and merits investigation. Frequently a buildup of cerumen in the external auditory canal will produce a "sudden" conduction hearing loss that resolves after removal of blockage.

The physiologic, anatomic, and functional changes that accompany normal aging predispose the mature adult to certain hazards and pathologic conditions. Many of these common hazards and conditions affect, directly or indirectly, basic activities of daily living in general and mobility in specific. Epidemiologically, a limited number of age-related problems predominate and account for the majority of acute and chronic orthopaedic conditions. These problems include (1) falls, (2) fractures, and (3) degenerative problems (e.g., osteoporosis and arthritis).

FREQUENT AGE-RELATED PROBLEMS

Alcohol Abuse

Alcohol abuse is a problem most prevalent in young and middle-aged adults, but one that affects a significant number of mature adults. In 1983 alcohol use was reported in more than 70% of persons ages 20 to 34 years, in 42.5% of those ages 65 to 74 years, and in only 30.1% of those age 75 years and older (Schoenborn and Cohen, 1986). Heavy drinking, defined as more than 2 drinks/day, was reported in 8% of those ages 65 to 74 years and in 4.7% of those 75 years and older. And, as with younger adults, significantly more older men than older women use, and abuse, alcohol.

Regardless of gender, two patterns of alcohol abuse predominate. Approximately two-thirds of elderly alcoholics began drinking at a young age and continued to drink heavily for decades. The other one-third did not drink heavily until middle age, often in response to the stresses and losses of aging or later (Scott and Mitchell, 1988). Fortunately, advanced age is associated with a decrease in alcohol consumption and alcoholism; but, assuming a 5% prevalence of alcohol abuse among mature adults, over 1.5 million mature adults are affected. Such factors as the normal physiologic changes of aging, the probability of these changes coexisting with chronic health problems and the use of medications mean that the consequences of such abuse for the elderly may be more detrimental than the consequences for young adults.

The normal changes in body composition that occur with aging (i.e., decreased total body water and decreased lean body mass) will cause a higher relative blood alcohol concentration in mature adults than in younger adults (Scott and Mitchell, 1988). The metabolism of alcohol by oxidation in the aging liver often is decreased, and the time until its elimination is prolonged. Thus older adults may experience toxic effects at lower doses, and for longer periods, than younger adults. Combined with "normal" gait changes and slowing of reflexes, alcohol use can be particularly hazardous and is often a factor contributing to falls. Alcohol-induced changes in liver enzyme systems may decrease the elimination of some drugs (e.g., chlordiazepoxide, diazepam, propranolol) while increasing the inherent toxicity of others (e.g., acetaminophen).

Many of the drugs frequently prescribed for older patients interact with alcohol, and this interaction results in a variety of deleterious effects. Alcohol increases the gastrointestinal irritation caused by aspirin and significantly prolongs bleeding time. It markedly potentiates the depressive effect of other central nervous system depressants such as benzodiazepines and antihistamines. Mature adults with Type II diabetes, for whom sulfonylurea agents like tolbutamide are prescribed, are at increased risk of hypoglycemia.

Alcohol, although a socially accepted drug, has many inherent dangers for older adults. In interactions with patients the nurse provider must be attuned not only to signs of alcohol abuse, but also to evidence of its use in an apparently "normal" manner. Patient education is indicated whether alcohol is used problematically or responsibly, frequently or rarely. Referral to a substance abuse counselor or mental health agency should be made without hesitation when appropriate.

Suicide

Although the continuing escalation of suicide rates for adolescents and young adults is well known, it is adults age 65 years and older who have a higher suicide rate than any other age group. Suicide is the ninth leading cause of death for this population. In 1980 17% of all suicides reported in the United States were committed by older adults (National Center for Health Statistics, 1985). Moreover, the actual incidence of suicide in the elderly may be significantly greater due to underreporting. Suicide prevention should be a concern for all nurses working with mature adults and begins by identifying those adults at greatest risk.

As with alcohol abuse, suicide is a predominant problem of older men. Men age 65 years and older have a suicide rate 6 times greater than that of women age 65 years and older. Although the suicide rate for women peaks at age 50, the rate for men increases linearly throughout life. This pattern is specific to older white men; the suicide rate for blacks, regardless of gender, is significantly lower than that for whites. Certain characteristics other than gender and race help to identify those at risk of suicide and provide the focus for prevention.

Regardless of age, depression is the most frequent precipitator of suicide (Blazer et al., 1986). In mature adults depression is not uncommon and is frequently related to the many losses associated with aging: loss of income, career, and self-esteem that accompany retirement; loss of spouse; physical health and functional abilities; and the narrowing sphere of social contacts and interactions. Loneliness is a common emotion that affects approximately 25% of all adults; loneliness also correlates with depression, particularly for older men (Ryan and Patterson, 1987). Feelings of helplessness, hopelessness, and haplessness (i.e., to experience a succession of losses over which one has no control) often accompany depression and are red flags indicating a mature adult at risk of suicide (Boxwell, 1988).

The most effective way to screen for depression and suicide risk is a direct one. Within the context of any patient encounter a brief but thorough psychosocial assessment can be completed. Questions to consider include: Is the patient expressing feelings of loneliness, helplessness, or hopelessness? Have there been any recent significant losses? Are effective support systems in place? Has the patient lost interest or demonstrated poor compliance with the treatment regimen? The responses to those questions will identify patients for whom direct questions are indicated: Are you depressed? How so, and what does it mean to you? Have you ever considered suicide? Have you thought about how you might take your life? Acknowledgment of depression or related symptoms mandates further evaluation and treatment. Patients with a history of attempted suicide or who admit suicidal ideation are at particular risk of suicide and demand immediate intervention. Referral to a physician, mental health worker, or crisis intervention team should be made. Informing the patient and family or significant other as to why measures are needed and how these individuals should participate in the plan of care is an integral part of crisis intervention.

Nurses spend considerable time with patients and therefore are in a unique position to screen for both alcohol abuse and suicide risk. The nurse provider must avoid attending only to the identified "chief complaint" or problem at hand and must always maintain a high index of suspicion for hidden and hazardous problems.

Falls

Falls are a leading cause of morbidity and mortality in the mature adult population and account for serious major problems with morbidity. Adults age 65 years and older account for more than 75% of the fatal falls in the United States annually (Waller, 1974). Of the 185,000 mature adults who fracture a hip as the result of a fall, more than 30,000 die within 6 months of the injury (Barclay, 1988). Not surprisingly, the death rate from falls increases with age.

The majority of falls are not fatal, but result in significant physical, psychologic, and economic trauma. Approximately one-third of the community-residing mature adult population will have at least one fall each year, with 1 of 40 falls resulting in hospitalization (Rubinstein and Robbins, 1984). Independence, self-esteem, and mobility are affected by a fall, and a fall often precipitates institutionalization. Effective primary and secondary prevention of falls requires an understanding of the characteristics of individuals at risk to fall; the multiple causes of falls; and the identification and implementation of appropriate preventive and corrective measures.

Mature adults at risk to fall are likely to:

Table 4.1
Causes of Falls in Mature Adults

I. *Host factors*
  A. *Normal Physiologic changes of aging*
     1. Impaired gait, balance, and righting mechanisms
     2. Decreased height of stepping
     3. Decreased flexibility of trunk and extremities
     4. Decreased muscle mass, strength, and tone, especially in lower extremities
     5. Sensory changes—impaired vision, hearing, proprioception, tactile sense
     6. Orthostatic hypotension
     7. Impaired mechanoreceptors in cervical facet joints
  B. *Pathologic conditions*
     1. Chronic conditions—e.g., DJD, RA, Parkinson's disease, dementia, peripheral neuropathies, depression, vertebral basilar insufficiency
     2. Acute and episodic conditions—e.g., cardiac dysrhythmia, syncope, drop attack, transient ischemic attack
  C. *Drug effects*
     1. "Normal" side effects—e.g., orthostatic hypotension
     2. Adverse reactions—electrolyte imbalance, secondary diuretics, digitalis toxicity
     3. Drug interactions—e.g., OTC anticholinergic drugs plus anxiolytic or antidepressant
     4. Alcohol

II. *Environmental factors*
  A. *Outside home*
     1. Community obstacles, high curbs without wheelchair type ramp; timing of traffic light "walk-don't walk" cycle; use of escalators over elevators in malls; mass transit vehicles with high steps; lack of wheelchair lifts; poor street lighting
  B. *Home hazards*
     1. Entrance ways—stairs in good repair and negotiable height?; hand rail sturdy?; adequate lighting?; path to/from driveway or garage unobstructed?
     2. Floors/hallways—slick?; scatter or throw rugs secured?; electric cords in pathway?; adequate lights?
     3. Kitchen—linoleum or waxed floor?; are top or high shelves used?

(1) be incontinent, (2) use several medications, (3) have impaired gait and balance, (4) have arthritis or past stroke, and (5) experience significant orthostatic hypotension.

Causes of falls are commonly divided into two main categories: host ("intrinsic") and environmental ("extrinsic") factors. Host factors include normal physiologic changes of aging, pathologic conditions, and drug effects. Environmental factors include both home and community hazards (Table 4.1). Rarely, can a fall be attributed to only one factor or cause; usually, falls result from the interaction of several factors. A thorough investigation into the circumstances of the fall is essential and will often explain the nature of this interaction. Adults who "simply tripped" on a throw rug when getting up at night to go to the bathroom may, upon closer questioning, recall that: (1) they did get up suddenly, experiencing some light-headedness (orthostatic hypotension); (2) they were not wearing their eyeglasses (visual impairment); (3) the night light was off (environmental hazard); and (4) they had taken a sleeping pill 3 hours earlier (drug effect). Each of these factors may be corrected through appropriate patient education and specific interventions.

Certain host factors are readily modified, and these modifications result in a significant risk reduction. Simple remedies are often the most important (e.g., assuring the use of appropriate shoes and keeping canes and walkers accessible and in good repair). Exercise influences many potentially deleterious normal physiologic changes by improving strength, flexibility, gait, and balance. Correction of sensory impairment through the appropriate use and maintenance of adaptive devices (e.g., eyeglasses) is a simple but crucial measure. Orthostatic hypotension, a significant risk factor for 33% of the mature adult population, frequently results in dizziness, altered balance, muscle weakness, and visual disturbances (Cunha, 1987). Adjustment or elimination of certain medications (e.g., antihypertensives, diuretics, and antidepressants) often is "curative." Patients with persistent orthostatic hypotension must be educated in methods to reduce the frequency and severity of disabling symptoms. Adaptive behaviors include rising slowly from a lying to sitting position, then sitting for a minute before standing, especially in the morning; remaining seated while dressing; and using a recliner chair when possible. Activities that result in vasodilation and venous pooling should be avoided (e.g., hot baths and prolonged exposure to hot or humid conditions, prolonged lying or standing, and very large meals). For some adults, the use of elastic support garments and drug treatment may be necessary.

Pathologic conditions often play a role in falls, and include the impact of chronic disease on mobility (e.g., Parkinson's disease), as well as impaired function due to acute episodic conditions (e.g., viral labrynthitis and dehydration secondary to gastroenteritis). Neurologic and cardiovascular conditions are often implicated in falls of acute or recent onset. Thorough medical evaluation is indicated to identify and correct the underlying disorder, which may be cardiac dysrhythmia, transischemic attack (TIA), or acute syncopal episode. With increasing age there is the probability of multiple etiologies, as in the elderly hypertensive with Type II diabetes who has significant retinopathy, autonomic dysfunction, and peripheral neuropathy; concurrently, the risk of drug effects as a contributing factor must be suspected and evaluated. The patient should be questioned in detail about the drug regimen, with particular emphasis on certain classes of drugs (diuretics, antidepressants, hypnotics, all central nervous system (CNS) drugs) and the use of over-the-counter drugs. Important questions to ask include: Are drugs being taken as directed? Are there deleterious drug interactions? The nurse should take advantage of this important opportunity to provide patient education and counseling.

As most falls occur in the home a home hazard assessment is mandatory. The assessment and interventions must be accomplished with considerable tact, a concerned objectivity, and unqualified respect for the autonomy of the resident (Table 4.2).

Fractures

Fractures are a common orthopaedic problem for mature adults, and the incidence of fractures increases with age.

Normal physiologic changes of aging, osteoporosis, and falls are the most important etiologic factors related to fractures. Loss of bone density, a stiffened and weakened musculoskeletal system, and impaired gait accompany normal aging and increase the risk of fractures. Osteoporosis is implicated in almost 1.5 million fractures each year. Bone demineralization is further accelerated by certain life-style behaviors, medications, and other pathologic conditions (Table 4.3). Secondary to aging and osteoporosis, alcoholism, estimated to affect at least 10% of adults age 65 years and older, exacerbates the decrease in bone density. Corticosteroids, often used in chronic lung disease and arthritis, and furosemide, often used in hypertension and heart disease, increase bone loss and urinary excretion of calcium, respectively. Metastatic disease from primary breast, prostate, thyroid, and kidney cancers, and multiple myeloma often result in lytic bone lesions.

Each encounter provides the nurse an opportunity to assess the patient's relative risk of fractures. All clients should be assessed for dietary deficiencies (e.g., calcium and vitamin D). Alcohol abuse remains underdiagnosed but, when recognized, mandates appropriate referral. A review of medications may identify the need for adjustment (e.g., reducing steroids or substituting hydrochlorothiazide for furosemide). The activity and functional level of all patients should be assessed, with the goal of establishing baseline data and developing an exercise program directed toward optimal function. Special attention should be directed to those with certain

Table 4.2
Home Hazard Assessment and Intervention

Hazard	Intervention
I. *Outside*	
Uneven, cracked, or cluttered walk	Repair; remove obstacles
Loose, slippery steps on porch	Repair; paint porch with nonskid paint
Inadequate lighting	Walk-way, porch, steps should be well lit
Loose or absent railing	Provide railing, well-secured to house or steps; one on both sides best
Tight, "sticky", or cumbersome storm or main door	Repair; lever-type handle superior to round-knob or push button
II. *Inside*	
Hallways	
Extension cords, furniture, or other obstacles	Remove
Loose scatter or throw rugs	Remove or secure to floor
Inadequate lighting	Ceiling or floor lighting with light switch at each end of hallway greater than or equal to 100 watt
No railing	Installation of railing secured to underlying wall studs
Living Area	
Furniture on castors	Remove castors or place furniture against wall
Low chairs without arms	Suggest chairs with arms and high seat; electric lift chair when appropriate (may be covered by Medicare)
Kitchen	
Linoleum or slick floors	Table, chairs with rubber nonskid tips; avoid waxing
High shelves	Move items to shelves preferably shoulder height or lower
Bathroom	
Low toilet seat	Raised toilet seat with arms
Slick tub, absense of mat or grab bars	Rubber nonskid mats; grab bars; bath seat or shower stool
Excessively-high hot water temperatures	Adjust hot water heater to temperature of 120 to 130°
Stairways	
No railing	Railing on both sides secured to underlying wall studs
Carpeting on floor same color as walls/ceiling	Red or yellow paint or reflection strip on first and last riser

chronic conditions (e.g., cancer, thyroid, and parathyroid disorders).

The most common fracture sites for mature adults are the hip, wrist, and vertebrae. Hip fractures predominate, with an annual incidence in the United States of more than 200,000. The mortality rate for hip fractures is 15 to 20% in the first 3 months postfracture and 50% in the 6 months postfracture (Consensus Conference on Osteoporosis, 1984). Death is more likely for men in the presence of other medical problems and if medical assistance is not provided

within 1 hour of injury (Barclay, 1988). Wrist fractures are generally of the Colles' type (i.e., fractures of the distal radius within 1 inch of the articular surface that result in the characteristic "silver fork" deformity with the wrist displaced dorsally and radially). Typically such a fracture occurs when the victim falls on outstretched arms. Vertebral fractures may also result from trauma, although the responsible event may be minor and unrecognized for some time.

The cardinal signs and symptoms of fractures include deformity, swelling, bruis-

Table 4.3
Chronic Conditions Affecting Skeletal Integrity

Osteoporosis
Hyperparathyroidism
Hyperthyroidism
Adrenal insufficiency
Alcoholism
Nutritional deficiencies (calcium, vitamin D)
Metastatic carcinoma
Hypogonadism
Diabetes mellitus
Immobility
Corticosteroids

ing, muscle spasm, tenderness, pain, impaired sensation, impaired function, crepitus, and abnormal mobility. Their presence and magnitude are a function of the site, type, and severity of the fracture; other structural injury; general physical condition; and psychologic factors (e.g., mental status). Compared to younger patients, mature adults are significantly more likely to present atypically, particularly with fractures of the hip and vertebrae. The arthritic, osteopenic 77-year-old who falls 7 times in 6 months, and for whom the constant but tolerable pain and the absence of bruising or other external sign of serious injury have become familiar sequelae, may have unknowingly sustained a serious hip fracture. The extent of injury may be disproportionately greater than the level of pain or initial functional limitation might indicate. Medical attention may not be sought for days when pain resulting from applying weight or the inability to sustain basic activities of daily living necessitates help.

The absence of obvious trauma does not exclude the possibility of fracture, particularly in the presence of advanced osteoporosis. Frequently, older adults, especially the "old old," may present with a gradual decline in specific functional abilities and a reluctance to perform what had been routine activities (e.g., dressing, grooming, or ambulation). There may be an associated complaint of arthritis "flaring up" or a similar attribution to some chronic condition which may or may not explain the behavioral change. Physical examination should

focus on the (apparently) involved extremity, assessing for any pain to palpation or with motion, range of motion, muscle strength and tone, and circulation and neurologic function. Any abnormal findings merit more thorough diagnostic evaluation, but especially erythema, swelling, pain with motion, or limitation in range of motion. A minor infection, monoarticular arthritis, or superficial soft tissue injury will often be a fracture in disguise.

The nurse provider should expect the presentation of fractures to vary greatly from person to person and according to site (Table 4.4). Fractures are often the first and most prominent clinical sign of osteoporosis. The majority of hip fractures result from falls, yet most falls do not result in a fracture. Hip pain following a fall (or any other traumatic event), no matter how benign the event may seem, should give rise to the presumption that a fracture has occurred, until an evaluation proves otherwise.

Table 4.4
Clinical Presentation of Fractures by Site

Site	Signs and Symptoms
Hip	—Pain on weight bearing and/or ambulation
	—Increased pain with percussion of sole of foot on involved side
	—Decreased ROM—but may be normal except for extremes of rotation, especially internal rotation
	—Point tenderness
	—Leg abducted, externally rotated, may be shortened compared to non-involved side
Vertebrae	—Sudden acute back pain or slow, insidious increase in chronic back pain
	—Usually thoracic or lumbar spine
	—Pain increased by sitting, relieved when lying supine
	—Alteration in respirations
	—Decreased bowel sounds, ileus
	—Silent progression of kyphosis and decrease in stature
Wrist (Colles' fracture)	—"Silver fork" deformity (acute)
	——Pain with all ROM, especially flexion and extension, supination and pronation
	—Decline in ADLS, such as personal hygiene
	—New onset of preferred use of non-dominant hand

When there is no apparent history of trauma and a patient complains of a gradual increase in pain over a period of days or weeks, the possibility of a metastatic or pathologic fracture must be considered. Multiple myeloma frequently presents with back pain secondary to a pathologic vertebral fracture. Over one-half of malignant bone lesions originate from primary carcinoma elsewhere, yet the bone lesion may be the presenting complaint. Such lesions are commonly located in the vertebrae and pelvis, and are rarely below the knee.

Following a fracture, the primary goal should be the earliest possible resumption of normal activities and ambulation. This is essential for the patient to achieve the highest possible level of functioning and independence, and to maintain muscle action and joint function. The approach to rehabilitation after a fracture will vary according to fracture site and severity; prefracture functional abilities; and coexisting medical problems. It is crucial to involve the patient and family (or support system) in planning the postfracture treatment and rehabilitation program, and in setting realistic and attainable goals.

The type of fracture and the method of repair will have the greatest impact in determining rehabilitative goals. Hip fractures almost always require some sort of surgical intervention and, particularly in the "old old," often necessitate use of a hip prosthesis. There usually will be a limited period of relative immobility postoperatively, which significantly increases the risk of such complications as pneumonia, pressure ulcers, generalized muscle weakness and atrophy, impaired bowel function, and changes in mental status such as acute confusional states. The physician, nurse, and patient must collaborate in actively preventing such complications by the implementation of a care plan that emphasizes early activity and control of pain and discomfort. From the onset patients must be encouraged to participate in self-care to the greatest extent possible.

The nurse must assume responsibility for anticipating potential obstacles to recovery and for adjusting the care plan accordingly. This responsibility presumes a thorough knowledge and understanding of the patient, especially prefracture physical, functional, and psychosocial characteristics.

Although rehabilitation and care plans must be different for each patient, certain guidelines can be applied to all patients. Such topics as cast care; potential complications and their signs and symptoms that must be reported (e.g., thrombophlebitis, compromised circulation); appropriate use of analgesics; comfort measures; correct use of mobility aids (crutches, canes, walkers; see Appendix I); and a thorough description of allowed and contraindicated activities should be reviewed. Caregivers should be present when possible, and written instructions should be provided. Sufficient time should be allowed for the patient and caregiver to express fears and concerns; acknowledge understanding of instructions; and have all questions answered. Arrangements for supportive services such as in-home skilled nursing care, physical therapy, or occupational therapy should be reviewed so that no misconceptions or misunderstandings occur.

Early resumption of normal activities and ambulation is extremely important. Although fractures often result in some residual functional impairment, the degree of such impairment can be minimized by appropriate rehabilitation so that the patient may continue to live independently.

Arthritic Disorders

No chronic condition affects more people than arthritis. Rare indeed is the mature adult who does not have symptoms of one of the arthritides: osteoarthritis (OA, or degenerative joint disease); rheumatoid arthritis (RA); gout; pseudogout; polymyalgia rheumatica; or soft-tissue rheumatism. Certainly osteoarthritis and rheumatoid arthritis predominate. All arthritic conditions can result in chronic pain, functional impairment, and complications resulting from treatment can be serious. Arthritis generally can not be prevented. The nurses' efforts will be most effective if aimed at limiting pain and disability and assisting patients in the implementation and maintenance of appropriate rehabilitative measures. These efforts require insight into the prevalence, clinical presentation, natural history, and clinical management of osteoarthritis and rheumatoid arthritis.

More than 80% of mature adults age 65 years and older demonstrate radiographic signs of osteoarthritis, but fewer than 10% have associated clinical symptoms (Fam, 1987). The clinical presentation is one of slowly progressive, intermittent aching joint pain, stiffness, and deformity primarily involving the cervical and lumbar spine, shoulders, hips, knees, proximal interphalangeal joints; and distal interphalangeal joints. In the absence of a history of trauma or fracture, involvement of the elbows, wrists, and ankles is rare (Spiera, 1987). The process is diffuse and generalized in women (women typically have multijoint involvement), but is usually localized in men to the hips and knees. There is no associated systemic process, and acute joint inflammation is rare. Pain is directly related to deterioration of articular cartilage, joint stress, and bone proliferation. Joint stiffness is common in the morning and after prolonged periods of sitting or standing, but rarely lasts more than 30 minutes. Treatment is symptomatic; most patients respond well to physical measures, mild analgesics such as acetaminophen or nonsteroidal anti-inflammatory drugs. Severely damaged joints may require surgical intervention.

Rheumatoid arthritis differs from osteoarthritis. Rheumatoid arthritis onset is typically acute or subacute; systemic illness is common; and some degree of inflammation is always present, usually involving the shoulders, elbows, wrists, metacarpophalangeal joints, proximal interphalangeal joints, knees, ankles, and feet (Spiera, 1987). Treatment is aimed primarily at reducing acute inflammation, usually through the use of nonsteroidal anti-inflammatory drugs or, on a short-term basis, corticosteroids. Physical therapy and the use of adaptive devices often result in marked improvement of functional abilities.

Patients with arthritis can and should assume primary responsibility for the management of their rehabilitation program. They are the experts in understanding how their condition affects them; what activities are most limited; the type and severity of pain and discomfort; and the relative success of different treatment modalities. Health care providers can best assist the patient by providing ongoing assessment, education, and consultation.

Assessment and education should occur simultaneously. The patient who presents with an arthritic complaint for the first time must have a thorough nursing and medical assessment to identify the nature of the problem. What appears to be "arthritic" back pain may be a vertebral compression fracture, peptic ulcer disease, pneumonia, or cardiac ischemia. Once the diagnosis is made, education should focus on the natural history, treatment options, and expected outcomes. The rehabilitative measures and goals should be addressed, both generally and specifically in terms of how they relate to the patient's particular manifestations of disease (Table 4.5). Based on the findings of the medical and nursing assessments, and the specific problems identified, the patient and nurse can develop a plan of care that is individualized, goal-directed, and flexible. Specific instructions must often be given and written guidelines may be necessary. Family members, or others involved in the provision of care, must be involved in all phases, from the initial history taking and physical assessment to the identification of short- and long-term goals. More than one perspective on a problem often facilitates its resolution. From a caregiver's perspective the patient who complains of intractable early morning stiffness and pain that "linger all day," despite apparent compliance with suggested therapeutic interventions, may be experiencing mild pain that is accentuated by social isolation or dysfunctional family dynamics. Until the psychosocial issues are addressed, pain control would be an unrealistic expectation from the patient.

Ongoing assessment and evaluation of the patient's condition and plan of care are necessary due to the chronicity of arthritic conditions and the potential for functional decline. With older patients it is often necessary for the nurse provider to inquire di-

Table 4.5
Rehabilitative Measures for Arthritis[a]

Intervention	Purpose/Goal
Rest	
Bed rest indicated only for acute phase of inflammatory arthritis; must be accompanied by ROM exercises and short periods of rest for DJD	Eliminate effects of gravity and weight bearing Minimize hazards of immobility Reduce stress on joints
Splinting	
Immobilization of inflamed or deformed joints	Mechanical support and stabilization
Optimal effect for acute inflammation requires continuous use for at least 24 hours	Maintain anatomic alignment Stretch joint, stimulate muscle activity
Exercise/Activity	
Slowly progressive isometric exercise	Muscle strengthening
Maintain physical activity and ADLs through work simplification and energy conservation	Maintain muscle strength and mass; joint flexibility; prevent/delay functional decline
Physical Therapy	
Active and/or passive ROM	Maintain joint flexibility Gradual release of contractures
Application of cold/heat	Cold to relieve acute pain, inflammation Heat to relieve chronic pain, inflammation

[a]From Portnow J, Helfgett S: Rehabilitation of the elderly arthritic patient. *Geriatr Med Today* 6(9):63, 1987.

rectly and explicitly about their status if "false negative" histories are to be avoided. Poor pain control, gradually declining self-care abilities, and social isolation may go unreported if patients fear that acknowledgment would signal the need for institutional care. Similarly, problems in paying for, taking, or tolerating medications may be an embarrassment or presumed sign of inadequacy that is difficult to verbalize. Patients recognize nurses as "experts" on drugs, and patients will share problems and concerns if encouraged and allowed to do so. The time spent reviewing the medication regimen is never wasted and, in the typical geriatric scenario of multiple medications and potentially adverse reactions, this time will often identify previously unrecognized, serious complications.

Medications and Associated Problems

For many reasons advancing age is associated with an increase in the use of both prescription and over-the-counter medications. Older adults usually have one or more chronic conditions that are managed in part by drug therapy (e.g., arthritis, hypertension, and heart disease). Normal changes of aging, such as impaired bowel function, result in the use of many nonprescription drugs. Receiving health care from more than one provider may result in drug duplication or polypharmacy. Drugs are not innocuous and are associated with frequent noxious or deleterious side effects and/or adverse reactions (Table 4.6). Independent of practice setting, nurses must be aware of the normal changes of aging that impact on drug therapy. These include both changes in body composition and functional decline in organ systems that alter drug absorption, metabolism, excretion, and distribution (Table 4.7). In general, older adults are more sensitive to drugs, require lower doses, are more likely to experience adverse reactions, and may react in a paradoxical or unexpected fashion. Therefore, the cliche "start low and go slow" is an important caveat when prescribing drugs for older patients. Equally important is careful attention to individual patient characteristics (such as presence of chronic disease) that may interact with normal changes of aging and result in a greater impact on pharmacokinetics and pharmacodynamics. The malnourished patient, with a greater than "normal" decrease in serum albumin, is likely to have higher

Table 4.6
Commonly Used Drugs and Related Problems

Drug	Problem
Digitalis	Cardiac dysrhythmias
	Nausea and vomiting
Diuretics	Dehydration
	Electrolyte imbalance
	Hyperuricemia
	Hyperglycemia
	Ototoxicity (furosemide)
Beta blockers	Orthostatic hypotension
	Depression
	Masked hypoglycemia
CNS drugs	
benzodiazepines	Oversedation
	Paradoxic response (agitation)
	Impaired gait/balance
	Altered sleep cycle
antipsychotics/	Oversedation
antidepressants	Paradoxic response
	Tardive dyskinesia
	Disturbed temperature control
	Orthostatic hypotension
	Constipation
	Urinary retention
	Dry mouth
NSAID	Nausea
	Diarrhea
	Constipation
	Stomatitis
	Gastritis
	Active peptic ulceration
	Sodium retention

serum concentrations of highly protein bound drugs.

Adverse drug reactions are a significant hazard for older patients. An adverse drug reaction (ADR) is defined as "any unintended or undesired consequence of drug therapy"; this reaction may be manifested in many ways (e.g., hypersensitivity, toxicity, idiosyncratic response, undesirable side effects, or deleterious drug interactions) (Trinca and Dickerson, 1979). It has been reported that almost one-third (30%) of outpatients experience ADRs, and that such reactions precipitate hospitalization for 10% of elderly inpatients (Nolan and O'Malley, 1988). Generally there is no single "cause" of an ADR; rather, an interaction of several factors results in increased susceptibility and probability (Table 4.8).

Despite the many potential hazards as-

sociated with their use, drugs are often essential in the management of chronic and acute conditions that accompany aging. Nurses should be instrumental in seeing that patients use their medication safely and appropriately. The patient's drug regimen should be reviewed at each visit, and particular attention should be paid to compliance; the patient should understand each drug's indications and potential side effects or adverse reactions; and the signs and symptoms of drug-related problems should be investigated, and the nurse should recognize that many patients may not acknowledge the extent of their use without prompting.

Table 4.7
Normal Changes of Aging Affecting Drug Therapy

Change	Consequences
Body composition:	
Decreased total body water	Increased sensitivity to water-soluble drugs
Decreased lean body mass/increased total body fat	Delayed onset and prolonged action of fat-soluble drugs (e.g., psychotropics)
Decreased serum albumin	Elevated serum levels of highly protein-bound drugs (e.g., warfarin, phenytoin)
Decreased homeostatic abilities	Increased risk of adverse reactions and side effects
Impaired baroreceptors	Orthostatic hypotension
Kidney function:	
Decreased ability to concentrate urine and conserve Na$^+$	Tendency to dehydration with diuretics
Decreased glomerular filtration	Delayed drug clearance longer half-life of *most* drugs
Decreased creatinine clearance	
G.I. function:	
Decreased bowel perfusion	Decreased drug metabolism by liver—increased serum levels (e.g., propranolol, acetaminophen, tricyclics)
Decreased motility	
Decreased hepatic perfusion and metabolism	
Decreased amount/ acidity of gastric secretions	Decreased absorption of weak acids (e.g., ASA, theophylline)

Table 4.8
Factors Associated with Adverse Drug
Reactions

Factor	Effect
Patient age	Incidence of ADR increases with age
Number of drugs used	Incidence of ADR increases exponentially with increasing number of drugs
Drug class	Drugs with highest incidence of ADRs: psychotropics antibiotics antihypertensives digitalis NSAID
Presence of pathologic condition	Altered drug disposition Increased risk of ADR
Normal changes of aging	Altered absorption, distribution, metabolism and excretion Altered pharmacokinetics and pharmacodynamics

Incidence of ADRs by Number of Drugs Used[a]	
Number of Drugs	Incidence of ADR
1–5	4%
6–10	7%
11–15	24%

[a]From Williams P, Rush D: Geriatric polypharmacy. *Hosp Pract* 21(2):1986.

Elderly patients are likely to have difficulty managing complicated drug regimens, although often they will not admit this unless specifically asked. This hesitancy should not be viewed as noncompliance but, rather, as an attempt to maintain independence and control in the face of growing dependence on others. Such mismanagement may present as poor control of chronic conditions (e.g., hypertension, diabetes, or chronic lung disease); presence of side or adverse effects that are dose-related (e.g., digitalis toxicity, gastritis secondary to nonsteroidal anti-inflammatory drugs); or inappropriate requests for refills indicating over- or underutilization. In some cases drug regimens can be simplified, (e.g., by using a NSAID with daily or twice a day doses and accepting the associated hazards of a longer half-life). For many patients the correction of minor problems may be all

that is needed to improve compliance. In prescribing medications it may be useful to specify nonchildproof containers, large-print labeling, and explicit instructions for drug use (e.g., not "take as directed," but "take 1 tablet every 4 hours as needed for pain, not to exceed 6 tablets in 24 hours"). A wide variety of "pill reminders" are available commercially and often result in improved "compliance." Finally, perhaps the most important intervention is to involve the patient's spouse, family, and support systems. Some patients will require minimal prompting and supervision, while others will require the implementation of elaborate systems or direct administration of drugs by others.

Exercise

Health professionals tout the benefits of exercise to all patients, regardless of age. Exercise is recommended as a means of becoming physically fit, of weight loss, and of "feeling better" physically and psychologically. The mature adult population can perhaps benefit most from exercise in terms of maintaining function and independence. Appropriate and effective education should focus on the specific benefits of exercise; the development of an exercise prescription or program; and individualized exercise recommendations based on specific chronic problems.

It is important for health professionals to convince patients that they will benefit in certain measurable, objective ways. Ironically, this may be easier with mature adults, who often have some degree of physical or functional limitation, than with younger patients, who generally are in good health. Life expectancy, a measurable criterion that older patients tend to pay more attention to, has been shown to correlate with exercise. In a prospective study of more than 16,000 Harvard alumni ages 35 to 74, physical activity was examined in relation to mortality and longevity (Paffenbarger et al., 1986). Exercise was found to have an inverse relationship to mortality, particularly to cardiovascular and respiratory disease. In general, the greater the level of exercise, as measured by the number of calories expended/week, the greater the decrease in death rates. Mortality rates were lower for those people who were physically active, regardless of the presence or absence of hypertension, cigarette smoking, or extremes of body weight. And by the age of 80 years, adequate physical activity and exercise were found to result in an increase in life expectancy of 1 to more than 2 years.

Exercise often will improve the quality of the patient's life by ameliorating physical and functional changes that accompany normal aging (Table 4.9). The degree of improvement clearly will be a result of the level, frequency, and type of exercise, as well as of the patient's general condition and physical capabilities. However, all patients can benefit from exercise if the program is geared to their capabilities and aimed toward realistic goals. A 67-year old retired businessman who is 15 kg over ideal body weight, has a 40 pack-year history of cig-

Table 4.9
Normal Changes of Aging and Related Benefit of Exercise

Aging Change	Exercise Benefit
Cardiovascular	
Decreased maximum cardiac output and maximum work capacity	Increased maximum aerobic capacity
Increased total peripheral, resistance	Decreased vascular resistance
Increased systolic BP	Decreased BP
Respiratory	
Decreased maximum ventilation	Increased maximum voluntary ventilation
Endocrine	
Impaired glucose tolerance	Improve glucose tolerance
Increased incidence of hypercholesterolemia and hyperlipidemia	Decreased serum lipid levels; increased HDL fraction
Increased total body fat	Decreased body fat
Musculoskeletal	
Decreased muscle mass/strength	Increased muscle strength
Decreased flexibility	Increased flexibility
Decreased bone density	Decreased involutional bone loss
	Increased bone mineral content

arette smoking, is being treated with medications for hypertension, and has a "game knee" from an old football injury would benefit from an exercise program. This program should include aerobic conditioning (e.g., walking or cycling), strengthening of specific muscle groups (i.e., those around the knee), and general stretching and flexibility exercises. Realistic, achievable 6 month goals include loss of 10 kg; a 10 to 20% decrease in resting heart rate; a reduction of dose frequency of hypertension drugs; and the resumption of activities that he had enjoyed in the past but had to discontinue due to his "unstable" knee. The 87-year-old widow who lives alone, has osteoarthritis of the hips and knees, and has not left her home for months due to dyspnea on exertion and fear of falling would also benefit from an exercise program. Realistic goals include increasing exercise tolerance, improving overall muscle strength and tone, and achieving greater independence and social interaction. The benefits of exercise for this woman include a reduction in the risk of falls and fractures, and improved self-esteem.

Prior to beginning an exercise program all patients should undergo a thorough medical evaluation. This is necessary to (1) document baseline level of fitness, (2) identify health problems that affect and will be affected by exercise (e.g., anemia, hypertension, coronary artery disease), (3) review the patient's medications and foresee possible adjustments (e.g., of insulin, beta blockers, calcium channel blockers), and (4) to identify patients for whom a strenuous conditioning program would be contraindicated (Lampan, 1987). Exercise tolerance testing using a bicycle ergometer or treadmill is essential to establish stress levels and to identify the maximum attainable heart rate (from which the exercise level of intensity is calculated) (Barry, 1986). During testing some patients will demonstrate signs and symptoms of exercise intolerance. For such patients the intensity of exercise should never exceed the level at which these signs and symptoms occurred.

The results of the exercise tolerance testing provide data to develop an exercise program or prescription. It is important to remember the primary purpose of such a program (i.e., "to improve movement (strength, flexibility, balance, and coordination) and fitness in a safe manner") (Barry, 1986). This necessitates patient education about several topics related to their exercise program (Table 4.10).

Exercise, while beneficial, does have some risks and complications. Older patients are more prone to develop problems of dehydration, heat intolerance, cardiac ischemia, and musculoskeletal injuries from overuse than younger patients. They should be instructed about the signs and symptoms of exercise intolerance and complications that indicate the need to stop the associated activity. Dehydration and hyperthermia are of particular concern. Due to normal changes of aging (i.e., a 15 to 20% decrease in total body water; impaired heat dissipation; and altered hemodynamic response to exercise and heat stress) older patients are at significant risk of rapid dehydration (Eisenmann, 1986). Moreover, clinically significant dehydration often occurs long before the onset of thirst. Specific guidelines for exercising in hot and/or humid conditions should be provided (Table 4.11). The exercise program should specify what types of activity are permissible (e.g., walking and cycling). The type of activity should be based on patient preference and abilities, cost, and the goal of the program. If exercise is to become a routine part of the care plan it should be enjoyable and should fit into the patient's pattern of daily living.

Instructions should be given on the purpose and methods of warming-up before, and cooling-down after, exercise. A gradual stretching of muscles and supporting structures, particularly those muscle groups most involved in the specific activity, can prevent injuries such as sprains and strains. Rhythmic, repetitive exercises, beginning at a slow pace that is gradually increased, will allow the cardiovascular system to adjust to the increased functional demands put on it and will optimize vasodilation. In general, warming-up and cooling-down involve the same activities. If walking is the main exercise activity, the pace should be slow at first and be gradually increased during the first 10 to 15 minutes to the desired maximum pace, then gradually decreased over 10 to 15 minutes at the end of the session. Stretching exercises should precede the warm-up and follow the cool-down periods.

Specific guidelines should be provided on the intensity, duration, and frequency of exercise activities. The intensity of ex-

Table 4.10
Components of Patient Education Related to Exercise: Signs and Symptoms of Exercise Intolerance and/or Complications[a]

Exercise Program Guidelines	
Types of exercise	
Warm-up purpose and methods	
Intensity	
Duration	
Frequency	
Cool-down purpose and methods	

Symptoms	Signs
Dizziness/vertigo	Irregular pulse
Chest pain/angina	Tachycardia greater than target heart rate
Dyspnea disproportionate to exertion	Systolic BP 250+ or 10 mm + drop in systolic BP
Nausea	Diastolic BP 120+
Muscle cramps	
Muscle/joint pain weakness	
Impaired cognition	

[a]From Barry, H: Exercise prescriptions for the elderly. *Am Fam Phys* 34:1986.

Table 4.11
Guidelines for Exercise in Hot Weather[a]

Avoid hottest part of day—exercise early in a.m. or late p.m.

Drink appropriate fluids in advance of and during exercise—16 to 32 ounces of water 30 to 60 minutes before, then 6 to 8 ounces every 15 minutes during exercise.

Wear proper clothing—loose fitting; light-colored; porous; include hat.

Be alert to symtoms/signs of heat stress—dizziness, weakness, nausea, headache, cognitive impairment.

Stop activity, pour water on head/neck/limbs, go to cool area.

Seek medical assistance if symptoms worsen or do not abate.

[a]From Eiserman P: Hot weather, exercise, old age and the kidneys. *Geriatrics* 41(5):1986.

ercise is most practically measured and defined in terms of the exercise heart rate (i.e., the heart rate to be reached and maintained in order to achieve the greatest conditioning effect while avoiding complications or excessive stress) (Table 4.12). Obviously, patients must be taught to take their pulse and calculate their heart rate. For older patients, the intensity level should be based on attaining between 65 to 75% of the maximum heart rate (Lampman, 1987). Lower levels of intensity may be required in some patients, and a conditioning effect can still be achieved by increasing the duration of activity. Each exercise session should last from 30 to 60 minutes; the patient should begin with shorter periods and slowly increase the duration over the course of several weeks. Optimal conditioning is achieved by exercising three to 5 times/week. However, a flexible schedule should be encouraged; it might consist of daily exercise sessions of alternating vigorous and less-intense activities. On a daily basis, vigorous exercise is potentially harmful and should be avoided.

The presence of activity-limiting chronic diseases, such as coronary artery disease (CAD), chronic obstructive pulmonary disease (COPD), or end-stage renal disease (ESRD), does not preclude exercise. Rehabilitation programs for patients with these diseases should include exercise as a means of optimizing function, preventing disability, and adapting to the chronic illness (Painter and Blackburn, 1988). The type, intensity, duration, and frequency of exercise must be individualized. Patients with advanced rheumatoid or osteoarthritis may need to avoid weight bearing and would benefit from such activities as swimming, ambulating in water, or cycling. The duration and intensity of exercise is likely to be limited in patients with advanced CAD, COPD, or ESRD. The use of an exercise target heart rate may be inappropriate for these patients. Brief periods of activity at the desired intensity level, alternating with periods of rest, will result in some conditioning effect. Alternative methods of monitoring intensity include the assessment and monitoring of signs and symptoms (e.g., by using angina and dyspnea scales).

Clearly, many older patients can not engage in vigorous or strenuous exercise. But virtually all patients can benefit from exercise if realistic and attainable goals are developed. Remind these patients that exercise can make everyday life easier and more enjoyable; Exercise will be a part of the patient's daily routine as long as it is "dynamic, interesting, fun, varied, easily accessible, and without adverse sequelae" (Larson and Bruce, 1986). Exercise should not be done on a "p.r.n." basis.

NUTRITIONAL NEEDS OF THE ELDERLY

Improved nutrition has been suggested as a means of decreasing illness and morbidity associated with aging. Despite this appealing claim, nutrition research has shown that up to 50% of elderly people consume less than two-thirds of the currently recommended dietary allowances for several nutrients (Burns, 1986).

The problem is not that nutritional needs increase in the elderly population. Nutrient requirements for the elderly are no different than adult requirements, except that the requirements for calcium increase and the overall caloric requirements decrease. However, the multiple effects of physiological, social, psychological, and economic changes that impact nutritional status are different.

Furthermore, the key to understanding nutrition in the elderly is to recognize the extreme heterogeneity among the aging population. The healthy elderly tend to have a better nutritional intake and fewer physiologic changes than the frail elderly. The

Table 4.12
Calculating Exercise Target Heart Rate (ETHR)

$$ETHR = P \times (MHR-RHR) + RHR$$

P = % of MHR desired (usually 60–90%)

MHR = Maximum heart rate as measured during exercise tolerance testing, or 220 minus age in years

RHR = Resting heart rate

economically advantaged elderly have a significantly different nutrient intake than the economically disadvantaged. An assessment of all areas affecting nutrition is crucial to developing a dietary approach.

The complex interrelations of these factors on the overall nutritional status of the elderly will be considered next.

Physiologic Changes

Not only may essential nutrients be in short supply in the elderly, but also impaired absorption and utilization may actually dictate that increased amounts are needed to prevent disease (Hickler and Wayne, 1984). Impaired absorption is caused by a decrease in the secretion of gastric acid and digestive juices and primarily impacts iron, vitamin B_{12}, and lactose.

In addition to impaired absorption, a decreased gastrointestinal motility is found in the aging population. Complaints of frequent constipation and should be treated with dietary modification rather than laxatives. The emphasis should be on fiber-rich foods and an adequate fluid intake. A decreased sensitivity to thirst accompanies aging, so the older client must be instructed to consume 6 to 8 glasses of fluid/day. Foods such as fresh fruits and vegetables, prune juice, high-fiber cereals, and bran are recommended.

The intake of high-fiber foods in the form of fruits and vegetables is often complicated by poor dentition, which makes it difficult or unpleasant to chew (Fuller, 1986). People who wear dentures have reduced masticatory efficiency, and those with seriously compromised natural dentition or ill-fitting dentures tend to alter their food choices to reduce chewing (Burtis et al., 1988). Loss of teeth is secondary to periodontal disease but may be partially related to concomitant osteoporosis.

Energy expenditure decreases with aging and therefore requires a decrease in caloric intake. Failure to modify the caloric intake downward contributes to the high incidence of weight control difficulties in the elderly. On average, caloric consumption decreases by 200 kcal/day after age 51 and by 500 kcal/day after age 75 years (Fuller,

1986). The necessary caloric reduction is probably due to the concomitant decrease in activity level.

The caloric intake recommended to maintain a desirable body weight for the elderly, moderately active client is approximately 25 to 35 kcal/kg (approximately 1700 to 2380 kcal/day for a 150-lb person). This figure must be decreased for those requiring weight loss or those with minimal activity levels and increased for those requiring weight gain. The caloric intake should be approximately 12 to 15% protein, 50 to 60% carbohydrate, and 20 to 30% fat.

Maintenance of an ideal weight is not only necessary for optimum health but is a significant factor in preventing adult onset, Type II diabetes. Elderly persons have an altered glucose metabolism. Insulin resistance increases postprandial blood glucose levels and contributes to a slower return to fasting blood glucose levels. The risk of developing diabetes in the overweight, elderly client increases with age.

Renal and hepatic function are also impaired with aging, and this impairment has the overall affect of impairing the metabolism of foods and drugs and impeding the excretion of food waste products and drug metabolites. Attention to nutrient-drug interactions and drug excretory routes is important for this age group.

Sensory changes in the elderly client can also effect nutritional status. The sense of taste and smell gradually declines with aging, and this decline may be exacerbated by medications commonly taken by the elderly client, such as antihypertensive drugs, anti-Parkinson drugs, and hypoglycemic agents; this decline also may result in a decreased desire to eat. The altered perception may make the individual unable to recognize tastes and smells indicative of spoilage. Decreased vision may make food preparation difficult as well as hazardous, and assistance with meal planning and preparation may be necessary.

Mobility deficits are a common problem in the aging adult not only because of generalized energy reductions, but also because of concomitant medical problems found in this age group. Mobility deficits related to osteoporosis, arthritis, and poststroke deficits limit the person's ability to shop, use transportation, and stand for long periods, all of which may impact dietary practices.

Social/Psychological Changes

After physiologic changes have been assessed, it is important to determine key social and psychological concerns that may influence dietary practices. The quantity and quality of foods purchased can be influenced by changing social status, availability of storage facilities for food, and the person's method of transportation to markets. It is important to determine if the individual has the resources to get to the grocery store. Transportation may be limited for some elderly clients; driving licenses may be revoked because of visual or mobility deficits. The nurse needs to assess the reliability of transportation, whether it is independent or via community resources.

Assess who prepares the patient's food. Is this individual reliable? Are there adequate food storage and cooking facilities? Does the person live alone? Thirty-six percent of elderly women and 15 % of elderly men live alone; this factor has been correlated with inferior nutritional status (Hickler, 1984). Munro (1982) noted an increased incidence of anemia and a diet low in vitamin C in elderly men living alone. Clients living alone can be considered at risk and should be encouraged to take meals with nearby friends and relatives to provide social stimulation and change of environment (Kandzari and Howard, 1981).

Loneliness and depression, common in the elderly, are frequently associated with either undernutrition or overnutrition. The phenomena of loneliness and depression may cause a lack of motivation to interact with friends and relatives as well as a lack of motivation to remain healthy. These individuals are not concerned with a balanced diet, and this can result in either a loss or gain of weight. Increased social stimulation needs to be recommended for these clients and may be all that is necessary to remedy the eating problem.

Nutrition programs for the elderly to provide RDAs of essential nutrients as well as opportunities for socializing. Meals in a group setting are encouraged, and meals are delivered to those who are homebound because of illness, handicap, or transportation problems.

Economic Considerations

The nurse must determine if the client can afford to eat an adequate diet. Fifteen to 20 percent of Americans 65 years of age and older are at, or near, the poverty level. The amount of money allocated for appropriate nutrition is apt to be less than optimal (Hickler and Wayne, 1984). The cost of medication and rent may leave inadequate funds for food; in these cases the client should be referred to public assistance and community programs such as the Food Stamp Program and Senior Nutrition Program (Kandzari and Howard, 1981).

Table 4.13 details nutritional bargains from the basic four food groups. General guidelines for nutrition for people with a limited income include: (1) purchase the least expensive items in each food group and rely on store brands and generic products if possible; (2) eat minimal servings of meats and utilize meat substitutes such as legumes, cheese, and peanut butter; (3) serve larger quantities of grains, cereals, and pasta products; (4) prepare most foods from scratch rather than buying convenience foods; (5) eliminate processed foods that have poor nutrient contents such as carbonated beverages and potato chips; and (6) void snack foods and sugar-coated breakfast cereals because of their low-nutrient values (Burtis, 1988). Nutrient dense foods include spinach, beef liver, tomatoes, tuna, nonfat and low-fat milk, tofu, dry-roasted peanuts, eggs, and fresh carrots (Schaus and Briggs, 1983).

Nutritional Recommendations

Prior to discussing the common nutrient deficiencies found in the elderly, it must be reemphasized that of all age groups, the elderly represent the most heterogeneous in terms of nutritional patterns and deficiencies. Elderly individuals most likely to

Table 4.13
Nutritional Bargains from the Basic Four[a]

Food Group	More Economical	More Expensive
Milk	Skim and 2% milk	Whole milk
	Nonfat dry milk	Whole milk
	Evaporated milk	
Cheese	Cheese in bulk	Grated, sliced, or individually wrapped slices
	Cheese food	Cheese spreads
Ice cream	Ice milk or imitation ice cream	Ice cream or sherbet
Meat	Home-prepared meat	Luncheon meat, hot dogs, canned meat
	Regular hot dogs	All beef or all-meat hot dogs
	Less tender cuts	More tender cuts
	U.S. Good and Standard grades	U.S. Prime and Choice grades
	Bulk sausage	Sausage patties or links
	Pork or beef liver	Calves liver
	Heart, kidney, tongue,	
	Bologna	Specialty luncheon meats
Poultry	Large turkeys	Small turkeys
	Whole chickens	Cut-up chickens or individual parts
Eggs	Grade A eggs	Grade AA eggs
	Grade B eggs for cooking	
Fish	Fresh fish	Shellfish
	Chunk, flaked, or grated tuna	Fancy or solid-pack tuna
	Coho, pink, or chum salmon (lighter in color)	Chinook, king, and sockeye salmon (deeper red in color)
Fruits and vegetables	Locally grown fruits and vegetables in season	Out-of-season fruits and vegetables or those in short supply and exotic vegetables and fruits
	Grades B or C	Grade A or Fancy
	Cut up, pieces, or sliced	Whole
	Diced or short cut	Fancy-cut
	Mixed sizes	All the same size
	Fresh or canned	Frozen
	Plain vegetables	Mixed vegetables or vegetables in sauces
Fresh fruits	Apples	Cantaloupe
	Bananas	Grapes
	Oranges	Honeydew melon
	Tangerines	Peaches
		Plums
Fresh vegetables	Cabbage	Asparagus
	Carrots	Brussels sprouts
	Celery	Cauliflower
	Collard greens	Corn on the cob
	Kale	Mustard greens
	Lettuce	Spinach
	Onions	
	Potatoes	
	Sweet potatoes	
Canned fruits	Applesauce	Berries
	Peaches	Cherries
	Citrus juices	
	Other juices	
Canned vegetables	Beans	Asparagus
	Beets	Mushrooms
	Carrots	
	Collard greens	
	Corn	
	Kale	
	Mixed vegetables	
	Peas	
	Potatoes	

continues

Table 4.13—*Continued*

Food Group	More Economical	More Expensive
Canned vegetables —*continued*	Pumpkin Sauerkraut Spinach Tomatoes Turnip greens	
Frozen fruit	Concentrated citrus juices Other juices	Cherries Citrus sections Strawberries Other berries
Frozen vegetables	Beans Carrots Collard greens Corn Kale Mixed vegetables Peas Peas and carrots Potatoes Spinach Turnip greens	Asparagus Corn on the cob Vegetables, in pouch Vegetables, in cheese and other sauces
Dried fruits and vegetables	Potatoes	Apricots Dates Peaches
Breads and cereals	Day-old bread White enriched bread Cooked cereal Regular cooking oatmeal Plain rice Long-cooking rice Graham or soda crackers	Fresh bread Rolls, buns Whole grain Ready to eat cereals Quick cooking or instant oatmeal Seasoned rice Parboiled or instant rice Specialty crackers

[a]From Green ML, Harry J: *Nutrition in Contemporary Nursing Practice.* Copyright © 1981, John Wiley & Sons, Inc. Reprinted by permission of John Wiley & Sons, Inc.

be at risk for nutritional deficits include women, poorly educated persons, those who have recently experienced a drastic social change (the death of a loved one or a move from a lifelong residence), persons with chronic illness, and persons with financial burdens. However, most of these individuals can achieve the recommended daily allowances by ingesting a variety of foods from the basic four food groups (see Appendix M).

Protein

Protein intake should be 12 to 15% of the entire caloric intake. Inadequate protein intake is common in the chronically ill and economically deprived client. Hypoproteinemia may be accompanied by symptoms of edema, muscular weakness, and wasting. It should be emphasized that the mus-

cle wasting occurs in vital muscle (such as intercostals and cardiac muscle) as well as in strength skeletal muscle. Burtis (1988) suggests that inadequate protein intake is probably related to lack of money to purchase the best sources of protein: red meat, fish, poultry, eggs, and milk. Clients should be encouraged to obtain protein from leguminous plants (dry beans, dry peas, lentils, nuts, peanut butter, and soybeans); these sources are economical and provide valuable nutrients (Burtis, 1988, p. 315). To insure quality alternative protein ingestion, it may be necessary to refer the individual to a dietitian. An average intake of 2 servings from the meat group/day should assure attainment of the RDA for protein as well as iron, vitamin B_{12}, and niacin. More than 4 servings/day do not signal a problem from a protein viewpoint but may indicate an excessive fat intake.

Carbohydrates

Carbohydrate intake should account for 50 to 60% of the caloric intake. Carbohydrate sources are by the milk, fruit/vegetable, and grain groups. Complex carbohydrates, or starches, are provided by grain products and some vegetables such as corn, potatoes, beets, carrots, and peas. Starchy foods have an unwarranted negative reputation (high in calories and unhealthy) when in fact they provide essential carbohydrates, fiber, and bulk; some are also excellent sources of incomplete proteins. Deficiencies in carbohydrate intake are frequently accompanied by corresponding B vitamin deficiencies. These deficiencies are seen in individuals with extreme reduced caloric intake. At least 4 servings/day from the bread group provide adequate carbohydrate.

Fats and Vitamins

Fats serve as an important energy source and are a carriers for fat-soluble vitamins. Fat intake in the elderly should be 20 to 30% of the caloric intake. Fats are supplied primarily from meat, whole milk products, and added fats, such as margarine and salad dressings.

Fat-soluble vitamins include vitamins A, D, E and K. Vitamin A and D intakes have been found to be deficient in this age group. Although absorption of vitamin A is increased with age, the elderly generally consume fewer fruits and vegetables, and these individuals may be vitamin A deficient. Vitamin D deficiency may result from dietary insufficiency and kidney disease, as well as decreased exposure to sunlight in the homebound individual. Dark green or yellow vegetables at least 3 times/week should prevent deficiencies in vitamins A, E, and K.

Deficiencies in water-soluble vitamins have also been reported in this age group. Many elderly patients are deficient in vitamin C. Vitamin C requirements are increased with the stress of aging and the stress of illness. In addition many drugs such as corticosteroids, aspirin, indomethacin, and phenylbutazone impair absorption and utilization of ascorbic acid. Vitamin C deficiencies are associated with gum lesions, poor wound healing, and frequent bouts of respiratory infections. One serving/day of a citrus fruit (oranges, tomatoes, strawberries, cantaloupe) or cruciferous vegetable (cauliflower, broccoli) should avoid deficits.

Vitamin B deficiencies have been commonly reported in both the healthy and the frail elderly. Patients with impaired cognitive function should be assessed for low blood levels of vitamins C and B_{12}, riboflavin, and folic acid (Ludman and Newman, 1986). Alcoholics are at great risk for B vitamin deficiencies, and alcoholism is estimated to occur in 2 to 10% of the population 60 years of age and older (Hickler and Wayne, 1984). An average of 2 servings/day from the dairy group and 4 servings/day from the bread group should prevent any deficiencies.

The media have made "iron-poor blood" a household term. It must be stressed that iron deficiency is not a normal physiologic alteration with aging but represents a pathology. Iron-deficiency anemia is suggestive of gastrointestinal bleeding either from cancer or large dosages of drugs such as aspirin or other anti-inflammatory agents. Self-medication with vitamin E may also cause bleeding as vitamin E antagonizes vitamin K (Fuller, 1986). Individuals should be counseled to avoid indiscriminate doses of vitamin E in favor of moderate multivitamin dosages.

Calcium

Calcium intake is consistently low in both the healthy and frail elderly. Postmenopausal and older women receiving estrogen need approximately 1000 mg of calcium/day for calcium balance. Postmenopausal women who are not on estrogen require 1500 mg of calcium/day. Men also require 1000 mg of calcium/day to prevent bone loss. Dairy products are the major dietary source of calcium followed by dark green vegetables. Four servings of milk or yogurt/day will generally supply the needed calcium. Insufficient calcium can be a significant problem in the elderly because many are lactose deficient. The most common carbohydrate malabsorption problems are caused by lactose intolerance. Lactose intolerance is generally treated by decreasing the input of dairy products. The elderly lactose intolerant individual may be helped by Lactaid, a product that increases the ability of the body to utilize the ingested milk product. Generally, yogurt can be tolerated by lactose deficient individuals and is one of the best sources for calcium. Dry powdered milk can be added to foods without a significant change in taste and provides an excellent source of calcium. Orange juice fortified with calcium and cereals high in calcium may contribute to calcium intakes (see Appendix M).

Calcium carbonate supplements may be indicated for clients unable to ingest sufficient quantities of dietary calcium. Absorption of calcium carbonate from supplements may be impaired if there is decreased stomach acid; therefore to improve absorption it is recommended that the supplement be taken with meals.

In addition to dietary intake of calcium, exercise is a crucial part of the osteoporosis prevention and treatment plan. Inactivity leads to bone loss and weight bearing exercise reduces bone loss. Walking for at least 30 minutes 3 times/week is highly recommended not only for bone health but for general wellness.

REFERENCES

Barclay A: Falls in the elderly: is prevention possible? *Postgrad Med*, 83(2):241–248, 1988.

Barry H: Exercise prescriptions for the elderly. *Am Fam Phys* September:155–161, 1986.

Beard O: Age related physiological changes in the cardiovascular system. In Cape R, Coe R, Rossman I (eds): *Fundamentals of Geriatric Medicine*. New York, Raven Press, 1983.

Bellantoni M, Blackman M: Osteoporosis: diagnostic screening and its place in current care. *Geriatrics* 43(2):63, 1988.

Berman R, Haxby J, Pomerantz R: Physiology of aging. Part I. normal changes. *Patient Care* 22(1):15–21, 1988.

Blazer D, Bachar J, Manton K: Suicide in late life: review and commentary. *J Am Geriatr Soc* 34:519–525, 1986.

Boxwell A: Geriatric suicide: the preventable death. *Nurse Pract* 13(6):10–19, 1988.

Burns R, Nichols L, Calkins E, Blackwell S, Pragay D: Nutritional assessment of community living well elderly. *J Am Geriatr Soc* 34(11):781–785, 1986.

Burtis G, Davis J, Martin S: *Applied Nutrition and Diet Therapy*. Philadelphia, WB Saunders, 1988.

Cunha UV: Management of orthostatic hypotension in the elderly. *Geriatrics* 42(9):61–66, 1987.

Eisenman P: Hot weather, exercise, old age, and the kidneys. *Geriatrics* 41(5):108–114, 1986.

Erikson R: *Childhood and Society*, ed 2. New York, WW Norton, 1963.

Fam A: Osteoarthritis in the geriatric patient. *Geriatr Med Today* 6(4):71, 1987.

Fitzsimmons V: Maintaining a positive environment for the older adult. *Orthop Nurs*, 4(3):45–51, 1985.

Fuller E: What's a "sound diet" for the elderly? *Patient Care* June 15:90–106, 1986.

Goldman R: Aging changes in structure and function. In Carnevali D, Patrick M (eds): *Nursing Management for the Elderly*. Philadelphia, JB Lippincott, 1979.

Hickler R: Nutrition and the elderly. *Am Family Pract* 29(3):137–145, 1984.

Kandzari J, Howard J: *The Well Family: a Developmental Approach to Assessment*. Boston, Little, Brown, 1981.

Lampman R: Evaluating and prescribing exercise for elderly patients. *Geriatrics* 42(8):63–76, 1987.

Lappe J: Reminiscing: the life review therapy. *J Gerontol Nurs* 13(4):12–16, 1987.

Larson E, Bruce R: Exercise and aging. *Ann Intern Med* 105(5):783–785, 1986.

Ludman E, Newman J: Frail elderly: Assessment of nutrition needs. *Gerontologist* 26(2):198–201, 1986.

Munro H: Nutritional requirements in the elderly. *Hosp Pract* 17(8):143–154, 1982.

National Center for Health Statistics: Vital and Health Statistics of the United States. 1980. Vol 2, Mortality (Part B). *DHHS. (PHS)*. 85–1102, 1985.

National Center for Health Statistics: Health statistics on older persons, United States, 1986, Havlik RI, Liu BM, Kovar MG, et al (eds): 1986. Vital and Health Statistics. Series 3, No 25. *DHHS*. Pub. No. (PHS) 87-1059, 1987.

Nolan L, O'Malley K: Prescribing for the elderly. Part I. Sensitivity of the elderly to adverse reactions. *J Am Geriatr Soc* 36(2):142–148, 1988.

Paffenbarger R, Hyde R, Wing A, Hsieh C: Physical activity, all-cause mortality, and longevity of college alumni. *N Engl J Med* 314:605–613, 1986.

Painter P, Blackburn G: Exercise for patients with chronic disease. *Postgrad Med* 83(1):185–195, 1988.

Preston D, Grimes J: A study of differences in social groups. *J Geriatr Nurs* 13(2):10–16, 1987

Ryan M, Patterson J: Loneliness in the elderly. *J Geriatr Nurs* 13(5):6–12, 1987.

Schaus E, Briggs G: Naturally economic foods. *J Nutr Educ* 15(4):130, 1983.

Scott R, Mitchell M: Aging, alcohol, and the liver. *J Am Geriatr Soc* 36(3):255–265, 1988.

Spiera H: Osteoarthritis as a misdiagnosis in elderly patients. *Geriatrics* 42(11):37–42, 1987.

Stoller E, Earl L: Help with activities of everyday life: sources of support for the non-institutionalized elderly. *Gerontologist* 15(6):64–69, 1983.

Storey J: *Older Americans in the Reagan Era: Impacts of Federal Policy Changes.* Washington, DC, Villers Foundation, 1983.

Townsend P: Isolation, desolation, and loneliness. In Shanes E, Atherton, Townsend P, Wedderburn D, et al (eds): *Old People in Three Industrial Societies.* New York, Atherton, 1968.

Trinca C, Dickerson J: Adverse drug reactions. In Wiener M, Pepper G, Kuhn-Weisman G, Romano J (eds): *Clinical Pharmacology and Therapeutics in Nursing.* New York, McGraw-Hill, 1979.

U.S. Dept. of Commerce, Bureau of the Census. *Money, income, and Poverty Status in the U.S.: 1985.* (Advance Data from theMarch 1986 Current Population Survey). Series P-60, No. 154, 1986.

Villers Foundation: *On the Other Side of Easy Street: Myths and Facts about the Economics of Old Age.* Washington, DC, Villers Foundation, 1987.

Vitale J, Santos J: Nutrition and the elderly. *Postgrad Med* 78(5):79–81, 1985.

Waller JA: Injury in the aged: clinical and epidemiological implications. *NY State J Med* 12(12):10–16, 1974.

Walther R, Harber L: Expected skin complaints of the geriatric patient. *Geriatrics* 39(12):67–79, 1984.

Whipple RH, Wolfson RI, Amerman RM: The relationship of knee and ankle weakness to falls in nursing home residents: an isokinetic study. *J Am Geriatr Soc* 35(1):13–20, 1987.

chapter 5

The Spine: Cervical, Thoracic, and Lumbar

SHARON J. GATES, R.N., M.S.N., C.R.N.P., A.N.P.C.

Back and neck pain occur commonly in the general population. Patients with back pain are seen only slightly more frequently than those with neck pain (Bland, 1987). Often, patients present with confusing symptoms, making the diagnosis difficult. A systematic approach to problem solving ensures the best possible clinical outcome. Neck and back problems are often enigmatic, therefore they require a trusting patient/provider partnership for a successful clinical conclusion.

In early life, the spine is a straight column. As the developing child sits and walks this straight column develops three separate curves: the lordotic curves of the cervical and lumbar spine and the kyphotic curve of the thoracic or dorsal spine. This curved column is comprised of 24 individual vertebrae that rest on a bony base called the sacrum (Fig. 5.1). The motion provided by the cervical and lumbar spine is flexion, extension, lateral bending, and rotation. The primary motion of the thoracic spine is rotation. The facet joint functions to limit motion, restricting movement beyond the normal range.

Between the vertebrae are intervertebral discs. The disc is comprised of two parts. The outer portion, the annulus, consists of concentric rings of fibrocartilage. The central portion, called the nucleus, is comprised of a hydrophilic, gelatinous substance that distributes applied stresses to the annulus, allowing the disc to function as a shock absorber. The disc also aids the glid-ing movement between each of the vertebrae. As part of the normal aging process, the nucleus becomes less hydrophilic and is less able to resist compressive and torsional forces. The smooth gliding motion of the vertebrae over the disc is disrupted. The disc space narrows, altering the mechanics of the posterior facet joints. Osteophytes (bone spurs) form on the facet joints and vertebral bodies in response to the altered mechanics. The combination of a narrowed disc space and osteophytes in the intervertebral foramen can cause nerve root impingement (Fig. 5.2).

Disc degeneration can begin as early as adolescence in the cervical spine, and usually occurs in the lumbar spine after age 25. By middle age most individuals will have radiograph changes demonstrating this phenomenon (Won, 1984). These aging changes in the disc can result in pain and limited mobility.

THE CERVICAL SPINE

History

Observe the patient during the history taking. Posture, facial expression, eye contact, and clothing are clues to a differential diagnosis. Establishing the location of the pain is critical (Table 5.1). Be careful not to lead the patient, but if necessary, offer hints of description. Does the pain feel aching and dull, hot and bursting, or lancinating, knife-like? Was there a precipitating event?

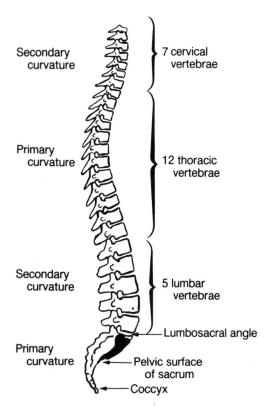

Secondary curvature

7 cervical vertebrae

Primary curvature

12 thoracic vertebrae

Secondary curvature

5 lumbar vertebrae

Lumbosacral angle

Primary curvature

Pelvic surface of sacrum

Coccyx

Figure 5.1. The cervical, thoracic, lumbar, sacral, and coccygeal regions of the vertebral column. (From Draves DJ: *Anatomy of the Lower Extremity.* Baltimore, Williams & Wilkins, 1986, p 18.)

Neck pain following trauma may develop within several hours, or it may be delayed 24 to 48 hours (Rothman and Marvel, 1975). Nontraumatic neck pain is felt upon arising in the morning. Patients complain of neck stiffness and aching. Is there associated pain? If arm pain is associated with neck pain, determine the nature of this pain, the location, and intensity. Patients with degenerative neck conditions rarely complain of neck discomfort. Their chief complaint is of shoulder pain that may or may not radiate down the arm. Are there paresthesias (tingling sensations) associated with the pain? If so, determine the duration, the location, the nature, and timing. Ask about specific activities that aggravate the pain. Is the pain worse with motion? If worse with movement, determine whether the pain increases on the ipsilateral or contra-

lateral side. The pain of cervical disc degeneration typically *follows* activity. Rotator cuff tendinitis is worse *with* activity (MacNab, 1975). Is the pain worse following rest? When neck pain increases following supine lying, suspect injury to the supporting musculature. Careful symptom analysis directs the physical examination and aids in a differential diagnosis (Table 5.2).

Physical Examination

Observation

The physical examination begins with the initial observation.

Ask the patient to point to the area of pain. Differentiate shoulder lesions due to rotator cuff tendinitis from neck pain. Patients with pain originating in the cervical spine will point to the trapezius muscle. Patients with shoulder tendinitis will place their hand over the deltoid muscle (MacNab, 1975). Examine the position and posture of the head. Normally the head is held erect, perpendicular to the floor (Hoppenfeld, 1976). A forward flexed posture may be observed in normal individuals, but it can also represent a soft tissue injury to the neck.

Have the patient disrobe to the waist to allow observation of the neck and upper extremities. The arc of motion during the process of undressing should be unrestricted. The patient with significant muscle spasm splints the neck and leans towards the spasm to avoid pain. With the patient seated comfortably on the examining room table, inspect the neck for scars, blisters, and discoloration.

Examine the spine for symmetry of the cervical musculature and for the normal cervical lordosis. A loss of lordosis can indicate paravertebral spasm, degenerative changes related to normal aging, or prior injury.

Palpation

It is essential to have muscles relaxed to differentiate between soft tissue and skeletal pain. With the patient supine, palpate the anterior bony structures, and with the

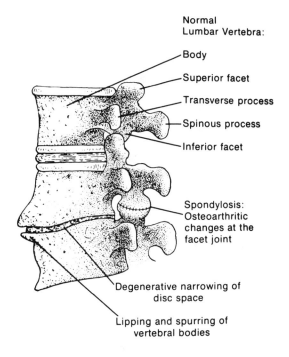

Normal
Lumbar Vertebra:

Body

Superior facet

Transverse process

Spinous process

Inferior facet

Spondylosis:
Osteoarthritic
changes at the
facet joint

Degenerative narrowing of
disc space

Lipping and spurring of
vertebral bodies

Figure 5.2. Degenerative spondylosis. (From Reilly BM: *Practical Strategies in Outpatient Medicine*. Philadelphia, WB Saunders, 1984, p 48.)

head cradled in one hand use the other hand to palpate the posterior bony structures. Identify the area of maximal tenderness.

Palpate the anterior and posterior soft tissues, including the paracervical musculature, the cervical nodes, and the thyroid gland.

Palpate the carotid pulse and listen for bruits. Examine the shoulder girdle and arm.

Upon direct pressure certain areas are normally tender. These may include the trapezius muscle, the superior medial angle of the scapula, the insertion of the deltoid, and the origin of the common extensors of the elbow. Painful neck lesions may increase this tenderness (MacNab, 1975).

Gross neck tenderness can be related to emotional or functional factors. Tenderness of the triceps occurs with C6–7 problems. Tenderness of the biceps and pectoralis major is associated with C5–6 lesions. This is often associated with tenderness of the costochondral junction of the first six ribs at the origin of the pectorals, imitating Tietze's syndrome (costochondritis). Tenderness of the sternocleidomastoid muscle may be associated with hyperextension injuries of the neck.

Paravertebral muscle spasm occurs with soft tissue injury and cervical disc herniation. Enlarged lymph nodes resulting from upper respiratory infection can cause wryneck (torticollis).

Range of Motion

With the patient sitting and facing the examiner, check for active and passive range of motion. Active motion should be recorded in flexion, extension, lateral flexion, and rotation; note the painful range. To test active flexion have the patient touch the chin to the chest. This is the normal range of flexion. Extension is tested by asking the patient to look directly at the ceiling. This is the normal range of extension.

Individuals with degenerative neck disease frequently have a decrease in the normal range of extension. Patients with a herniated disc have resticted lateral flexion and extension. Soft tissue trauma can result in a decrease in both flexion and extension.

Test rotation by having the patient turn to the right and then to the left. Normally the chin should line up with the shoulder; note any restriction in the arc of motion.

To test lateral flexion have the patient touch the ear to the shoulder. (Caution the

Table 5.1
Eight Critical Questions for Data Gathering

1. Was there a precipitating event?
   A. Trauma
   B. Lifting
   C. Bending

2. What was the onset?
   A. Gradual?
   B. Sudden?

3. How long has the pain persisted? (duration)

4. Where exactly is it? (location)
   A. Neck, back, buttocks
   B. Extremities

5. What is the nature of the pain?
   A. Aching
   B. Burning
   C. Radiating

6. What are the aggravating and relieving factors?
   A. Worse with coughing, sneezing, straining, and sitting
   B. Relieved by lying down

7. Are there associated complaints?
   A. Paresthesias of extremities
   B. Weakness or numbness of extremities
   C. Bowel or bladder dysfunction

8. Occurrence: when is the pain worse?
   A. Morning
   B. Afternoon/evening
   C. Night

patient against bringing the shoulder up to the ear.) Normal lateral bend is 45°. Compare the left side to the right side. Enlarged cervical lymph nodes may limit the motion of lateral bend.

Some examiners prefer to examine for passive range of motion with the patient supine. With the muscles supported and relaxed the range of motion is increased. Caution: Do not attempt passive range of motion with a suspected unstable neck (i.e., fracture).

To test passive range of motion during flexion and extension, place your hands on either side of the head and bend the head forward and then backward. Normally the chin should touch the chest during flexion, and the patient should see the ceiling above during extension. Test right and left lateral bend by gently moving the head so the ear approaches the shoulder. Move the head

from side to side in a "no" motion to test rotation. Compare the left motion with the right motion (Hoppenfeld, 1976).

Neurologic Examination

Motor strength: To test neck flexion (sternocleidomastoids) stabilize the sternum with one hand, and with the opposite hand placed against the patient's forehead, offer resistance as the patient flexes the neck forward. Record the result, using the 0 to 5 motor grading scale (Table 5.3). To test neck extension (paraspinals and trapezius) stabilize the posterior thorax and scapula with one hand and place the opposite hand over the occiput and gently offer resistance as the patient extends the neck. Record the strength results. For lateral bending (scalenus) place one hand on the patient's right shoulder and offer resistance with the palm of the opposite hand placed on the the patient's temple. As the patient brings the ear to the shoulder, note maximum resistance. To test lateral rotation (sternocleidomastoid) place the left hand on the patient's left shoulder and with the right hand placed on the right side of the mandible offer resistance as the patient rotates the head in a "no" motion (Hoppenfeld, 1976).

Neurologic level: In a systematic manner with the patient seated on the edge of the examination table, legs dangling over the side, evaluate the neurologic levels from C5 to T1 (Fig. 5.3).

C5 level: The deltoid is examined along with the biceps, which has both C5 and C6 innervation for motor function. Test deltoid strength by offering resistance against the shoulder motions of flexion, abduction, and extension (see Chapter 6). Test biceps strength by offering resistance against elbow flexion. The biceps is examined for reflex, and the lateral arm over the lateral deltoid muscle is examined for sensation (axillary nerve).

C6 level: The wrist extensors and the biceps are examined for motor function. Evaluate the wrist extensors by offering resistance and comparing the strength of both extremities. The brachioradialis and biceps are examined for reflex, and the lateral forearm, thumb, index finger, and one-half the middle finger are examined for sensation.

Table 5.2
Differential Diagnosis of Cervical Spine Problems

Cervical strain/sprain ("whiplash")
    This pain is dull and aching in nature. It may begin gradually following trauma and is often associated with a burning, throbbing headache. This may be accompanied by visual symptoms (blurring vision) and auditory symptoms (either increased or decreased sensitivity to noise). If arm pain is present it is not localized to a dermatome. The pain may be vague or aching and does not increase with coughing or sneezing. It may be worse with activity and improve with rest.

Cervical radiculopathy
    This pain is described as aching with stiffness. If associated with headache, the headache is described as sharp, splitting, or shooting. Associated shoulder and arm pain will follow a definable upper extremity dermatome. Symptoms will increase with coughing and sneezing. Activities will increase the pain, while rest will relieve the symptoms.

Brachial plexus injury
    This lesion may cause neck pain, but the prominent complaint is of a sudden, severe, burning pain along the shoulder that radiates down the arm to the hand and is associated with parathesias and motor weakness (Roy and Irwin, 1983).

Cervical myelopathy
    This chronic pain syndrome is variable. Symptoms are related to spinal cord compression. The pain is bursting, hot in nature. It may also be dull, aching, and poorly localized. It seldom radiates, but can be referred to the subcostal areas, anterior aspect of the thighs, or the buttocks. Weakness of the lower extremities with a sense of instability may be present, along with bowel or bladder dysfunction. Neck motion and straining do not increase the pain (Rothman and Marvel, 1975).

Table 5.3
Motor Grading Scale[a]

Muscle Grading Chart	
Muscle Gradations	Description
5—Normal	Complete range of motion against gravity with full resistance
4—Good	Complete range of motion against gravity with some resistance
3—Fair	Complete range of motion against gravity
2—Poor	Complete range of motion with gravity eliminated
1—Trace	Evidence of slight contractility. No joint motion
0—Zero	No evidence of contractility

[a]From Hoppenfeld S: *Physical Examination of the Spine and Extremities*. East Norwalk, CT, Appleton-Century-Crofts, 1976, p 161.

C7 level: The triceps, wrist flexors, and the finger extensors are examined for motor function. Test triceps strength by offering resistance against elbow extension. Have the patient begin with the arm in flexion, and as the patient begins to extend the elbow offer resistance. Test the wrist flexors by resisting against the palmar aspect of a closed fist. Test the strength of the finger extensors by asking the patient to resist downward pressure on the dorsum of the extended fingers. The triceps reflex is examined and the middle finger is tested for sensation.

C8 level: The finger flexors are examined for motor function. Test the strength of the finger flexors by placing your fingers inside the patient's flexed fingers and trying to force the patient's fingers out of flexion. At this level there is no reflex that is tested. The ulnar side of the distal half of the forearm, the ulnar side of the ring finger, and the small finger are tested for sensation.

T1 level: The finger abductors are examined for motor strength. Test finger abduction by having the patient extend and spread the fingers apart while the examiner tries to squeeze them together. At this level there is no reflex tested. The medial side of the upper half of the forearm is tested for sensation. Table 5.4 describes the symptoms associated with compromise of the nerve roots of C5, C6, and C7.

The patient with hyperreflexia should be examined for upper motor neuron pathology. Look for long tract signs (indicating cord compression) by testing for clonus, the Babinski reflex, the cremasteric reflex, and the abdominal reflex.

Distinguish cervical myelopathy from

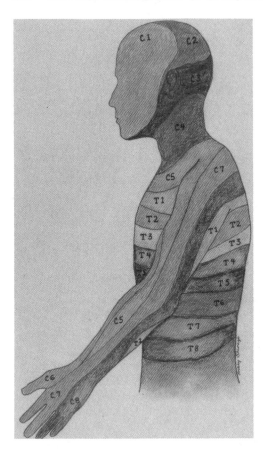

Figure 5.3. Sensory level by dermatome. (From Scott WN, Nisonson B, Nicholas, JA (eds): *Principles of Sports Medicine*. Baltimore, Williams & Wilkins, 1984, p 63.)

Table 5.4
Pain/Paresthesias[a]

C5 Root (C4–C5 Disc Level)

Symptoms
    Anterosuperior shoulder pain
    Anterolateral upper arm and forearm pain

Signs
    Decreased biceps reflex
    Weakness of arm and shoulder extension

C6 Root (C5–C6 Disc Level)

Symptom
    Dorsoradial aspect of forearm and thumb pain

Sign
    Decreased brachioradialis reflex and biceps reflex
    Weakness of wrist extension and biceps muscle

C7 Root (C6–C7 Disc Level)

Symptom
    Altered sensation in the middle finger, radiating
      pain to middle of forearm

Signs
    Decreased triceps reflex
    Weakness of elbow extension, wrist flexion,
      finger extension, weakness of triceps muscle

[a]Adapted from Rothman RH, Simeone FA (eds): *The Spine*, ed 2. Philadelphia, WB Saunders, 1982, p 454.

Special Tests

Compression: With one hand, press down upon the top of the patient's head. Note if neck pain increases and, if it radiates, note the dermatome. Increased neck pain, or reproduction of referred pain with compression, indicates a joint or bony injury, a narrowed foramen, or pressure on the facet joints or muscles.

Valsalva: Have the patient hold his/her breath and tighten his/her buttocks. This maneuver increases intrathecal pressure. Intrathecal pressure increases in the presence of a space-occupying lesion such as a tumor or a herniated nucleus pulposus. If the test is positive the patient will complain of neck pain or radiating pain that follows a definable dermatome.

Swallowing: Swelling of the esophagus from trauma, bony osteophytes, hematomas, infection, or tumor in the anterior portion of the cervical spine can sometimes cause difficult or painful swallowing.

Adson: Take the patient's radial pulse at the wrist. While you extend, abduct, and

cervical radiculopathy. Evaluate for long tract signs, lower extremity spasticity, and bowel and bladder control (Table 5.2). The pain of radiculopathy is described as aching and the pain follows a sensory dermatome. It may be accompanied by weakness, loss of tone and bulk of the upper extremity muscles, and absent or diminished reflexes. The signs and symptoms of myelopathy may be preceded by radicular symptoms with great variability. Paresthesias of the hands are common. There may be evidence of progressive lower extremity weakness. Ataxia and long tract signs may be present.

Examination of the radial, ulnar, median, axillary, and musculocutaneous peripheral nerves follows (see Chapter 7).

externally rotate the arm, have the patient take a deep breath and hold it while turning the head toward the arm being tested to determine if the pulse is still present. A diminished or absent pulse is a positive Adson's test. This evaluates the presence of compression of the subclavian artery (Hoppenfeld, 1976).

Evaluate associated areas that can mimic cervical spine problems: the upper extremities, lower jaw, teeth, temporomandibular joint, scalp, and shoulder (Won, 1984).

Guidelines for Diagnostic Tests

Several tests will assist in differentiating the causes of neck pain (Table 5.5).

Obtain cervical spine plain films: Routine views will include AP, LAT, and both obliques (odontoid views for axis/atlas evaluation) for the following: root pain, a neurologic deficit, patients involved in litigation and all patients over age 40. Add lateral flexion and extension views if the

Table 5.5
Differential Diagnosis of Neck Pain

Ligamentous/muscular disorders
  Spasm
  Strain/sprain
  Contusion
  Wryneck (torticollis)

Skeletal disorders
  Cervical disk degeneration
  Cervical disk herniation
  Shoulder joint (rotator cuff tendinitis)
  Fracture
  Atlantoaxial instability secondary to RA
  Discitis
  Cervical stenosis

Psychogenic
  Secondary gains
  Litigation pending

Neurologic disorders
  Nerve root lesions
  Brachial plexus lesions ("stingers")
  Thoracic outlet syndrome
  Neurogenic pain syndromes

Spinal cord/brain
  Meningitis
  Spinal cord compression
  Cervical myelopathy

Cardiac disorders
  Angina

patient complains of neck or arm pain with head motion in order to evaluate for the presence of a fracture, subluxation, ligament stability, narrow foramina, and soft tissue abnormalities. Provide a description of the clinical picture when requesting x-rays; interpretation must correlate with clinical findings. Some of the findings may include:
(1) Narrowing of the interspace with associated symptoms suggests acute disc syndrome;
(2) A vacuum disc (air in the disc space) indicates an acute degenerative process;
(3) Loss of normal cervical lordosis results from either paravertebral muscle spasm, restriction of motion secondary to neck pain, the result of soft tissue injury, musculoskeletal injury, or an acute or chronic disc syndrome;
(4) Cervical instability or injury to the supporting ligaments.
Obtain a bone scan: If a fracture is suspected, but it does not appear on plain film, or if a tumor or infection is suspected.

Obtain an electrocardiogram: If the patient complains of chest pain that radiates to the neck or jaw, or in any patient who is in a high-risk group for coronary disease.

Aids to diagnosis of persistent or worsening symptoms after 6 weeks include:
(1) Electromyography: For suspected cervical radiculopathy electromyography will evaluate for nerve root involvement. This distinguishes peripheral nerve involvement from nerve root involvement, and is diagnostic of either radiculopathy, a brachial plexus lesion, or peripheral neuropathy. Electromyography aids in the differentiation of organic from inorganic (functional) problems.
(2) Magnetic resonance imaging: For suspected nerve root or cord involvement;
(3) Computerized axial tomogram: For suspected herniated disc, for suspected stenosis, and patient reassurance;
(4) Laboratory studies: For hemoglobin, hematocrit, complete blood count with differential, urinalysis, erythrocyte sedimentation rate, blood chemistry

studies, immunologic studies, serum protein electrophoresis, and TB skin tests to rule out underlying systemic disease.

The Adolescent with Neck Pain

Neck symptoms in the adolescent are unusual. Complaints of neck pain need careful evaluation.

Predisposing factors

(1) Immaturity of the cervical spine;
(2) Mobility of the young cervical spine (under age 20);
(3) Congenital instability of C1–2, C4–5, C5–6 (that may occur with Down's syndrome);
(4) Long, thin necks (increased susceptibility to sports-related injuries);
(5) Participation in certain competitive and contact sports (wrestling, swimming, diving, football, rugby, and gymnastics) (Funk and Wells, 1975; Wroble and Albright, 1986);
(6) Motor vehicle accidents (all terrain, motorcycle, and automobile).

Etiology

(1) Acute or chronic muscle, tendon, or ligamentous strain that results from head-on tackling during football when trauma to the head is transferred to the neck. Athletes playing as defensive backs or wide receivers risk violent flexion (most dangerous), extension, and lateral stretch injuries (most common) (Funk & Wells, 1975).
(2) Localized acute muscle strain resulting from motor vehicle accidents.
(3) A direct blow to the cervical spine causing a contusion which can mimic cervical strain.
(4) Cervical disc herniation can occur on impact with sports or motor vehicle accidents, but is rare in this age group. Evaluate the athlete to distinguish cervical radiculopathy (nerve root compression) from a brachial plexus (stinger type) injury (Table 5.6).

Prevention

The injured athlete must be assessed immediately. The team physician or trainer must be drilled in the proper techniques for evaluation, on-field treatment, and transportation. Education is the key to preventing many of the cervical spine injuries in this age group. Prevention can be aided by:
(1) Preseason screenings of the cervical spine to identify high-risk individuals. These screenings should include determination of general fitness, strength testing, evaluation of range of motion, evaluation of cervical tenderness, axial compression test, and information about previous injury. Obtain cervical spine x-rays on all individuals with a history of pain or prior neck injury. An athlete with prior injury and a positive physical examination is at increased risk for injury (Wroble and Albright, 1986). Athletes with a normal examination and a history of prior injury have a slightly increased risk.
(2) Utilize a strict criterion for returning to competition.
(3) Establish a 12-month conditioning/training program to include neck exercises. Recommend isometric resistance and isotonic resistance (Nautilus) to build the strength of the supporting neck musculature.
(4) Bar trampolines from regular gymnastic classes.
(5) Educate the coaching staff and the athletes to the associated risks for injury and the prevention techniques.
(6) Insist that athletes wear seat belts at all times, adjust car headrests to protect the head and neck and do not drive under the influence of alcohol, sedatives, or tranquilizers.

Common Management Problems

Pinched Nerve Syndrome (Brachial Plexus Lesion, Stinger, and Burner).

Etiology.
Common football or wrestling injury. The head is forced to one side while the opposite shoulder is depressed.

Table 5.6
Radiculopathy Versus Plexus Injury[a]

Brachial Plexus	Nerve Root Compression
Sudden onset	Sudden onset
Paresthesias over 2 to 4 dermatomes	Paresthesias over definable dermatome
Complete transient paralysis of arm	Partial transient paralysis of affected arm
1. Sensation loss 2 to 4 dermatomes	1. Sensation loss to definable dermatome
2. Tenderness over brachial plexus	2. No tenderness over brachial plexus
3. Increased symptoms with passive movement of head and neck to the opposite side	3. Hyperflexion, extension, lateral flex toward the affected side may increase symptoms
4. No posterior neck tenderness on palpation	4. Posterior neck tenderness
5. No increased symptoms with compression test	5. May have positive compression test

[a]Adapted from Roy S, Irvin R: *Sports Medicine: Prevention, Evaluation, Management, and Rehabilitation.* Englewood Cliffs, NJ, Prentice Hall, 1983.

Symptoms.
(1) Sudden onset;
(2) Burning sensation in the shoulder;
(3) Paresthesias of entire arm, hand, and fingers;
(4) Possible pain and weakness in the arm and hand;
(5) Possible complete transient paralysis of affected arm.
Signs.
(1) Sensation loss over multiple (2 to 4) dermatomes;
(2) Tenderness over the brachial plexus;
(3) Increased symptoms with passive movement of head and neck to the opposite side;
(4) No posterior neck tenderness;
(5) No increased symptoms with compression test.
Treatment (Acute).
(1) Ice;
(2) Anti-inflammatory medications;
(3) Muscle relaxants;
(4) Splinting (rolled towel, soft collar, and sandbags).
Rehabilitation.
(1) Active range of motion exercises as soon as possible;
(2) Neck strengthening exercises for supportive musculature when symptoms subside;
(3) Education focusing on proper techniques to avoid injury;
(4) Use of a heavy roll or collar to prevent lateral motion of the head upon return to the game (Funk and Wells, 1975).
Referral.
(1) Immediate, if severe injury suspected;

(2) Seven days, if symptoms do not subside;
(3) Three to 6 weeks if sensation does not return for EMG, bone scan, medical evaluation;
(4) As needed follow-up office visits.
Outcome. Return to play criteria:
(1) No pain with full active neck range of motion;
(2) No pain during resistance testing of neck movements;
(3) Full motor power of shoulder shrugs, abduction, elbow flexion and extension, and grip;
(4) Normal sensation along all dermatomes (Roy and Irvin, 1983).

The Adult with Neck Pain

Degenerative change in the cervical spine is a part of the aging process. This phenomenon can begin in adolescence and can affect the discs and/or the facet joints. By age 40 some individuals have narrowing of the interspace between C5–6 and C6–7, osteophyte formation, and sclerosis of the facet joints. These changes can be seen on the x-ray and can compress and irritate the nerve roots, the spinal cord, and the vertebral arteries.

Adult problems may originate in the workplace. The worker with a neck injury loses more work time than the worker with a back injury, although neck injury occurs only 20% as frequently. The most common cause of upper extremity pain in middle age is the result of osteoarthritis of the cervical spine (Wiesel et al., 1985).

Predisposing Factors

(1) Static arm postures, such as those used by dentists, hairdressers, and bike riders;
(2) Repetitive arm movements such as those used by coal miners, assembly line packers, meat cutters, and swimmers;
(3) Static sitting postures assumed by computer terminal operators and secretaries;
(4) Motor vehicle accidents.

Etiology

(1) Acute or chronic muscle, tendon, or ligamentous strain that results from work-related postures or recreational activities;
(2) Localized acute muscle strain resulting from motor vehicle accidents;
(3) Cervical disc herniation occurring as a result of the impact on the aging spine following a fall or motor vehicle accident. Most herniations will resolve with conservative management within 6 weeks, although the patient may be left with residual aching and limitation of movement.
(4) Changes associated with aging, a sedentary life style, work-related postures, and recreational activity. The "weekend athlete" syndrome presents as either overuse (acute), degenerative, or chronic pain.

Prevention

(1) Identifying at-risk groups in the work environment. Conduct educational programs targeting at-risk occupational groups to emphasize the importance of alleviating static postures. Workers should be able to change their postures at least every hour. On-site institutional aerobic programs are effective in promoting fitness to reduce injury.
(2) Fostering the wearing of seat belts at all times, and adjustment car headrests to protect the head and neck.
(3) Educating posttrauma victims about the long-term nature of their illness and the need for protracted treatment. Provide continuous support through active listening and encourage patients to return as soon as possible to normal activities to promote a successful outcome.
(4) Educating patients about the decreased risk of injury with proper training techniques, including a regular exercise regimen for 30 to 40 minutes 5 times/week. Each exercise session should begin with 15 minutes of warm-up and end with 15 minutes of cool-down.

Common Management Problems

Cervical Spondylosis (Degenerative Arthritis and Osteoarthritis)

Commonly found at C4–5, C5–6, and C6–7, cervical spondylosis affects more males than females, usually between the ages of 40 and 70. The problem can follow a precipitating event and cause sudden, severe pain with splinting of the neck, or it can begin gradually without a precipitating event and become chronic over a period of months or years. Patients complain of pain and neck stiffness that is localized in the middle or upper neck and radiates to the occiput area and shoulder (the levator scapulae muscles), causing headache and pain. Motion, especially extension, increases the pain, and the pain is worse at the end of the day.

Etiology.
(1) Excessive axial loading of the head and neck;
(2) Static postures;
(3) Repetitive movements;
(4) Extreme movements;
(5) Minor injuries;
(6) Chronic strain of ligaments or joints.

Symptoms.
(1) Recurring neck stiffness;
(2) Mild aching of the neck musculature and associated structures, especially in the cervical scapular region;
(3) Limitation of neck motion that the patient has noticed for months or years;
(4) Headache (migratory, with a typical pattern from the temple to the forehead) or sensory dermatome of the first trigeminal nerve, accompanied by discomfort behind the eye, dizziness, visual blurring, alteration in hearing, dissociation from the environment;
(5) Vertigo;
(6) Radicular pain, pain radiating to the

arms, back, and head, and associated with tingling, numbness, and weakness; the pain pattern typically proceeds along the ulnar side of the upper extremity, posterior aspect of the forearm, or radial side of the hand;

(7) Spastic weakness of the legs, which could indicate silent cord involvement;

(8) Possible complaints of neck constriction, difficulty swallowing, and voice changes as a result of swelling of the esophagus and associated structures.

Signs.

(1) Limitation of cervical flexion, rotation, and extension;

(2) Tenderness/pain with anterior palpation;

(3) Crepitus;

(4) Reproduction of pain in the upper- to mid-cervical spine with movement;

(5) Long tract signs indicating cord compression (i.e., hyperreflexia).

Treatment (Acute). Diagnostic tests (see chapter introduction for indications).

(1) Initial weekly appointments to help develop trusting provider/patient relationships, lessen anxiety, and foster early return to normal activities. Maintain communication with the employee's supervisor as an early return to work is encouraged.

(2) Education using a 3-dimensional model increases knowledge of spinal structure, the disease process and its causes, and the potential long-term treatment and chronic nature of the problem. Increased knowledge decreases apprehension. Distinguish between hurting and harm; teach that all pain does not necessarily mean permanent damage. Underscore the need to increase physical fitness and avoid postures or movements that increase risks.

(3) Decreased inflammation resulting from immobilization with a soft cervical collar continuously (including during sleep) from several days to weeks, if it relieves the symptoms.

The neck must be maintained in a neutral position with the head held in slight to moderate flexion. The usual collar height is 3½ inches. If the collar is too high the neck will be forced into hyperextension; if too low there will be no support. During

the acute phase collars are to be worn 24 hours/day for 2 to 3 weeks or until the pain subsides. Rigid supports are contraindicated; they can increase muscle stiffness and result in muscle atrophy. Nonsteroidal anti-inflammatories ice or heat, phonophoresis (ultrasound with cortisone cream), and cervical traction for 2 to 3 months at home for 20 minutes 3 times/week are helpful for many patients.

Rehabilitation.

(1) Physical therapy for instruction in isometric exercises to strengthen paravertebral musculature, and modification of home/work environment to reduce the chances of exacerbations. *Note*: Prolonged physical therapy promotes the sick role and can foster long-term disability.

(2) Reviewing activities of daily living with specific advice on how to avoid extension-producing strain. Do not restrict activities unnecessarily, but base restrictions on personal tolerance. General guidelines to avoid increasing neck pain follow.

(a) Avoid reaching overhead or looking up at the ceiling.

(b) When driving an automobile adjust the seat and headrest to keep the spine in proper alignment; the seat should be close to the steering wheel to avoid craning the neck. Driving should be avoided with acute pain.

(c) Avoid lifting or carrying packages over 10 lb; avoid moving heavy loads and wearing heavy overcoats.

(d) When sitting avoid resting the chin on the hand.

(e) Sleep either with several pillows to keep the head supported or with a cervical neck roll.

(f) Sports should be avoided with severe symptoms; golf, bowling, and swimming (except on the back) aggravate neck pain.

Be sure the patients understand what has been taught, and provide patients written instructions to eliminate confusion. Keep a copy of instructions with patient's record (see Appendix K.).

Referral.

(1) Intractable pain;

(2) Signs of extremity weakness;
(3) Indications of cord compression (long tract signs);
(4) Meningeal signs (fever, stiff neck, severe occipital headache, positive Brudzinski, positive Kernig);
(5) Suspected cardiac or thyroid disease;
(6) Lymph node involvement;
(7) Vertebral artery insufficiency (dizziness, diplopia, syncope that is induced by head movements of rotation, extension, and lateral flexion) (Bland, 1987).
Outcome.
(1) 60% will improve with resolution in 3 to 4 months;
(2) 20% will have symptomatic relief;
(3) 20% no improvement.

Cervical Disc Disease (Cervical Radiculopathy)

This is part of the syndrome of cervical osteoarthritis. Faulty forward head posture can be contributory. It can be acute or chronic.

Acute Symptoms.
(1) Sudden, severe pain along the involved sensory dermatome;
(2) Radiation of pain to the neck, shoulders, or down the arm, forearm, and to the fingers;
(3) Possible anterior or posterior chest pain;
(4) Possible paresthesias along the involved sensory dermatome.

Acute Signs.
(1) Pain that increases with all movement, especially rotation, lateral flexion, and extension;
(2) Possible loss of motor strength;
(3) Possible diminished or absent reflexes;
(4) Muscle atrophy with fasciculations may be present.

Chronic Symptoms.
(1) Insidious pain, usually following repetitive work or exercise that is performed in an awkward position;
(2) Symptoms similar to those of acute disc disease.

Chronic Signs.
(1) Possible loss of cervical lordosis;
(2) Mild muscle atrophy;
(3) Loss of motor strength (rarely);
(4) Limitation of motion to the affected side in rotation and lateral flexion;

(5) Increased pain with extension, lateral flexion, and rotation toward the affected side;
(6) Increased pain with palpation of the cervical muscles;
(7) Increased pain with bony palpation of the spinous process over the affected disc;
(8) Possible pain that radiates in the distribution of the affected nerve root;
(9) Possible leg weakness.

Treatment.
(1) Patient education regarding probable, usually good, outcome;
(2) Ice/heat to affected area;
(3) Physical therapy for instruction in gentle stretching, strengthening, and range of motion exercises;
(4) Immobilization with a soft collar;
(5) Nonnarcotic analgesics (aspirin);
(6) Anti-inflammatory drugs;
(7) Cervical spine pillow;
(8) Therapeutic massage by either a physical therapist, massage therapist, or nurse.

Referral. (See Cervical Spondylosis.)

Outcome. Prognosis is good, usually with improvement in 3 to 4 months.

Stiff Neck, Acute Torticollis (Wryneck)

This usually occurs in individuals age 21 and older, but may occur in adolescents as young as 15 years. It involves muscles, ligaments, tendons, and probably a cervical spine joint (Bland, 1987). The differential diagnosis includes spinal cord or cerebellar tumors, lymphadenitis, herniated disc, rheumatoid arthritis, typhoid fever, tuberculosis, and fractures, subluxations, and dislocations of the cervical spine, especially C1–C2.

Etiology.
(1) Trauma;
(2) Awkward positions held for many hours (especially those sleeping positions where the neck is unsupported and tilted toward one side);
(3) Occupational postures of secretaries and computer terminal operators who glance to the side;
(4) Recreational stressors such as following a ball during a tennis match, overuse syndrome (particularly in

swimming), and playing tennis when out of shape or without warming up;

(5) Occurrence prior to the onset of an upper respiratory infection.

Symptoms.

(1) Awakening with a "crick" in the neck (stiff neck);

(2) Pain, usually unilateral and constant, that increases with rotation toward painful side;

(3) Neck fixed to the side (may be either toward or away from the affected side) and held rigid;

(4) Patient looking sideways by turning body or eyes, not the neck.

Signs.

(1) Exquisite tenderness of the sternocleidomastoid, levator scapulae, and trapezius muscles;

(2) Restricted rotation and flexion with pain at the end point of movement;

(3) Possible flattening of the normal cervical lordotic curve;

(4) Possible limitation of shoulder motion.

Treatment. Patients who have experienced trauma or have had a prior malignancy should undergo definitive testing, particularly cervical spine films, with open mouth view (if pain worsens or does not improve after 2 weeks), a bone scan (if there is a high suspicion of infection, fracture, or tumor) and a CBC with differential, SMA 12, ESR, SPEP, and tine test (if infection or tumor is suspected).

(1) Initial rest (in a supine position with the head on a small pillow or in a semi-reclining position with head and neck supported by several large pillows) alleviates the muscles from supporting the head.

(2) Ice application with massage or ice pack to the painful area 15 to 20 minutes several times/day for the first 48 hours.
   (a) Freeze water in a paper cup.
   (b) Position patient lying on the unaffected side, with a small pillow supporting the head.
   (c) Peel down the top of the cup.
   (d) Using a circular motion, apply to the painful neck area.

(3) After 72 hours, moist heat may be applied for 20 minutes/hour; caution the patient not to lie on the heating pad.

(4) Gentle stretching exercises several times daily promote the return to normal function by decreasing stiffness (Fig. 5.4**B**). Physical therapy may be indicated for passive exercises, and if the patient is reluctant to exercise.

(5) Medications including nonnarcotic analgesics (aspirin 2 to 3 tablets 4 times/day with meals), or nonsteroidal anti-inflammatories. Muscle relaxants are centrally acting and tend to produce unpleasant side effects, such as drowsiness. It is unclear whether or not the various drugs effectively relax the muscles; however, they do help the patient remain on bed rest.

(6) A 3-dimensional model and an illustration of the supporting musculature to increase the patient's understanding of the injury and treatments. Educate the patient in methods to decrease side effects of medications (i.e., take anti-inflammatories with meals); review the importance of proper posture, especially during sleep; adjust the height of chairs, work surfaces, and keyboards to reduce strain (see Chapter 3). Instruct the patient to continue exercises indefinitely, and to take a rest period after work if aching persists. Instruct the patient to apply warm moist heat or ice to the affected area as needed at the end of the work day.

Referral.

(1) Failure to respond to therapy;

(2) Trauma;

(3) Suspected fracture;

(4) Suspected infection;

(5) Suspicion of a tumor.

Outcome.

(1) Seven to 15 days complete resolution;

(2) Return to work as soon as the pain subsides, or as able.

Muscle Strains. Tension Neck (Middle and Lower Trapezius Muscle)

Etiology. Continuous contraction of the muscle, combined with poor posture, results in a rounded upper back. This commonly occurs as a result of leaning forward during sitting at or standing over a desk, or using a microscope. Heavy breasts that are poorly supported are also a contribut-

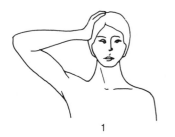

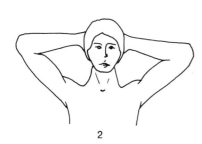

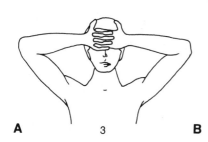

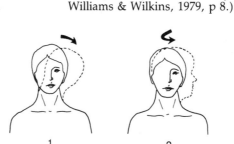

A 3   **B** 1   2   3

Figure 5.4. Exercises for cervical pain syndromes. **A,** Isometric exercises. **1,** Press head sideways against the heel of the hand (place the heel of the hand just above the ear), tense, relax, repeat. **2,** Clasp hands behind head (over large bony prominence), tense head backward with chin tucked in, relax, repeat. **3,** Press forehead against clasped hands, tense muscles without moving head, relax, repeat. **B,** Range of motion exercises. Sit in a comfortable chair and take a moment to relax. Shrug shoulders in all directions, both together and alternately, until you relax. Shrug between exercises if you need to relax more. **1,** Tip ear toward shoulder, turn to midposition, relax, tip to opposite side, relax, repeat. **2,** Turn head and chin toward shoulder, return to midposition, relax, turn toward opposite shoulder, return to midposition, relax, repeat. **3,** Tip head forward, return to erect position, relax, repeat. (From Ramamurti CP (Tinker RV, ed): *Orthopaedics in Primary Care.* Baltimore, Williams & Wilkins, 1979, p 8.)

ing factor. Tension neck is usually seen after the age of 30 years.

Symptoms.
(1) Soreness and fatigue along the muscle;
(2) May be accompanied by a burning pain;
(3) Intermittent pain;
(4) Relief with position change or lying down.

Signs.
(1) Point tenderness where the trapezius muscle attaches to the thoracolumbar spine, pectoral muscles, and tendons;
(2) Adaptive shortening of the pectoral muscles;
(3) Rounding of the upper back (may have thoracic kyphosis);
(4) Pain in posterior neck;
(5) Forward head posture;
(6) Hyperextension of the cervical spine.

Treatment.
(1) Ice/heat to painful area;
(2) Emphasis on correct posture that maintains the normal spinal curves;
(3) Correction of round shoulder posture with following exercise. Stand erect with the back to the wall. To improve posture, abduct both shoulders, pressing elbows against the wall; to strengthen the trapezius, pull arms back against the wall in a diagonal overhead position. Hold for a count of 10, release; repeat 5 times twice/day;
(4) Instruction of female patients in wearing properly fitted bras;
(5) Reviewing patient's job-related activities, and if necessary, referring the patient to an occupational rehabilitation specialist for job retraining.

Outcome. Relief of symptoms with readjustment of occupational movements or correction of other underlying problems.

Strain of the Upper Trapezius Muscle

Etiology. Overstretching of the trapezius muscle while reaching for an object with the head tilted in the opposite direction. This condition may be acute or chronic.

Symptoms.
(1) Pain in the posterolateral portion of the neck (from the occiput to the acromial process of the scapula);
(2) Tenderness of the muscle;
(3) Excessive spasm and contraction of the muscle.

Signs. The muscle may be tight, tense, or very tender along its insertion, from the occiput to the acromion.

Treatment.
(1) Massaging with an upward stroke. (Downward stroking increases tension.)
(2) Wearing a soft collar.

Outcome. Resolution in 2 to 7 days.

Acute Cervical Strain/Sprain (Whiplash)

Whiplash is a soft tissue injury of the neck involving a sudden acceleration of the head and neck into hyperextension, followed by hyperflexion beyond the normal range of motion. This results in a tear of one of the musculotendinous units in the neck: the trapezius, sternocleidomastoid, erector spinae, scalenes, levator scapula, or rhomboids (Hohl, 1975).

Etiology.
(1) Motor vehicle accident, especially a rear end collision;
(2) Competitive sports, especially wrestling, football, and gymnastics;
(3) Work-related accidents.

Symptoms. Onset may be delayed from 2 to more hours following the precipitating event.
(1) Headache;
(2) Aching neck pain, soreness, stiffness;
(3) Pain that radiates to the upper shoulder, scapula, occiput, or eyes;
(4) Possible difficulty with swallowing;
(5) May be associated with visceral symptoms, dizziness, ringing or buzzing in the ears, blurring of vision.

Signs.
(1) Spasm and pain of the paravertebral muscles;
(2) Restricted range of motion;
(3) Flexion of the neck to the contralateral side producing pain;
(4) Local tenderness and swelling;
(5) Numbness and radiating pain (if present, does not follow a dermatome);
(6) Head may be tilted toward the affected side.

Treatment (Acute). In order to promote an active patient role, involve the patient in the recovery process and avoid passive treatment such as massage. This can cause further irritation of the muscles and promote the sick role. The management regimen should be based on a careful evaluation of the nature and severity of the injury, the magnitude of the symptoms, the physical findings, the emotional make-up of the patient, and the psychosocial environment. Additional diagnostic tests should be performed on victims of trauma, occupational, or sports-related injuries, or if there is potential for litigation. Patients with suspected fracture, nerve root pain, and/or a neurological deficit also should have definitive testing.

(1) Reassurance, support, active listening with a relaxed manner;
(2) Explanation of the problem, its course, and expected outcome in detail;
(3) Application of ice to the painful area for 15 minutes several times/day, until symptoms subside. After 72 hours, ask the patient to stand under a warm shower to increase muscle relaxation. Avoid deep radiating heat as it can increase muscle and ligament irritation (Hohl, 1975).
(4) Immobilization that allows soft tissues to heal by decreasing the work of the head's supporting musculature. This is initially accomplished with 2 to 4 days of bed rest, soft collars, or intermittent traction.

If cervical traction is indicated for severe injury, use 6 to 10 lb applied in a sitting position for 20 to 30 minutes 2 to 4 times/day. Initial instructions should be given by a physical therapist; the traction is then applied at home. Additional physical therapy should be avoided unless nerve impingement is suspected or the therapy reduces the symptoms, as it promotes the sick role.

(5) Medication as indicated under stiff neck, decreasing medication as symptoms subside.

Rehabilitation. The patient can increase activity as tolerated and can be encouraged in early return to normal activity and work.

When the patient is asymptomatic for 2 weeks it is time to begin isometric exercises (Fig. 5.4**A**) and gradually to wean the patient from the collar, by omitting daytime wear. The patient may perform range of motion exercises and isometric exercises twice a day beginning with 5 repetitions of each exercise and increasing to 10 with tolerance. A warm shower or warm moist towel should be used to warm the neck before exercising. It is important to bear in mind that exercises are to increase the strength of the cervical musculature, not to increase the range of motion.

Referral.

(1) No improvement within 10 days;
(2) Neurologic symptoms;
(3) Intractable pain;
(4) Significant weakness;
(5) Pressure on spinal cord as indicated by long tract signs on physical examination;
(6) Meningeal signs;
(7) If there is no improvement in 6 weeks and x-rays are normal, a bone scan, medical evaluation, and a psychosocial evaluation should be done.

Outcome.

(1) Most patients respond to treatment within 10 days. Allow 6 weeks for healing; at 6 weeks most symptoms are relieved. Most patients return to normal activity within 2 months (Wiesel, Feffer, and Rothman, 1985). Occasionally patients exhibit a reluctance to return to normal activities with no evidence of objective findings.
(2) Symptoms may return with fatigue. Daily rest periods lessen chances of exacerbation.
(3) Return to light duty work, if pain is tolerable in 0 to 7 days. Return to non-

competitive sports when pain is tolerable and activity does not increase pain (usually 10 to 14 days). Return to competitive sports when full painless range of motion in all planes and strength have returned (usually by 6 weeks).

Thoracic Outlet Syndrome (TOS)

TOS describes a group of symptoms caused by compression of the brachial plexus and the subclavian artery and vein (usually between the clavicle and first rib). It can be associated with a cervical strain.

Occurring between the ages of 30 and 50 years, this syndrome is most common among women with an asthenic body type.

Etiology.

(1) Bony abnormality of the first rib;
(2) C7 elongated transverse process;
(3) Overuse related to athletics (basketball and swimming);
(4) "Whiplash" injury;
(5) Occupational postures, especially those requiring overhead work;
(6) Postural fatigue;
(7) Emotional stress (sagging shoulders);
(8) Carrying heavy shoulder loads.

Symptoms.

(1) Pain in the arm in certain positions;
(2) Color changes in the hand;
(3) Aching pain across the shoulder;
(4) Pain may be felt in the side of the neck and down the arm;
(5) Pain may be associated with heaviness, sensation of weakness, and fatigue when using the arm, especially above shoulder height (i.e., when combing or washing the hair);
(6) A sensation of cold, pallor, and swelling of the hand (less common).

Signs.

(1) Sensory loss of the fourth and fifth fingers of the affected hand (ulnar nerve);
(2) Weakness of the fourth and fifth fingers (ulnar nerve);
(3) Positive Adson's test;
(4) Possible reflex changes;
(5) Possible bruits heard over the subclavian artery.

Treatment. Care must be taken to differentiate TOS from Raynaud's phenomenon, ulnar nerve entrapment at the elbow, pulmonary tumor (compression of the brachial plexus can result from neoplasm or fibrosis due to radiation), or Horner's syndrome. Definitive diagnostic tests for TOS are plain cervical spine films, EMG, and ultrasound of the subclavian artery.

At the initial office visit carefully explain the source of the symptoms. Use line drawings of the anatomy to increase patient understanding. Listen carefully to the patient to allay anxiety, fear, and frustration. Teach progressive relaxation. Provide shoulder exercises (see Chapter 6).

Outcome. Early recognition and treatment of TOS results in a better outcome; after 2 years little improvement can be expected.

Temporomandibular Joint Dysfunction

This muscular disease involves the cartilage (meniscus) and related structures of the temporomandibular joint (TMJ). Symptoms can begin many years after the incident.

Etiology.
(1) Malocclusion that causes overstretching of the lateral pterygoid and the mastication muscles;
(2) Overstretching that results from sports or motor vehicle trauma;
(3) Stress manifested by clenching or grinding of the teeth.

Symptoms.
(1) TMJ pain (most common complaint is tired jaw);
(2) Occipital headache;
(3) Neck pain;
(4) Dizziness;
(5) Arm/shoulder pain;
(6) Clicking sound with jaw movements;
(7) Earaches;
(8) Sinus pain.

Signs.
(1) Bilateral or unilateral TMJ tenderness;
(2) Limited neck motion;
(3) Tension, anxiety, depression, and passive hostility.

Treatment.
(1) Prosthetic dental appliance;
(2) Physical therapy;
(3) Meniscectomy;
(4) Relaxation techniques.

Referral.
(1) Dentist;

(2) Orthopaedic surgeon.
Outcome. Treatment alleviates discomfort and in some instances provides a cure.

The Mature Adult with Neck Pain

Chronic degenerative changes account for most of the neck problems encountered by the older adult.

Predisposing Factors

(1) Aging spine;
(2) Increased susceptibility to injury and strain from lack of muscle strength and flexibility;
(3) Decreased mobility that increases the risks for accident-related trauma;
(4) Lack of energy to participate in a regular exercise program;
(5) Lack of understanding of the importance of physical fitness;
(6) Lack of financial resources and fear of the environment that may keep the mature adult homebound and unable to join in group activities that may aid prevention.

Etiology

(1) Chronic degenerative disease such as osteoarthritis of the facet joints, discogenic syndrome, and cervical stenosis;
(2) Episodes of torticollis that occurred when patient was a young adult.

Prevention

Instruction focuses on recognition by the mature adult that aches and pains are not normal expectations of aging and that simple remedies such as regular exercise and aspirin (taken on a regular basis) will help to foster a sense of wellness and improve or maintain function.

Common Management Problems

Cervical Osteoarthritis (Discogenic Syndrome)

Etiology. Etiology is the degeneration of the cervical discs.

Symptoms.
(1) Constant aching in the scapular area;
(2) Most intense pain in the morning;
(3) Painless restriction of motion (stiffness);
(4) May have paresthesias in the hands;
(5) May have pain in both upper limbs.

Signs.
(1) Limitation of cervical spine movement, especially extension; severe pain with hyperextension;
(2) Preservation of forward flexion;
(3) Tenderness on compression of the facet joints.

Treatment.   See patient at 6-week intervals and monitor for myelopathy (may present as ataxia or difficulty in walking)
(1) Soft collar as needed with neck in 15° of flexion, avoid hyperextension, try narrow part of collar anteriorly to increase comfort;
(2) Nonnarcotic analgesics (aspirin), or nonsteroidal anti-inflammatories;
(3) Neck exercises (Fig. 5.4**A, B**);
(4) Patient reassurance;
(5) Develop short-term, easily attainable goals that will encourage compliance with suggested regimen.

Referral.
(1) Physician referral for local anesthetic and steroid injection into trigger points;
(2) When there is progressive neurologic deficit a referral is required.

Outcome.   This is a chronic problem, and the patient needs constant supervision and interaction with the health management team nurse.

THE THORACIC SPINE

The thoracic spine, due to its bony attachment to the ribs and sternum, is the part of the spine least vulnerable to trauma or to the problems of aging. Muscle strains from overuse are the frequent problems in this region. Athletic participation in contact sports and gymnastics increases the risk for injuries. Vertebral fractures can occur from direct or indirect blows, or as a result of osteopenia (osteoporotic fractures) or metastatic disease (pathologic fractures); herniated discs are rare. Differ-

ential diagnosis is critical to the evaluation of the thoracic spine. The clinician must distinguish between musculoskeletal problems, cardiac problems, and pulmonary problems.

History

Musculoskeletal problems in the chest are described as sharp, aching, or dull. The pain can last from seconds to days to months. It increases with deep inspiration and coughing, is localized, and can be precipitated with direct palpation, movement, and exercise. Costochondritis (Tietze's syndrome) can present with unilateral anterior chest pain that can be confused as cardiac pain. The patient with costochonditis presents with localized tenderness and swelling over the costal cartilages.

Cardiac pain can occur suddenly or gradually. The pain of a myocardial infarction is described as heaviness or tightness in the chest. The pain is usually substernal and may extend to the arms, neck, jaw, or back. Often it is associated with weakness, diaphoresis, nausea, or vomiting.

The sudden, severe pain of aortic dissection is described as knife-like. Patients report a sense of impending doom. The pain can occur in the anterior chest, the lower chest, the interscapular region, the back, flank, or abdomen. Symptoms suggestive of dissecting aortic aneyurism are neurologic (i.e., syncope) vascular (i.e., absent pulses) or cardiac (i.e., diastolic murmur and blood pressure greater in left arm than right arm). This patient requires *immediate* medical referral.

Pulmonary pain can be distinguished from skeletal pain as pulmonary pain is localized anteriorly, increases with inspiration, and the patient is able to relieve the pain by leaning forward while sitting. Costovertebral joint dysfunction can mimic pleuritic chest pain.

Physical Examination

Have the patient stand with the disrobed back facing the clinician. Inspect the skin for any abnormal markings (café au lait) or tags that could indicate an underlying bony abnormality. Note the posture. What is the position of the head in relation to the floor? Normally it should be aligned directly above the shoulders. Look for the normal outward kyphotic, dorsal curve. An increased curve or round shoulders are symptomatic of Scheuermanns' disease, scoliosis, degenerative disc disease, a compression fracture, the kyphosis of old age suggesting osteoporosis, or long-standing poor posture. A lateral curve is suggestive of scoliosis; note the convexity of the curve and the level of the shoulders and iliac crests. Normally both should be level.

Unequal shoulders are observed in scoliosis; note which shoulder is higher and whether there is a compensatory or second curve. An unequal pelvis can reflect a true leg length discrepancy. With the patient supine and knees straight, place a measuring tape from the anterior iliac crest to the medial malleolus to measure leg lengths. Compare right leg with left leg. A significant discrepancy is greater than ½ to ¾ inch.

Look for symmetry of the spinal musculature. Palpate bony structures of the spinous processes and the costovertebral joints for areas of tenderness. Palpate the soft tissues in the midline from the level above the iliac crests. Examine the rhomboids, the trapezius, and the latissimus dorsi muscles and note areas of spasm and tenderness. Observe the motion of flexion as the patient bends forward and then returns to erect posture. Bend the patient forward and look from head to tail to evaluate for a rotational spinal curve; note the convexity of the curve if present. Examine chest expansion with the patient facing the examiner. Place a tape measure around the largest diameter of the chest. Have the patient inhale and measure the chest. Ask the patient to exhale and measure the chest. Note the difference between inspiration and expiration. Normally it is between 6 and 10 cm. Patients with ankylosing spondylitis have a decreased ability to expand their chests.

Perform the neurologic examination with the patient seated on the examining room table. Figure 5.3 depicts the thoracic dermatomes. Ask the patient to twist at the waist; note any restriction of movement. Evaluate for sensation, motor strength, and reflex. Examine the medial forearm (T1), medial side of upper arm (T2), medial side of upper arm and axilla to the nipple line (T3), umbilicus (T10), triceps (C7), upper abdominal (T8, T9, T10), and lower abdominal (T11, T12). Examine for long tract signs: hyperreflexia in the upper or lower extremities; a positive Babinski sign (upgoing toes); the presence of clonus; the absence of the abdominal or cremasteric reflex indicating cord compression or upper motor neuron disease. The differential diagnosis of upper back pain is found in Table 5.7.

Guidelines for Diagnostic Tests

All patients presenting with upper back pain need x-ray evaluation. Obtain thoracic spine films (AP/LAT) during the first visit. If there is no improvement in symptoms in 6 weeks, obtain a bone scan. If a tumor or neurologic symptoms are suspected refer the patient to an orthopaedic surgeon or neurosurgeon.

The Adolescent with Upper Back Pain

Predisposing Factors

(1) Adolescent or second growth spurt;
(2) Increased susceptibility of the growth tissues to injury;
(3) Sports, especially skiing, football, rugby, and wrestling.

Etiology

(1) Acute muscle strains (pectoralis minor/major), contusions, or hematomas that result from compression of the chest during contact sports. Treatment consists of ice, analgesics (aspirin or acetaminophen), and avoidance of the sport until the pain subsides.
(2) Stitch, a sudden catching pain in the side of the competing athlete attributed to an intercostal muscle spasm. The treatment consists of extension and elevation of both arms above the head for 10 to 15 minutes (Scott et al., 1984).

Table 5.7
Differential Diagnosis of Upper Back Pain

Ligamentous/muscular disorder
　Costochondritis
　Strain/sprain syndrome
　Overuse syndrome
　Poor posture

Neurologic disorders
　Herpes zoster
　Intercostal neuralgias
　Nerve root compression

Skeletal disorders
　Scheuermann's disease
　Metastatic disease
　Thoracic disc herniation
　Compression fractures
　Metabolic bone disease (osteoporosis, Paget's disease)
　Ankylosing spondylitis
　Scoliosis
　Thoracic spondylosis

Spinal cord
　Intramedullary and extramedullary tumors

Cardiac disorders
　Myocardial infarction
　Aortic dissection
　Angina pectoris
　Mitral valve prolapse
　Coronary insufficiency

Pulmonary
　Acute pulmonary embolism
　Pleurisy

GI
　Hiatal hernia
　Peptic ulcer
　Cholecystitis
　Pancreatitis

Renal disease

(3) Localized injury to the thoracic facet joints; either the costovertebral, costosternal, or costochondral junctions. Athletes are injured during "pile on" in football and during wrestling when the chest is compressed by the opponent. Obtain chest and thoracic spine films to differentiate joint injury from fracture. Carefully review the history for the mechanism of injury.

(4) Rib fractures occur following blunt trauma. The pain is localized and severe and increases with inspiration. The treatment is analgesics, rest, and avoidance of sports for 4 to 6 weeks to allow for healing. Note: Do not strap the chest. This will restrict respiratory excursion and may result in atelectasis and pneumonia.

Prevention

(1) A preparticipation sports screening examination identifies physical maturation, skill level, muscular endurance, power and flexibility, and nutritional status. Reduce risks by tailoring educational and body conditioning regimens to individual need (see Chapter 2 for guidelines). Coaches and trainer must be in agreement to ensure the best outcome for the athlete. The training techniques must continue for 12 months.

(2) Sound nutritional education, especially for wrestlers (see Chapter 2 for dietary recommendations).

(3) Initiate a rehabilitation exercise program for at-risk athletes.

Common Management Problems

Costochondral Junction Syndrome (Tietze's Syndrome)

This is an inflammation of the costocartilage typically occurring in the young and midadult years.

Etiology.　Unknown, but possibly:
(1) Repetitive movements (overuse);
(2) Virus.

Symptoms.
(1) Anterior chest pain (usually unilateral but may be bilateral);
(2) Pain may mimic angina;
(3) A precipitating event, such as overstretching, that may cause symptoms to begin 12 to 24 hours later.

Signs.
(1) Tenderness over area of symptoms;
(2) Localized swelling may be present;
(3) Increased pain upon rotation;

Treatment.
(1) Obtaining an ECG if there is a suspicion of angina pectoris or other cardiac disease, or if the patient is in a high-risk group for an early cardiac death. Obtain a chest x-ray if there is a suspicion of pulmonary disease such as a pulmonary tumor.
(2) Carefully explaining the disease process, including the anatomy;

(3) Reassuring the patient, including elimination of causative motion;

(4) Allowing patient time to express fears and concerns;

(5) Applying ice or heat to the affected area until symptoms subside;

(6) Anti-inflammatories for 10 days may be helpful.

Outcome. Complete resolution in 2 to 3 days, but may persist for 6 to 8 weeks.

Scheuermann's Disease (Juvenile Kyphosis) or Postural Roundback Deformity

Young people who present with a severe kyphotic thoracic curve and a compensatory increase in the lumbar lordotic curve may have Scheuermann's disease, and should be carefully screened for organic roundback deformity. Differentiating postural roundback from Scheuermann's is difficult. Patients with Scheuermann's disease will have a fixed (no movement) deformity, which may be accompanied by vertebral wedging, end plate irregularity on x-ray, or symptoms of disc protrusion. A referral to an orthopaedic spine specialist for a complete evaluation is necessary to prevent back pain and severe deformity if Scheuermann's disease is suspected. (Bradford et al., 1982).

Scoliosis

See Chapter 2.

The Adult with Upper Back Pain

Predisposing Factors

(1) The aging spine, degenerative changes resulting from prolonged abnormal disc stress that are most noticeable in individuals with kyphosis or scoliosis;

(2) Menopause;

(3) Repetitive work-related movements such as lifting, bending, and reaching;

(4) Certain recreational activities that require repetitive arm movement, such as swimming the freestyle stroke;

(5) Poor posture.

Etiology

(1) At menopause, bone mass diminishes, bones become weaker and thinner, and the risks for fracture increase.

(2) Acute or chronic muscle or ligament strain from improper posture, failure to warm up before heavy labor or recreational activity, and overuse related to employment activity.

Prevention

(1) It is important to increase the individual's awareness of the risks. A preexercise evaluation based on age, the level of competition, and the sport, and that includes a cardiovascular assessment for all individuals in a known high-risk group and all those more than 40 years of age. A specific exercise prescription to increase muscle strength, flexibility, and overall physical fitness is recommended.

(2) For the worker, pay attention to the environment to identify risks and eliminate injury through education, proper stretching before work, and initiation of a regular weekly exercise regimen.

(3) For perimenopausal women a risk assessment for osteoporosis and the elimination of identified risks is encouraged (see Chapter 3).

Common Management Problems

Rhomboid Strain

Common in occupations requiring static postures (i.e., secretaries and sewing machine operators); the patient complains of a chronic aching pain in the midback.

Etiology. Static posture (the back is partially flexed while the arm is held forward and downward) and a stooped-forward position.

Symptoms.

(1) Burning and aching pain over the rhomboid muscles;

(2) May complain of shooting or stabbing pains;

(3) Pain that increases with rest, and increased muscle stiffness after rest.

Signs.

(1) Tenderness over the muscle;

(2) Trigger points;
(3) Reproduction of symptoms when the arm is held in the position of maximum rhomboid strain.

Treatment.
(1) Increase the patient's understanding of the positions that cause the strain. Offer suggestions to modify incorrect posture. If necessary, alter the height of work surfaces to relieve rhomboid strain.
(2) Ice/heat as necessary to relieve symptoms;
(3) Anti-inflammatories until symptoms subside;

Outcome.
(1) Complete relief will be hindered if the posture continues.
(2) Even with postural changes, recovery is often slow.

Adult Scoliosis

The adult with scoliosis may have been aware of the problem since adolescence. If the scoliosis has existed since childhood, determine the age of onset. Ask female patients if onset occurred before or after the start of menses. Determine if the spinal deformity has worsened. Back pain in this individual may or may not be related to the preexisting curvature. Determine the severity of the back pain, and if there is pulmonary impairment. Eliminate other causes of back pain, such as disc syndrome, osteoarthritis, degenerative joint disease, ankylosing spondylitis, and rheumatoid arthritis.

Obtain a standing single cassette AP and lateral thoracolumbar scoliosis series and compare with previous films. It is essential that a determination of the degrees of curvature be made. Refer the patient to an orthopaedic specialist for a complete evaluation and the development of an individualized treatment plan. Conservative management is directed toward relieving the pain with nonnarcotic analgesics and anti-inflammatories. If these measures are not successful in reducing the discomfort, then alternative treatments, which may include physical therapy modalities, facet joint blocks with steroids, and a body cast/plaster jacket, are instituted. If conservative management fails, then surgery to fuse the spine is recommended. This will correct the deformity, prevent further progression of the curve, and reduce pain.

The Mature Adult with Upper Back Pain

Predisposing Factors

(1) Chronic illness;
(2) Decreased muscle flexibility and strength;
(3) Facet joint dysfunction resulting from normal aging.

Etiology (see The Adult with Upper Back Pain)

Spinal stresses that began in adolescence and continued into adulthood.

Prevention

Educate the at-risk group to the importance of remaining physically active. Instruction focuses on decreasing spinal stresses and developing an exercise program for the ambulatory as well as the chair-bound mature adult. A weight bearing exercise such as walking helps to prevent bone loss and to decrease the risk for fracture. A preexercise examination will identify muscle strength and flexibility, chronic illness, and individual goals. The exercise prescription is tailored to individual needs, and includes a progressive walking or swimming program for the ambulatory, and weight lifting, stretching, and flexibility for the chair-bound (see Chapters 1 and 4).

Common Management Problems

Thoracic Spondylosis

Secondary degenerative changes in the aging thoracic spine cause pain and stiffness that are worse upon arising in the morning. This pain may or may not be related to a strain from a sudden and unexpected movement. Patients have limitation of thoracic rotation that is associated with an increased dorsal curve.

This problem is self-limiting and rarely causes disability.

The treatment goals are to decrease pain

and increase function. These goals are reached by instructing the patient in the disease process, using aspirin on a regular basis 3 times/day until the symptoms subside, and instituting a regular exercise regimen (swimming is preferred). Spinal manipulation may be beneficial.

THE LUMBAR SPINE

History

Meticulous history taking will lead to accurate diagnosis. Have the patient clearly describe the nature of the pain and determine if associated pain is present. If leg pain is associated with back pain, determine the nature of the leg pain, the location, and the intensity and compare it to the back pain. If paresthesias are associated determine the location, the nature, and the timing. Ask about specific activities that aggravate the pain. Inquire about bowel or bladder problems. Ask if the pain increases or decreases upon lying down. Mechanical back pain is aching in nature, worse toward the end of the day, localized to the lower back or buttocks, does not radiate below the knee, and is better with rest. Discogenic pain is often burning and aching in nature, may be constant, radiates below the knee, may be coupled with numbness and/or pins and needles sensation of the leg, and improves with rest. Discogenic pain is aggravated by sitting, sneezing, coughing, climbing stairs, walking, and lifting. The ominous pain of the tumor may or may not radiate, is boring in nature, worse at night, unrelieved by bed rest, and relieved by sitting. Pain of infection is characterized by severe muscle spasms of the back. Back pain of lymphoma may be vague, not well localized, and be accompanied by intermittent paresthesias and/or weakness of the lower extremities. Inquire about recent weight loss, chills, fever, night sweats, and diarrhea. Intense, unremitting pain across the saddle area accompanied by pins and needles sensation, weakness of the lower extremities, and incontinence or constipation of either bowel or bladder is an emergency and requires immediate referral. The diagnosis of cauda equina syndrome is made

when a significant neurologic deficit is present on physical examination. Careful symptom analysis will direct the physical examination (Table 5.8).

Physical Examination

Try to develop a standard pattern of examination and evaluation. Examine the mechanics of gait and posture when the patient enters the examining room and when the patient stands, walks, and sits. For a thorough examination of the lumbar spine, it is essential that the patient completely disrobe. Observe the mechanics of the lumbar spine as the patient undresses. The patient with significant back trouble avoids painful bending and twisting motions. While the patient is standing, inspect the skin for any abnormal markings or tags, such as hairy patches, lipomas, or neurofibromas. Look for symmetry in the spinal musculature. Examine for the normal lumbar lordosis and look for loss of lumbar lordosis that may indicate paravertebral muscle spasm (Fig. 5.5). An exaggerated lumbar lordosis is characteristic of weak anterior abdominal wall musculature or compression fractures. Palpate bony structures as the patient stands. Palpate the spinous processes for tenderness. Examine for sacral and coccygeal tenderness. Palpate the soft tissues in the midline and over the iliac crests. In the midline, the supraspinous and interspinous ligaments are palpated for tenderness (Fig. 5.6). Only the superficial paraspinal musculature is palpable when examining for spasm. The iliac crest is palpated for tenderness. The sciatic nerve is the largest nerve in the body and runs down the posterior aspect of the thigh. It exits the pelvis through the greater sciatic foramen under the piriformis muscle. The sciatic nerve can be located midway between the greater trochanter and ischial tuberosity; it is palpated with the hip flexed. Ask the patient to stand and place the patient's foot on a stool to facilitate palpation. With the patient's back to you, observe flexion, extension, lateral bending, and rotation (Fig. 5.7). To test flexion, the patient should bend forward as if to touch the toes with the knees straight. If the patient can-

Table 5.8
Physical Examination of the Lumbar Spine

Patient standing	Patient sitting	Patient lying
1. Inspection of skin and spinal curves	1. Evaluate for motor strength	1. Evaluate for sensory function
2. Palpation of soft tissues and bones	2. Evaluate for DTR reflexes, clonus, Babinski	Pin prick
3. Evaluate for ROM	3. Evaluate for tension signs	Soft touch
Flexion	Valsalva	2. Evaluate for tension signs
Extension	Sitting Root	Straight leg raising
Lateral Bend		Passive dorsiflexion
Rotation		Bowstring
4. Evaluate for motor strength		Femoral nerve stretch
Heel walking		3. Evaluate for muscle atrophy
Toe walking		4. Leg lengths
Hopping on one leg		5. Associated areas
5. Chest expansion		Abdominal exam
		Hip and pelvic
		Vascular
		Rectal

not touch the floor, measure the distance from the fingertips to the floor with a tape. This is an accurate reproduction of the limitations of flexion. To assist in testing extension, place your hands on either side of the patient's hips. Support and stabilize the pelvis to allow maximal extension. Spondylolisthesis, spondylolysis, and spinal stenosis cause increased back pain with extension.

Using the same technique, stabilize the pelvis during lateral bending. Compare right lateral bending to left lateral bending. Record any limitations by noting restriction of motion and measure the distance of the fingers in relation to the knee on the same side. Normal lateral bend is to the knee and is equal on both sides. Test rotation by stabilizing the pelvis and asking the patient to twist around to face you. Normal rotation is 35°.

The Neurological Examination

The neurological examination of the lower extremities as they relate to the lumbar spine consists of examinations of reflexes, motor strength, sensation, and evidence of tension signs. For each neurologic level there are specific localizing tests for motor, reflex, and sensation. Motor testing is recorded using a five-point scale (see Cervical Spine).

For the upper lumbar region (Ll, L2, L3) there are no specific reflexes. The sensory examination is an essential component for evaluating for nerve root compression at these levels. While the patient is seated on the edge of the examination table with the legs over the side, test the strength of the iliopsoas (T12, Ll, L2, L3) by having the patient flex the knee against resistance. Test quadriceps (L2, L3, L4) strength by having the patient squat and return to the upright position. Test the strength of the hip adductors (L2, L3, L4). Stabilize the pelvis by placing one hand on the iliac crest and the greater tubercle and have the patient turn on the side and abduct the leg as you offer resistance against the lateral thigh by attempting to force the leg into adduction. All these muscle groups contain multiple innervations, so identifying loss of specific muscle strength may be difficult. At the L4, L5, and S1 levels, the examination is more specific. At the L4 level, the tibialis anterior is examined for motor function (have the patient walk on his/her heels with the feet inverted). The knee jerk is examined for reflex, and the medial side of the leg for sensation. At the L5 level, the extensor hallucis longus is examined for motor function (have the patient walk on his/her heels). At this level, there is no reflex. The dorsal aspect of the foot is tested for sensation. At the Sl level, peroneus, longus, and brevis are examined for motor function (have the patient walk on the medial border of his/her feet). The ankle jerk is examined for reflex; the lateral aspect and the plantar

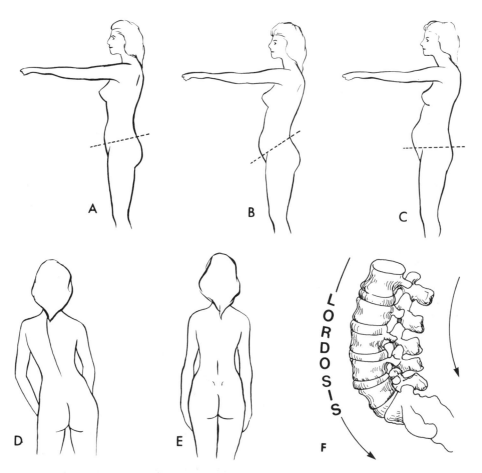

Figure 5.5. **A**, Normal posture with normal lumbar lordosis. **B**, Exaggerated lumbar lordosis due to pelvic tilting. **C**, "Paunchy" posture. **D**, Spastic scoliosis due to muscle spasm. **E**, Normal posture without scoliosis. **F**, The normal orientation of the lumbar spine is that of mild lordosis. Exaggerated lordosis may predispose the patient to mechanical back pain. (From Reilly BM: *Practical Strategies in Outpatient Medicine*. Philadelphia, WB Saunders, 1984, p 6.)

surface of the foot are tested for sensation (Fig. 5.8). The patient with a hyperreflexia should be examined for upper motor neuron pathology. In the normal individual, excessive reaction to deep tendon reflex testing is prevented by the higher cerebral centers. With loss of this inhibition, there is an exaggerated deep tendon reflex. Confirmatory tests for upper motor neuron lesions include an absence of the superficial abdominal reflex, the superficial cremasteric reflex, and the superficial anal reflex. The Babinski is the traditional test for upper motor neuron lesions. Dorsiflexion of the great toe with fanning of the other toes upon stroking the outer sole of the foot indicates upper motor neuron disease.

Examination for Tension Signs

There are a number of tests designed to stretch the spinal cord and sciatic nerve to test for nerve root compression. The straight leg test is performed with the patient supine while the leg is lifted upward by the foot and supported by the heel. The knee should be kept straight. The angle between the table and the extended leg at which pain is produced is the measure of positive straight leg raising. The pain of a positive

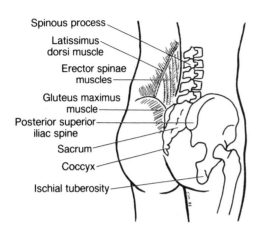

Spinous process
Latissimus dorsi muscle
Erector spinae muscles
Gluteus maximus muscle
Posterior superior iliac spine
Sacrum
Coccyx
Ischial tuberosity

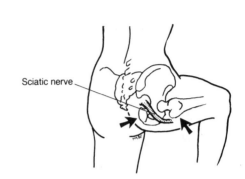

Sciatic nerve

Figure 5.6.   Left, Bony and muscular landmarks. **Right,** The *small arrows* point to the two landmarks, the ischial tuberosity and the trochanter, which help you to identify the location of the sciatic nerve. With the patient resting his foot on a stool, place your thumb on the trochanter and your index finger on the ischial tuberosity. With firm pressure, palpate the sciatic groove between these landmarks. (From Burnside JW, McGlynn TJ: *Physical Diagnosis,* ed 17. Baltimore, Williams & Wilkins, 1987, p 262.)

test should extend below the knee. Perform on both the affected and unaffected leg. Radicular pain in the affected leg during straight leg raising of the unaffected leg is a positive cross leg test (Fig. 5.9). The test should become negative when the knee is flexed and then become positive again when the knee is extended. Raising the leg to the area of pain, then backing off and dorsiflexing the foot should also produce pain. A variation of this test is the sitting root test. With the patient seated, the knee is extended while the patient grips the side of the examination table. The test is positive if the patient leans backwards and complains of radicular pain. Evaluation of the fourth lumbar nerve root is performed with the femoral nerve stretch test. With the patient prone the affected leg is elevated so the hip is extended and the knee is slightly flexed. The test is positive if the patient complains of radiating anterior thigh pain. Remember that lesions above and below can refer pain; therefore, diseases of the hip, rectum, and sacral iliac joints may refer pain to the lumbar region.

Associated Tests

Assess the abdomen for bruits that may indicate an aortic aneurysm; aortic aneu-

rysms can present as low back pain. Evaluate for CVA tenderness to rule out kidney disease. Rectal and pelvic examinations should be done when there is no mechanical stress associated with the pain or when the patient is elderly. Prostatic or rectal cancer may present as low back pain.

Guidelines for Diagnostic Tests

Several tests will assist in differentiating the several causes of lower back pain (Table 5.9).

Lumbar/Sacral Spine X-ray

Obtain five views: AP, LAT, and both obliques. Research indicates that spine films provide little information regarding muscle strains and disc herniations. These should be ordered when structural abnormalities (metastatic disease, fracture, scoliosis, spondylolysis, or spondylolisthesis) are of concern.

Bone Scan

Obtain a full or limited bone scan if there is a suspicion of fracture, Paget's disease, tumor, or infection, or with persistent symptoms after 4 to 6 weeks of conservative management.

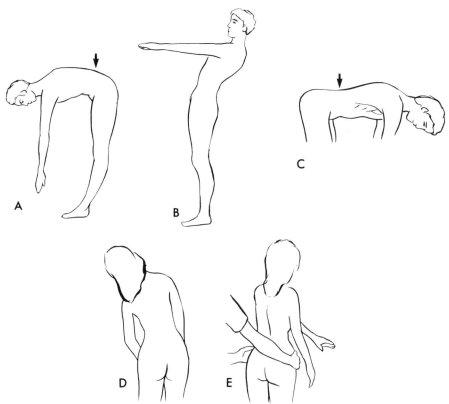

Figure 5.7. Back range of motion. **A**, Flexion—note the normal reversal of lumbar lordosis during flexion (*arrow*). **B**, Extension. **C**, Persistent lordosis during back flexion due to muscle spasm (*arrow*). **D**, Lateral flexion. **E**, Lateral torsion (rotation). (From Reilly BM: *Practical Strategies in Outpatient Medicine*. Philadelphia, WB Saunders, 1984, p 7.)

Laboratory Tests

Perform any time an underlying medical problem is suspected (tumor, infection, or multiple myeloma). Suggested screen: CBC, UA, SMA 12, acid P'tase, SPEP, ESR.

Electromyography (EMG)

Distinguishes peripheral nerve deficits from spinal nerve root compromise. Changes can be seen 10 days following episode of leg pain. Do not order an EMG before 10 days have elapsed.

CAT Scan

Obtain after 4 to 6 weeks with persistent symptoms to evaluate the spinal canal and associated structures for the presence of a herniated nucleus pulposus, tumor, or spinal stenosis. Best test to evaluate bony abnormalities.

MRI

Obtain after the patient complains of leg and back pain for 4 to 6 weeks or at any time the patient's conditions warrants. Evaluates the spinal canal and associated structures. The sagittal views of this non-invasive study aid in confirming the diagnosis of a herniated nucleus pulposus (Fig. 5.10).

Myelogram

Obtain prior to surgery and for progressive neurologic deficit.

The Adolescent with Low Back Pain

Predisposing Factors

(1) The adolescent or second growth spurt;
(2) Increased susceptibility of the growth tissues to injury;

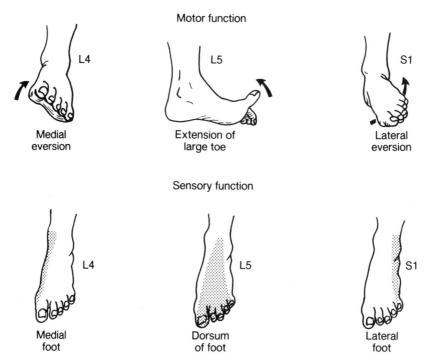

Figure 5.8. The neuromuscular control and function of the lower extremity. Disc L3–L4, nerve root L4: motor—anterior tibialis, medial eversion of the foot; sensory—medial leg and foot; reflex—patellar. Disc L4–L5, nerve root L5: motor—extensor hallucis longus, extend large toe; sensory—lateral leg and dorsum of foot; reflex—none. Disc L5–LS1, nerve root S1: motor—peroneus longus and brevis, lateral eversion of foot: sensory—lateral foot; reflex—Achilles. (From Burnside JW, McGlynn TJ: *Physical Diagnosis*, ed 17. Baltimore, Williams & Wilkins, 1987, p 262.)

(3) Participation in contact sports (football, rugby, soccer, basketball, hockey, and lacrosse) and sports that require weight training to maximal effort (bodybuilding, football, and competitive weight lifting.

Etiology

(1) Acute or chronic muscle, tendon, or ligamentous strain, which results from hyperlordotic postures during standing, gymnastics, and football. This occurs during the second growth spurt it may be accompanied by weakened abdominal muscles, tight hamstrings, and mild roundback posture. Treatment consists of flexibility exercises for the hamstrings and strengthening exercises for the abdominal muscles.

(2) A discrete localized injury to the vertebral end plates. This occurs at the thoracolumbar junction in young athletes. These athletes usually have tight lumbar dorsal fascia and are involved in repetitive flexion and extension activities such as rowing, gymnastics, and diving.

(3) Discogenic back pain differs in presentation from the adult. *Adolescents can have minimal back pain without radiculopathy.* They may have a thoracolumbar scoliosis, tightness of the lumbar dorsal fascia, and tight hamstrings as the only significant findings on physical examination. Asymmetric hamstring tightness may indicate herniated nucleus pulposus (HNP) (Micheli, 1979). The correct diagnosis can be determined by EMG, CAT scan, and MRI.

(4) Spondylolysis/Spondylolisthesis. Spondylolysis is an acquired or stress fracture of the pars interarticularis. At risk are female gymnasts as well as football linemen who must assume a hyperlordotic posture before the ball is snapped. Conservative management consists of

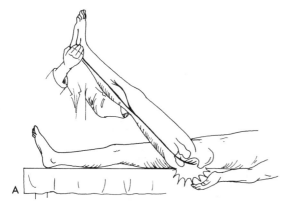

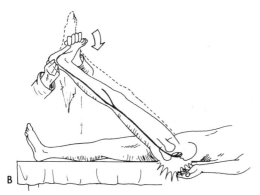

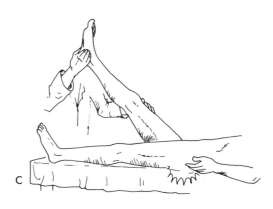

Figure 5.9.   Straight leg raising. **A**, Radicular symptoms are precipitated on the left with the straight leg raised to 45°. **B**, Dorsiflexion of the foot sometimes exaggerates straight leg raising responses. **C**, Crossed straight leg raising—pain on the left side is precipitated by straight leg raising on the right side. (From Reilly BM: *Practical Strategies in Outpatient Medicine*. Philadelphia, WB Saunders, 1984, p 10.)

rest, no sports until the pain subsides, and anti-inflammatories. For very severe pain, a low-profile brace may be used during acute episodes. Spondylolisthesis, a slippage of one vertebra on another, is classified in grades I through IV according to the degree of the slippage. Plain radiographs may be helpful in aiding diagnosis, but often a bone scan is needed for developmental spondylolisthesis. Treatment is aimed at relieving the symptoms and prevention of further slipping. This consists of rest, stretching of the hamstrings, abdominal strengthening exercises, and bracing. Patients may return to sports as long as they are asymptomatic and flexible, and the slippage does not progress. A 6-month follow-up that includes thoracolumbar x-rays is used for evaluation. If the spondylolisthesis is grade II or greater, participation in skiing, contact sports, and gymnastics is contraindicated. Grades I

and II can usually be managed by conditioning exercises, anti-inflammatories, and observation or bracing depending on the amount of pain. If the pain does not respond or the slippage progresses, surgical stabilization with an in situ fusion may be necessary. Grades III and IV require surgical stabilization with an in situ fusion or, in some cases, with fusion and instrumentation. A low-profile brace is used for 6 months after any surgical intervention.

(5) Direct blows to the back either during sports or due to a fall can cause pain and spasm (Micheli, 1979).

Prevention

In this age group it is important to prevent back pain before it occurs. This can be achieved by:

(1) Preseason screening of the lumbar spine. This should include postural observa-

Table 5.9
Differential Diagnosis of Low Back Pain[a]

Differential Diagnosis
1. Lumbosacral sprain/strain syndromes
   A. Acute
   B. Chronic/recurrent
   C. Early disc herniation

2. Visceral referred pain
   A. Renal lesions
   B. Intra-abdominal or pelvic disease (ovarian)
   C. Aneurysms
   D. Retroperitoneal mass or abscess

3. Condition or structural abnormalities of the
      vertebral column
   A. Degenerative disease of the spine
      (spondylosis)
   B. Osteoporosis
   C. Ankylosing spondylitis, rheumatoid arthritis
   D. Spondylolisthesis
   E. Lumbosacral transitional vertebrae
   F. Fractures

4. Invasive diseases of the spine
   A. Neoplastic
   B. Infections

[a]Adapted from Branch WT Jr: *Office Practice of Medicine.* Philadelphia, WB Saunders, 1982, p 772.

tion and flexibility and abdominal strength testing (Wooden, 1981).
(2) Appropriate training techniques. The training program must be followed for 12 months and includes stretching, flexibility, and strengthening exercises, isometrics, and swimming.
(3) Use of proper protective gear—gymnastics: proper thickness and placement of mats, elimination of the board during initial vaulting training, and avoidance of the trampoline (the trampoline should not be used in regular gym classes); football: proper equipment and careful instruction in techniques.

The Adult with Low Back Pain

Predisposing Factors

(1) Age 30 to 50;
(2) Repetitive movements such as lifting, pulling, bending, and twisting;
(3) Job-related activities that involve prolonged sitting, the constant vibration of long-distance driving;

(4) Recreational activities (jogging and skiing);
(5) Personal behavior (sedentary life-style, cigarette smoking, emotional stress, poor posture, and obesity) (Frymoyer, 1983).

Etiology (Unknown)

(1) Acute or chronic muscle, tendon, or ligamentous strain resulting from work-related postures or recreational activities;
(2) Lumbar disc herniation resulting from excessive loading of the spine or from a sudden unexpected force or blow to the spine;
(3) Degenerative changes that begin after the age of 25;
(4) Metabolic diseases that weaken the bone and result in mechanical failure;
(5) Facet joint dysfunction.

Prevention

Prevention focuses on education and screening. Educational programs increase the awareness of the problem, provide the necessary facts to identify which individuals are at greatest risk, and teach the skills that minimize the risks for lower back pain. Educational programs have the greatest success when participants are actively involved in protective back care. On-site instruction in proper body mechanics (individualized and job specific) followed by employee demonstration with immediate critique and reinforcement aids retention and adaptation of the newly learned skills. Screening programs in the work environment are cost effective. They identify individuals with a history of previous injury (past injury increases the risks for future injury) and those personal behaviors that are associated with back pain. Classes in stress management, weight control, and modification of the work and home environment provide the opportunity for employees to change at-risk behavior (Gates and Starkey, 1986).

Acute Mechanical Low Back Strain/Sprain

Refer to Table 5.10 for the etiology, symptoms, and signs of low back pain.

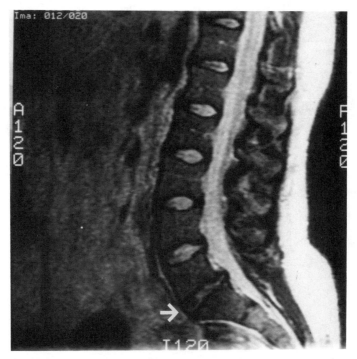

Figure 5.10.   MRI of the lumbar spine illustrating a L5-S1 disc herniation.

Treatment (Acute).

(1) Bed rest 2 to 5 days; avoid prolonged bed rest, as it increases muscle stiffness, lengthens healing time, promotes the sick role, and increases dependence. Rest in a firm bed on a firm mattress.

Bed Position:

(a) On the back with knees flexed on a pillow;

(b) On the side with a pillow between the knees;

(c) On the stomach with a small pillow under the lower abdomen to prevent hyperextension of the back (avoid prone lying);

(2) For the first 72 hours avoid heat (initially, heat increases the inflammatory response), apply ice as a pack or massage to the painful area for 15 to 20 minutes several times each day.

The Ice Massage:

(a) Lie prone and support abdomen with a small pillow.

(b) Freeze water in a paper cup.

(c) Peel down top of cup.

(d) Apply to painful lower back area using a circular motion.

(3) After 72 hours, heat may be applied using a moist heating pad for 20 minutes out of each hour; avoid prolonged lying on the pad.

(4) Avoid sitting during the acute period.

(5) Gentle stretching exercises several times a day (after the acute pain subsides), as exercise promotes flexibility and decreases stiffness.

(6) Medications (see Appendix A):

(a) Nonnarcotic analgesics.

(b) Non steroidal anti-inflammatories.

(c) Muscle relaxants (only if severe spasm is present). Muscle spasm is a result of the inflammatory process; once the inflammation has subsided, the spasms stop (all muscle relaxants are centrally acting and tend to produce unpleasant side effects).

(7) Abdominal supports are particularly helpful for short-term use for those who do heavy lifting or have weakened abdominal muscles, or for those who need

Table 5.10
Overview: Low Back Pain

Mechanical back pain Age 30 to 55	Discogenic back pain Age 30 to 55	Spinal stenosis Above age 50
Etiology	Etiology	Etiology

Improper posture
Trauma
Lifting
Bending
Twisting
Prolonged standing
	Repeated minor stresses
	A discrete injury (may sense a
	  snapping in the back)
	Trauma following bending
	Degeneration of the disc as a
	  part of normal aging
		Constriction and bony compres-
		  sion of nerve roots as osteo-
		  phytes form on disc margins
		  or facet joints.

Symptoms	Symptoms	Symptoms

Aching pain in the lower back
  that may or may not radiate
Radiation into the thigh but
  never below the knee
Restriction of spinal motion
Sudden onset
Increased pain with walking,
  bending, and sitting
Decreased pain with rest
	Similar to those reported with
	  low back pain
	Leg pain that radiates below
	  the knee, dull or burning in
	  nature with pins and needles
	  quality
	Altered sensation in the lower
	  extremities described as
	  numbness or tingling
	Leg pain may be worse with
	  coughing, sneezing, or bear-
	  ing down during defecation
	Weakness or giving way sensa-
	  tion of the knee
		Backache, backache with radiat-
		  ing leg pain below the knee
		Leg pain without back pain
		Bilateral leg pain "claudicant"
		  in nature
		Increased with walking and as-
		  sociated with pins and nee-
		  dles sensation and a sense of
		  weakness in the calf and foot
		Claudicant pain relieved with
		  lying down

Signs	Signs	Signs

Spasm and tenderness of para-
  vertebral muscles
Restricted spinal movement
Local tenderness over the spi-
  nous process may be present
Abnormal gait with hips flexed
Sciatic list (listing away from
  the pain) may be present
Difficulty with sitting (sits on
  the edge of the chair with
  legs extended)
	Limitation of spinal movement
	  may be present
	Increased pain during spinal
	  flexion
	Antalgic gait
	Sciatic list
	Hip and knee flexed while
	  standing
	Absent or diminished reflexes
	Motor weakness
	Decreased sensation along a
	  dermatome
	Positive straight leg raising test
	Positive tension signs may be
	  present
		Full range of motion may be
		  present
		Increased pain during spinal
		  extension
		May have normal exam

Treatment	Treatment	Treatment
Bed rest 2 to 5 days Ice massage Anti-inflammatories Education Exercise/fitness	Bed rest 7 to 14 days Ice massage Anti-inflammatories Education Exercise/fitness	Bed rest rarely employed Ice/heat Anti-inflammatories Education Exercise/fitness

reinforcement of good body mechanics. Supports provide a sense of security and diminish pain through a placebo effect.
(8) Education (instruction/evaluation):
   (a) Teach form and function of the spine using a three-dimensional model (this will make the back more understandable to the patient).
   (b) Teach the rationale for treatments.

The well-informed client experiences less anxiety, is able to formulate realistic goals, and complies more often with the recommended regimens (Table 5.11).
   (c) Teach the expected outcome. Discussing the short-term limitations of the disability and the undulating nature of the disease reduces the

Table 5.11
Nursing Care Plan for the Patient with Acute Low Back Pain

Possible Nursing Diagnosis	Goals	Interventions	Rationale
1. Knowledge deficit related to low back pain	Decrease anxiety, increase cooperation Formulation of realistic goals	Review patient's understanding of lumbar sacral anatomy and teach if necessary Mutually develop realistic expectations Provide reassurance	The well-informed patient, possessing realistic expectations, can cooperate fully with the treatment plan
2. Activity intolerance related to low back pain	Return to optimal functional ability	Teach the rationale for treatment Teach the undulating nature of the disease	The well-informed patient understanding the reasons for the treatment and nature of the disease will comply with the recommended regimen
3. Alteration in comfort, pain related to low back pain	Decreased pain Understanding the methods to control pain Redemonstration of relaxation techniques and instructed exercises	Teach the importance of NSAI, teach relaxation technique, teach flexion, extension, flexibility exercises Evaluate for pain responses; alter therapeutics as necessary	Pain control increases compliance with the treatment program
4. Potential for reinjury	Demonstration of proper body mechanics	Teach proper care of the back; arrange for rehabilitation at back school to include alteration of work environment to minimize risk; encourage regular exercise regimen	Understanding the importance of proper back care will assist in protecting the spine and preventing reinjury
5. Potential disturbance in self-concept	Preservation of family role and self-esteem as demonstrated by active participation in self-care	Arrange teaching environment to foster independent decision-making	Active involvement in decision-making preserves self-esteem and independence

fear that the treatment will fail. Use positive reinforcement, reassurance, and active listening.

(d) Teach the side effects of medications and appropriate dosages.

(e) Counsel on injury prevention, the use of proper body mechanics, and the importance of general fitness programs (Fig. 5.10).

Goals of the Educational Program:

(a) Foster active participation in addressing own health problem;

(b) Promote independence;

(c) Reduce chances of long-term disability;

(d) Preserve self-esteem;

(e) Promote early mobility;

(f) Promote return to work/home responsibilities in a shortened period of time.

Retraining/Rehabilitation.

(1) Graduated mobility program (3 to 10 days following episode).

(a) Stretching/flexibility exercises;

(b) Strengthening exercises (Fig. 5.11).

(2) Establishment of aerobic exercise rou-

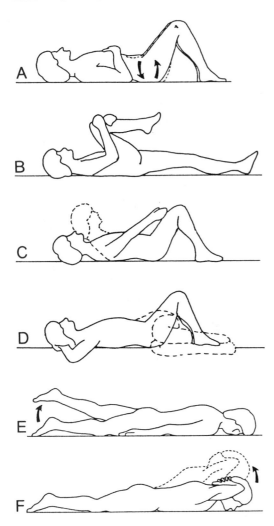

Figure 5.11. **A**, Isometric pelvic tilt. **B**, Lower back stretch. **C**, ½ curl situp. **D**, Lower back stretch. **E** and **F**, Active lumbosacral extension exercise. (From Ramamurti CP (Tinker RV, ed): *Orthopaedics in Primary Care.* Baltimore, Williams & Wilkins, 1979, p 158.)

tine 5 times/week for 40 minutes (2 to 6 weeks following episode):
   (a) Swimming;
   (b) Walking;
   (c) Bicycling.
(3) Back School (classroom education for patients with back pain) (Simon et al., in press).
   Referral to Orthopaedic or Neurosurgical Specialist.
(1) Failure to respond to therapy;
(2) Lack of specific diagnosis;
(3) Associated GI or GU symptoms;
(4) Neurological symptoms;
(5) Litigation pending;
(6) Suspected disc herniation;
(7) Fever;
(8) Suspicion of a tumor.
   Outcome (Based on the Natural History of Low Back Pain).
(1) Resolution should occur within 3 to 21 days (with or without treatment based on the natural evolution of the disease process).
(2) May return to work as soon as acute phase subsides (2 days); return to work with light duty restriction helpful. The industrial back injury work restriction classification was developed by Wiesel, Feffer, and Rothman (1985) to provide standardized guidelines to aid medical evaluation of the injured worker (Table 5.12).
(3) May take 4 to 6 weeks for return to full work/home responsibilities.
(4) The patient may have intermittent aches during the 2 to 6 week period following the initial bout. These aches can be relieved by brief rest periods (after work) and aspirin.
(5) Occasionally patients fail to respond to therapy and the pain persists, and they are reluctant to resume activities of daily living or to return to work. If there is no response to treatment after 3 to 6 months, consider a chronic pain syndrome. The etiology is complex and may be related to compensation claims or pending litigation (or other secondary gains), depression, lack of compliance with recommended regimen, or undetected disease process. All require appropriate intervention and investigation. Refer the patient to a physician for complete medical work-up if not already done. (see Chronic Low Back Pain).

Discogenic Low Back Pain

This is low back pain that radiates below the knee. The leg pain is significantly more bothersome than the back pain. Ten percent of all back aches are related to some form of nerve root irritation, and of those 10% only 2 to 3% require surgical intervention.

Table 5.12
Industrial Back Injury Work Restriction Classification
(As adapted from Social Security Regulations)[a]

Work Classification	Work Restrictions	PPPI[b]	Relevant Diagnoses
VERY HEAVY WORK	Occasional lifting in excess of 100 pounds Frequent lifting of 50 pounds or more	Zero	Recovered acute back strain Herniated nucleus pulposus treated conservatively with complete recovery
HEAVY WORK	Occasional lifting of 100 pounds Frequent lifting of up to 50 pounds	Zero	Healed acute traumatic spondylolisthesis Healed transverse process fracture
MEDIUM WORK	Occasional lifting of 50 pounds Frequent lifting of 25 pounds	Less than 5%	Chronic back strain Degenerative lumbar intervertebral disc disease under reasonable control Herniated nucleus pulposus treated by surgical discectomy and completely recovered Spondylolysis/spondylolisthesis under reasonable control Healed compression fracture with 10% residual loss of vertebral height
LIGHT WORK	Occasional lifting of no more than 20 pounds Frequent lifting of up to 10 pounds	10% to 15%	Degenerative lumbar intervertebral disc disease with chronic pain and restriction Herniated nucleus pulposus treated conservatively or operatively, but left with some discomfort, restriction, and neurological deficit Acute traumatic spondylolysis/ spondylolisthesis, treated conservatively or operatively, but with residual discomfort and restriction Lumbar canal stenosis Moderately severe osteoarthritis accompanied by instability Healed compression fracture with 25% to 50% residual loss of vertebral height
SEDENTARY WORK	Occasional lifting of 10 pounds Frequent lifting of no more than lightweight articles and dockets	20% to 25%	Multiply operated back (failed back syndrome)

[a]From Feffer HL: Evaluation of the low back diagnosis related impairment rating. In Wiesel SW, Feffer HL, Rothman RH (eds): *Industrial Low Back Pain.* Charlottesville, VA, The Michie Co., 1985.
[b]PPPI, permanent partial physical impairment.

Pathology. Nuclear material either bulges, protrudes, or extrudes, causing pressure on the ligaments and the nerve roots. In disc protrusion the annulus bulges beyond the rim of the vertebral bodies. While in disc herniation, there is a seepage of disc material through a disruption in the annular wall (Fig. 5.12). Both protrusion and herniation can cause alteration in neurological status and pain (Fig. 5.13).

Etiology. The molecular changes of the aging disc alter both the nucleus and annulus. The disc becomes dry, cracks, and is unable to withstand physical stressors.

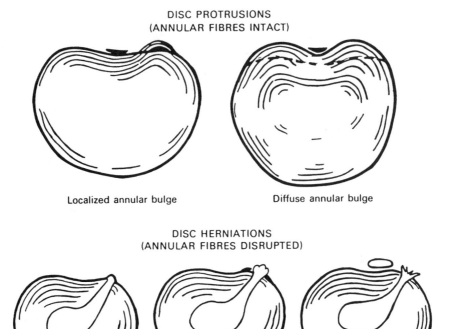

Figure 5.12. **Top**, In disc protrusions the annular fibers are not disrupted. The distortion of the normal configuration of the annulus may be confined to one side (a localized annular bulge) or the protrusion may be bilateral being constrained to some extent in the midline by the posterior longitudinal ligament. **Bottom**, In disc herniations the annular fibers are disrupted. Under such circumstances the nucleus pulposus may be confined solely by the outermost fibers of the annulus (prolapsed intervertebral disc); the nucleus may break through the outermost fibers of the annulus and come to lie underneath the posterior longitudinal ligament (extruded intervertebral disc); or a free fragment of nuclear material may break through the posterior longitudinal ligament and lie free in the spinal canal (sequestrated intervertebral disc). (From MacNab I: *Backache*. Baltimore, Williams & Wilkins, 1977, pp 93, 94.)

Symptoms.
(1) Initially, symptoms may be similar to those reported with acute low back strain.
(2) Leg pain of a lancinating or "pins and needles" quality (sciatica) which is dull or burning in nature.
(3) Altered sensation in the lower extremities described as either "numbness" or "tingling."
(4) The pain may be worse with maneuvers such as coughing, sneezing, or bearing down during defecation.
(5) Weakness or giving way at the knee.
(6) *Note*: Central disc herniations can pres-

ent as back pain without leg pain, especially in individuals less than 30 years of age. Other patients with a central disc herniation may complain of bilateral leg pain and paresthesias.
Signs.
(1) Possible limitation of spinal motion;
(2) Antalgic gait;
(3) Sciatic list (functional scoliosis secondary to a unilateral muscle spasm).
(4) Hip and knee flexed while standing;
(5) Reproduction of radicular symptoms during flexion;
(6) Absent or diminished reflexes;

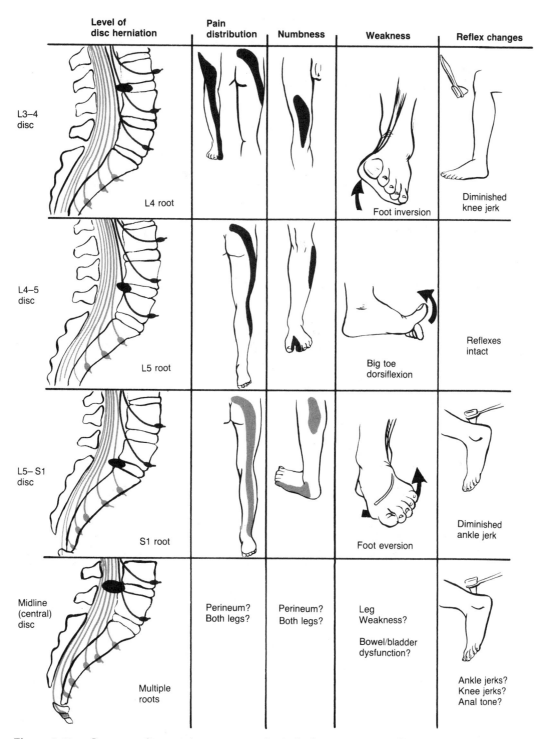

Figure 5.13. Common disc syndromes: neurologic findings. (From Reilly BM: *Practical Strategies in Outpatient Medicine*. Philadelphia, WB Saunders, 1984, p 15.)

(7) Motor weakness;
(8) Decreased sensation along a sensory dermatome;
(9) Positive straight leg raising test;
(10) Reproduction of sciatic symptoms during forced passive ankle dorsiflexion;
(11) Positive sitting root test.
Treatment.
(1) In the early stages of management it is sometimes difficult to differentiate a herniated intervertebral disc from degenerative disease (including spinal stenosis, displacement of facet joints related to disc degeneration, foraminal narrowing caused by osteoarthritic spurring) and other causes (i.e., diabetes and other neuropathies, spinal neoplasms, or psychogenic back pain). Diagnostic testing aids diagnostic decision making. Obtain as previously indicated if any of the following are present: positive tension signs, loss of a reflex, a sensory loss that follows a dermatome pattern, motor weakness or progressive neurologic deficits, or if surgery is contemplated.

Explicit instructions and explanations of treatments increase understanding and reassurance; they also promote patient participation in self-care and encourage transfer of control to the patient. Refer to the treatment section on acute low back pain for specific interventions. Treatment of disc herniation may be either conservative or surgical.
(2) Conservative:
(a) Bed rest usually 10 to 14 days (see Acute Low Back Pain). For every 3 hours of daytime bed rest a 20 minute walk is recommended (except in the very acute), but *no sitting*. Prolonged bed rest deconditions the body and fosters calcium loss. Once calcium is lost it does not return. This increases the risk for osteoporosis.
(b) Prescribe anti-inflammatory drugs (see Appendix A).
(c) Encourage decision making.
(d) Encourage the patient to participate actively in management.
(e) Gradually return to normal activities with planned rest periods.
Patients may return to work in 3 to 4 weeks if able and if the job does not require heavy lifting. If recovery is complete they may return to normal work activities. However, even in this case frequent lifting should be evaluated on an individual basis. Generally, frequent lifting should be limited to less than 50 lb for 3 to 6 weeks (Table 5.12).
Referral.
(1) Persistent symptoms after 4 to 6 weeks of conservative management;
(2) Progressive neurologic deficits;
(3) Litigation pending;
(4) Lack of a specific diagnosis;
(5) Associated GI or GU symptoms;
Outcome.
(1) Relief of sciatica:
(a) 60% in 4 weeks;
(b) 90% in 3 months;
(c) 96% in 6 months (Rowe, 1969).
(2) Persistence of low back pain;
(3) Intermittent relief of pain;
(4) Preservation of family role;
(5) Increased understanding of the nature of the problem and the need for personal control;
(6) Surgical intervention with progression of neurologic deficits, positive objective findings, and unrelenting lower extremity pain;
(7) Occasionally symptoms persist regardless of treatment. Consider chronic pain syndrome.

Cauda Equina Syndrome

This is a rare condition in which a large midline disc herniation can compress several nerve roots of the cauda equina. This usually occurs at the L4 and L5 level. Symptoms can vary, back or perianal pain predominate, and the patient may or may not complain of bowel or bladder dysfunction. The dysfunction can be either the loss of bowel or bladder control (incontinence) or the inability either to defecate or urinate (males may report a recent onset of impotence). This may be followed by leg pain, numbness of the legs or feet, and difficulty with walking. This is an emergency requiring immediate referral (Rothman, et al., 1982).

Chronic Low Back Pain

This is traditionally defined as pain that has continued for more than 6 months. More recently, chronic back pain has been defined as pain that has continued for more than 3 months.

Etiology.

(1) History of mechanical stress that has failed to respond to traditional regimens;

(2) Lack of compliance with therapeutic recommendations;

(3) Depression;

(4) Environmental reinforcement that provides either psychologic or monetary secondary gains.

Symptoms.

(1) Back pain described as knife-like and unbearable;

(2) If leg pain present, is always less than back pain.

Signs.

(1) Abuse of medications (suspect if patient shows familiarity with many drugs, requests special medications, or develops drug allergies, slurred speech, hostility, or defensiveness);

(2) Obvious depression (flat affect, "blue moods," inappropriate crying, lack of sexual desire, appetite changes, disturbance in sleep patterns, or expressed attitude that the patient "never has fun");

(3) Amplification of symptoms;

(4) Excessive dependence on others;

(5) Manipulative behavior;

(6) Lack of motivation or interest in own management of symptoms;

(7) Lack of objective findings.

Treatment.

(1) If the patient describes disproportionate pain, pain that disturbs sleep, or migratory pain, rule out underlying causes with the following diagnostic tests: blood and urine laboratory studies, TB skin tests, bone scan, CAT scan, or MRI.

(2) Retraining/rehabilitation includes goals for chronic low back pain that are the same as the goals for acute low back pain. The patient needs a therapeutic regimen that is directed toward maintaining normal relationships and activities of daily living.

However, the patient with chronic low back pain has special needs. Referral to an aggressive functional restoration program may offer the best outcome. This program includes psychological treatment (stress management), aggressive physical therapy (floor stretching and strengthening exercises, progressive weight training, and general endurance exercises, i.e., arm and leg cycling, and walking), occupational therapy with work simulation, and didactic programs to explain the anatomy and function of the spine and the rationale for treatments (Mayer et al., 1987).

(3) Prevention consists of developing strategies during the initial management phase of acute low back pain that reduce long-term disability.

(a) Allow time during the visit for the patient to express concerns.

(b) Help the patient to formulate reachable goals.

(c) Help the patient to identify past coping skills and strengths; review existing abilities and help the patient use them.

(d) Have patient plan daily rest periods; adequate rest/sleep increase coping skills and lessen frustration. Try nontraditional methods for pain control (acupuncture, progressive relaxation, therapeutic touch, or creative imagery). A TENS unit for pain control may be indicated (see Appendix G).

(e) Provide an atmosphere that maintains independence and accustomed family roles.

(f) Initiate steps that modify the work environment. If necessary, contact the employer or supervisor.

(g) Recognize that prevention might not be possible.

Referral.

(1) Psychologist;

(2) Exercise physiologist;

(3) Occupational rehabilitation specialist;

(4) Chronic pain program.

Outcome.

(1) Improvement;

(2) Withdrawal, loss of family and friends;

(3) Social isolation;

(4) Chronic pain syndrome that is refractory to all treatments;

(5) Severe depression/suicide.

Paget's Disease of Bone

In Paget's disease bone growth is abnormally regulated. Excessive resorption of bone is followed by uncontrolled osteoblastic new bone formation. The result is a bone that is mechanically defective, enlarged, and deformed. Paget's disease affects individuals after 40 years of age; the peak incidence is between 50 and 70 years of age.

Etiology. Unknown.

Symptoms.

(1) Most individuals are asymptomatic;
(2) Pain in the hip, sacrum, spine, pelvis, skull, femur, and tibia is worse with weight bearing and cold weather;
(3) Difficulty with walking;
(4) Increasing head size;
(5) Hearing loss;
(6) May have compromise of spinal cord and nerve roots;
(7) May have high-output cardiac failure.

Signs.

(1) The cardinal clinical finding is an elevated alkaline phosphatase as high as ten times the upper limits of normal;
(2) Hearing loss on audiograms;
(3) Pain on palpation over affected areas.

Treatment.

(1) Differentiate between ankylosing spondylitis and other rheumatic, metastatic, and metabolic diseases. The bone scan is the most sensitive screen, and will pick up skeletal changes before the standard x-ray. X-ray examination reveals osteolytic areas with new bone formation.
(2) Treat mild bone pain with salicylates or anti-inflammatory medications.
(3) Severe Paget's disease is treated with calcitonin, mithramycin, or diphosphonates that inhibit bone reabsorption.

Referral. If Paget's disease is suspected, refer the patient to an orthopaedic surgeon, rheumatologist, neurosurgeon, endocrinologist, or cardiologist for a complete evaluation.

Outcome.

(1) Mild Paget's disease needs annual follow-up.
(2) Severe Paget's disease requires routine office visits.
(3) Some patients will have complete remission with drug therapy.

The Mature Adult with Low Back Pain

In this age group the most common cause of low back pain is the degenerative changes that occur as the spine ages. However, back pain in this age group can be a clue to an underlying disease that may or may not be intrinsic. Careful screening is essential to rule out the extrinsic causes.

Degenerative Back Pain (Lumbar Spondylosis)

Etiology is a result of either facet joint dysfunction or arthritis, repeated episodes of acute low back sprain/strain, osteoarthritic spurring, or chronic disc degeneration.

Symptoms.

(1) Aching pain in lower back or buttock, which may or may not radiate;
(2) Radiation into the thigh, but never below the knee;
(3) Possible restriction of spinal motion;
(4) Gradual onset;
(5) Increased pain with walking and bending;
(6) Decreased pain with bed rest;

Signs. (See Mechanical Back Pain.)

Treatment.

(1) Education to increase knowledge and to decrease fear and pain;
(2) Patient identification of stressors that increase pain;
(3) Reduction of activities that increase the symptoms;
(4) Involvement in a protective back regimen, which includes back flexibility and strengthening exercises, aerobic exercises, and progressive relaxation;
(5) Planned periods of rest each day, an understanding of the need to get adequate rest and sleep;
(6) Short course of nonsteroidal anti-inflammatories;
(7) Office visits scheduled at 6-week intervals to reinforce treatment plan and modify if necessary;
(8) Back school (classroom education for patients with back pain) (Simon et al., in press).

Referral.

(1) Failure to respond to therapy;
(2) Lack of a specific diagnosis;

(3) Neurologic symptoms;

(4) Suspicion of a tumor;

(5) Suspicion of infection.

Outcome. Chronic. The goal is to maintain functional ability and to offer modification of treatment to increase the patient's comfort.

Spinal Stenosis

Etiology. Degenerative changes that result in osteophytes forming on the disc margins and facet joints, causing bony overgrowth that constricts the nerve roots. Ligamentous thickening and discogenic protrusion.

Symptoms.

(1) Claudication that is worse with walking (typically patients are unable to walk 100 yards before having leg pain) (Selby, 1983). If walking continues the patient may experience pins and needles sensation and a sense of weakness in the calf and foot (MacNab, 1975).

(2) Leg pain relieved by either sitting or lying down. Stopping does not relieve the pain.

(3) Possible sensory changes, that, if present, are described as a feeling of water or candle wax dripping down the leg (Selby, 1983, p 49).

(4) Back pain with or without leg pain; if leg pain present it radiates below the knee;

(5) Possible increase in back pain with descending stairs.

Signs.

(1) May have normal examination;

(2) May have increased pain during back extension;

(3) If permitted to walk to the point of claudicant leg pain, patient may present with neurologic deficits on examination.

Treatment. Differentiate neurogenic claudication from vascular claudication. Patients with vascular claudication cannot swim or ride a bike without leg pain.

(1) Anti-inflammatories;

(2) Education;

(3) Ice/heat;

(4) Exercise;

(5) Surgery to decompress the nerve root.

Referral. Orthopaedic surgeon.

Compression Fractures (see Osteoporosis, Chapter 3)

Tumor

Most tumors in this age group result from metastases. Primary spinal tumors are rare. Tumors are either intraspinal or extraspinal and may present like a herniated disc (Boyd, 1987).

Symptoms.

(1) Progressive low back pain;

(2) Inability to relieve the pain with rest;

(3) Night pain that awakens the patient from sleep; relief is achieved by either sitting upright or pacing the floor.

Signs (Dependent on the Location of the Tumor).

(1) Neurologic deficit may be present;

(2) Increased back pain on percussion of the spinous processes may be present.

Treatment.

(1) Referral to an orthopaedic surgeon, neurosurgeon;

(2) Plain films at first office visit;

(3) Immediate bone scan, MRI or CAT scan if patient presents with night pain, a history of previous carcinoma, or progressive unrelenting pain that is out of proportion, or if the patient fails 4 to 6 weeks of conservative treatment;

(4) Patient and family education;

(5) Support and reassurance.

Infection

Most infections occur after spinal surgery and are iatrogenic. They also can occur in individuals of any age who are intravenous drug abusers.

Symptoms.

(1) Dull, unrelenting back pain;

(2) Severe low back pain with leg pain;

(3) Pain increased by any jarring motion;

(4) Possible increased pain at night.

Signs.

(1) Low-grade fever;

(2) Spasm of the paraspinal muscles;

(3) Tenderness to percussion over the involved vertebral body.

Treatment.

(1) Immediate referral;

(2) Obtain the following diagnostic tests at the initial visit: ESR, CBC with differential, plain spine films (changes may

not be seen for 3 to 6 weeks and x-rays then will reveal disc destruction with early bony erosion of the end plates) (Selby, 1983). Bone scan is most sensitive;

(3) Identification through needle biopsy of the vertebral body of the specific organism;

(4) Antibiotics;

(5) Immobilization (bed rest until pain subsides).

References

Bland JH: *Disorders of the Cervical Spine*. Philadelphia, WB Saunders, 1987.

Bradford DS, Moe, JH, Winter, RB: Scoliosis and kyphosis. In Rothman RH, Simeone FA (eds): *The Spine*, ed 2. Philadelphia, WB Saunders, 1982.

Boyd RJ: Evaluation of back pain. In Goroll AH, May LA, Mulley AG Jr (eds): *Primary Care Medicine*, ed 2. Philadelphia, JB Lippincott, 1987.

Burnside JW, McGlynn TJ: *Physical Diagnosis*, ed 17. Baltimore, Williams & Wilkins, 1987.

Capistrant T: Thoracic outlet syndrome in cervical strain injury. *Minn Med* 69(10):13–17, 1987.

Deyo RA, Diehel AK, Rosenthal M: How many days of bedrest for acute low back pain? *N Eng J Med* 315(17):1064–1070, 1986.

Feffer HL: Evaluation of the low back diagnosis related impairment rating. In Wiesel SW, Feffer HL, Rothman RH (eds): *Industrial Low Back Pain*. Charlottesville, VA, The Michie Co, 1985.

Frymoyer JW, Pope MH, Clements JH, Wilder DG, Macpherson B, Ashikaga T: Risk factors in low-back pain: an epidemiological survey. *J Bone Joint Surg*, 65-A(2):213–218, 1983.

Funk FJ, Wells RE: Injuries of the cervical spine in football. *Clin Orthop* (109):50–58, 1975.

Gates SJ, Starkey RD: Back injury prevention: a holistic approach. *American Association of Occupational Health Journal* 4(2):59–61, 1986.

Hagberg M: Occupational musculoskeletal stress and disorders of the neck and shoulder: a review of possible pathophysiology. *Int Arch Occup Environ Health* 53:269–278, 1984.

Hohl M: Soft tissue injuries of the neck. *Clin Orthop* 109(4):42–49, 1975.

Hoppenfeld S: *Physical Examination of the Spine and Extremities*. East Norwalk, CT, Appleton-Century-Crofts, 1976.

Kendall FP, McCreary EK: *Muscles Testing and Function*, ed 3. Baltimore, Williams & Wilkins, 1983.

Linton SJ, Kamwendo K: Low back schools: a critical review. *Phys Ther* 67(9):1375–1383, 1987.

Loy TT: Electroacupuncture verus physiotherapy. *Med J Aust* 2(8):32–34, 1983.

MacNab I: Cervical spondylosis. *Clin Orthop* 109(l):69–77, 1975.

MacNab I: *Backache*. Baltimore, Williams & Wilkins, 1977.

Mayer TG, Gatchel RJ, Mayer H, et al.: A prospective two-year study of functional restoration in industrial low back injury: an objective assessment procedure. *JAMA* 258:1763–1767, 1987.

Micheli LJ: Low back pain in the adolescent: differential diagnosis. *Am J Sports Med* 7(6):362–364, 1979.

Mohindra Y, Agarwal RP, Kumar A, Kumar B: Clinical and occupational aspects of spondylosis. *J Indian Med Assoc* 77(l):8–9, 1981.

Rothman RH, Marvel JP: The acute cervical disk. *Clin Orthop* 109:56–68, 1969.

Rothman RH, Simeone FA, Bernini PM: Lumbar disc disease. In Rothman RH, Simeone FA (eds): *The Spine*, ed 2. Philadelphia, WB Saunders, 1982.

Rowe ML: Low back pain in industry. A position paper. *J Occup Med* 11:16l–169, 1969.

Roy S, Irvin R: *Sports Medicine: Prevention, Evaluation, Management, and Rehabilitation*. Englewood Cliffs, NJ, Prentice-Hall, 1983.

Selby DK: Conservative care of the spine in the elderly. *Geriatrics* 38(12):42–56, 1983.

Scott WN, Nisonson B, Nicholas JA: *Principles of Sports Medicine*. Baltimore, Williams & Wilkins, 1984.

Simon WH, Gates SJ, Crawford AG, Robinson D: The Graduate Hospital Back School: results from the first 100 consecutive patients. *Pa Med* (in press).

Spitzer WO, LeBlanc FE, DuPuis M: Scientific approach to the assessment and management of activity-related spinal disorders. A monograph for clinicians. Report of the Quebec Task Force on Spinal Disorders. *Spine* 12(7S):59, 1987.

Torg JS, Truex RC Jr, Quedenfeld TC: The national football head and neck registry report and conclusions. *JAMA* 241:1477–1479, 1979.

Travell JG, Simons DG: *Myofascial Pain and Dysfunction: The Trigger Point Manual*. Baltimore, Williams & Wilkins, 1983.

Waddell G, McCulloch JA, Kummel E, Venner RM: Nonorganic physical signs in low-back pain. *Spine* 5(2):117–125,1980.

Waris P: Occupation cerviobrachial syndrome. *Scand J Work Environ Health* 6(Suppl 3):3–14, 1980.

Weiner HL, Levitt LP: *Neurology for the House Officer*, ed 3. Baltimore, Williams & Wilkins, 1983.

Wiesel SW, Feffer HL, Rothman RH: The development of a cervical spine algorithm and its prospective application to industrial patients. *J Occup Med* 27(4):272–276, 1985.

Wroble RR, Albright JP: Neck and low back injuries in wrestling. *Clin Sports Med* 2:295–325, 1986.

Won WWT: Temporomandibular joint dysfunction masquerading as chronic cervical strain. *Hawaii Med J* 43(12):441–443, 1984.

Wooden MJ: Preseason screening of the lumbar spine. *J Orthop Sports Phys Ther* 3(1):6–10, 1981.

chapter 6

The Shoulder

WILLIAM H. SIMON, M.D., F.A.C.S.

The function of the shoulder joint represents a triumph of motion over stability. Instability is a common consequence of injury, and pain and limitation of normal motion are the sequelae. The prominent role that athletics (baseball, basketball, football, ice hockey) play in the adolescent's life predisposes him/her to significant problems (most unavoidable) with the shoulder joint. Other problems that occur are due to overuse syndromes that result from too vigorous training techniques. Patients presenting with the latter syndrome require follow-up with school athletic departments and/or athletic trainers to prevent repeated problems.

Adults also suffer from overuse syndrome, particularly in industry where repetitive motions in an over head position place undue strain on shoulder structures. These patients also deserve follow-up in the workplace in order to prevent the recurrence of problems. Degenerative changes in the shoulder are common in the elderly. These changes produce pain and limited motion. Frozen shoulder syndrome (the opposite of instability) may be the result of painful, restricted motion.

In an out-patient setting, the nurse or nurse-practitioner must have knowledge of the anatomy and function of the shoulder joint in order to diagnose and properly treat the joint or to refer patients for treatment. This chapter will provide such knowledge. The chapter is divided into the following segments: Anatomy and Function of the Shoulder Joint, History, Physical Examination, Diagnostic Guidelines, The Adolescent with Shoulder Pain, The Adult with

Shoulder Pain, The Mature Adult with Shoulder Pain, and Rehabilitation of the Injured Shoulder. Treatment recommendations are those expected of a nurse-practitioner, including first aid prior to referral for definitive treatment, either nonsurgical or surgical.

ANATOMY AND FUNCTION OF THE SHOULDER JOINT

The shoulder joint literally hangs from the axial skeleton. It is suspended by muscular attachments, and articulates with the body by means of a strut bone known as the clavicle. At either end of the clavicle is a joint. The more stable joint, the sternoclavicular joint, is the only direct connection between the shoulder and the axial skeleton. The less stable joint, the acromioclavicular joint, is at the distal end of the clavicle, is palpable subcutaneously, and is a major bony landmark about the shoulder. The clavicle is an S-shaped bone, and is subcutaneous throughout its length. It rotates during flexion and extension of the shoulder and it aids in the stability of the joint. The clavicle is not necessary for shoulder motion. Individuals who are born without this bone (a condition known as cleidocranial dysostosis) have shoulders that function perfectly well (Fig. 6.1).

The scapula is a complex bone. The major portion of the scapula is the blade. This is a triangular structure to or from which major muscles that control the strength, stability, and function of the shoulder mechanism attach or originate. It is divided by the spine into a smaller upper supras-

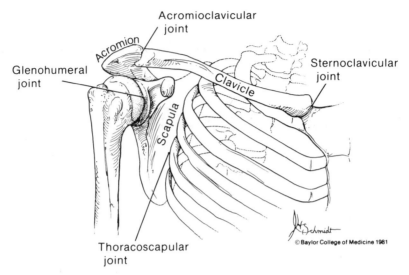

Figure 6.1. Bony anatomy of the shoulder girdle. (From Scott WN, Nisonson B, Nicholas JA (eds): *Principles of Sports Medicine*. Baltimore, Williams & Wilkins, 1984.)

pinatus portion and a larger infraspinatus segment. The supraspinatus muscle, the major component of the so-called rotator cuff, originates above the spine and attaches to the greater tuberosity of the humerus. It is a major stabilizer of the glenohumeral joint. The infraspinatus and teres minor muscles, two more components of the rotator cuff, originate below the spine. Both stabilize and externally rotate the humeral head in the glenoid cavity. The teres major muscle and internal rotator also originate on the scapula and attach to the humerus at the lesser tuberosity (Fig. 6.2). Also attaching to the scapula and acting as stabilizers and rotators of this bone are the rhomboids, the levator scapulae, and the trapezius muscles. The Latissimus dorsi muscle covers the tip of the scapula as it swings from the mid-back to attach on the lesser tuberosity of the humerus to depress and internally rotate the humerus. The undersurface or thoracic surface of the scapula is the site of origin of the subscapularis muscle—the fourth and final component of the rotator cuff—which is a depressor and internal rotator of the shoulder. In addition, the serratus anterior muscle comes off of the thorax and attaches to the undersurface of the scapula, thereby stabilizing the scapula against "winging"

out away from the thorax. All of the muscles attaching to the scapular blade aid in the complex coordinated movements of this bone including elevation, depression, rotation, abduction, and adduction (motion in the plane of the thorax). Many of these movements will occur in any complete movement of the shoulder joint, such as elevation of the arm from the side of the body to the overhead position.

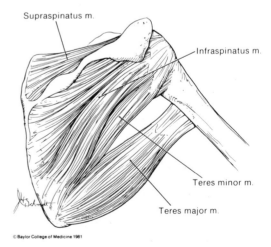

Figure 6.2. Posterior scapular musculature and rotator cuff. (From Scott WN, Nisonson B, Nicholas JA (eds): *Principles of Sports Medicine*. Baltimore, Williams & Wilkins, 1984.)

Other portions of the scapula, the acromion, the glenoid, and the coracoid process, each play a major role in the shoulder function (Figs. 6.3 and 6.4). The glenoid, the portion of the scapula that articulates with the head of the humerus, extends forward from the blade on a short neck of bone. It has a shallow, concave surface covered by articular cartilage and is deepened for stability by a fibrous ring known as the labrum or lip. Attached to the glenoid is the fibrous capsule of the shoulder, which also attaches to the neck of the humerus in order to contain the glenohumeral joint. The capsule is lax with the arm at the side and is taut in the overhead position. The capsule is reinforced anteriorly by three ligaments: superior, middle, and inferior. A relatively small gap between the middle and inferior ligaments acts as a *locus minoris resistentiae* (place of least resistance) with the arm overhead; this gap is the place through which anterior dislocations of the glenohumeral joint most typically occur. The biceps tendon (long head) attaches to the superior surface of the glenoid. It travels inside the shoulder capsule over the head of the humerus, into the bicipital groove, and thence down the shaft of the humerus

(Fig. 6.5). The long head of the triceps tendon attaches extracapsularly to the inferior surface of the glenoid (Fig. 6.4).

The acromion is the outrigger of the scapula. It is the main subcutaneous landmark of the lateral aspect of the shoulder. It acts as the "roof" of the shoulder, and the strong deltoid muscle (the major overhead rotator of the humerus) is also attached to it. Beneath the acromion, the rotator cuff tendons function, separated from the deltoid muscle by the subacromial bursa (an envelope of synovial tissue that allows one tendon to glide over the other). Extending from the anterior tip of the acromion to the coracoid process is a tough fibrous ligament (the coracoacromial ligament) that forms an arcade over the anterior aspect of the rotator cuff and the biceps tendon (Fig. 6.3).

The coracoid process is a finger-like anterior protuberance off of the scapular blade to which is attached the conjoined tendons of the short head of the biceps, the pectoralis minor, and the coracobrachialis muscles. In addition, the major stabilizing ligaments of the clavicle—the trapezoid and conoid ligaments—attach to the coracoid process (Fig. 6.3). The humeral head (a

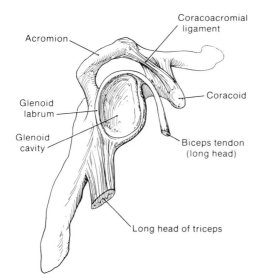

Figure 6.3.   Glenoid fossa and relationship to scapular structures. (From Scott WN, Nisonson B, Nicholas JA (eds): *Principles of Sports Medicine.* Baltimore, Williams & Wilkins, 1984.)

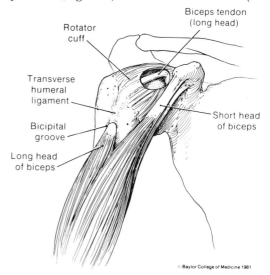

Figure 6.4.   Long head of the biceps tendon across glenohumeral joint. (From Scott WN, Nisonson B, Nicholas JA (eds): *Principles of Sports Medicine.* Baltimore, Williams & Wilkins, 1984.)

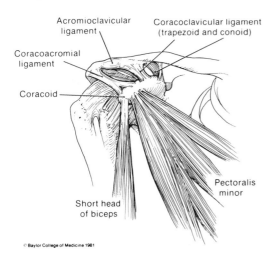

Figure 6.5. Anatomy of the coracoid and associated muscular and ligamentous attachments. (From Scott WN, Nisonson B, Nicholas JA (eds): *Principles of Sports Medicine*. Baltimore, Williams & Wilkins, 1984.)

spherical structure) is covered with articular cartilage and moves unimpeded on the glenoid surface. Its movements are tethered only by the capsular attachment at the anatomical neck, the biceps tendon, and the tendons of the rotator cuff (Fig. 6.6). The bony prominence lateral to the head (the greater tuberosity) is another shoulder landmark covered by the thick deltoid muscle.

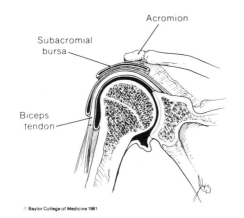

Figure 6.6. Cross-section of glenohumeral joint with tendinous and capsular relationships. (From Scott WN, Nisonson B, Nicholas JA (eds): *Principles of Sports Medicine*. Baltimore, Williams & Wilkins, 1984.)

The complex neurovascular supply of the shoulder will not be described here in detail. The major nerves and blood vessels enter the axilla just medial to the coracoid process and inferior to the glenohumeral joint. The musculocutaneous nerve runs under the coracoid process beneath the conjoined tendon. The axillary nerve runs from back to front about 1 inch below the acromion in the deltoid muscle, which it innervates. It is subject to injury in shoulder dislocations and by direct blows to the shoulder. The suprascapular nerve, supplying the rotator cuff muscles, runs in the supraspinatus portion of the scapula; it is subject to injury by blows to the top of the shoulder. The long thoracic nerve runs down the side of the thorax. An injury to this nerve, which supplies the serratus anterior muscles, produces winging of the scapula (Figs. 6.7 and 6.8).

The extreme mobility of the shoulder joint allows for 180° of motion in flexion and abduction away from the side of the body; 180° of rotation internal to external; 70° to 90° of backward extension; and 45° of adduction across the body. When viewed from behind, the synchronous function of the shoulder structures produces a smooth "scapulohumeral rhythm" when the arm is raised overhead. Any significant dysfunction in a major shoulder structure will disturb this rhythm, and dysfuction can be detected by comparing the appearance of shoulder elevation right to left. This is the simplest test of normal shoulder function. The gross observation of swelling, muscle atrophy, pain on motion, and point tenderness is the mainstay of a basic shoulder examination.

HISTORY

The most important aspect of the patient history as it relates to the shoulder is to obtain a clear and concise chief complaint. Questions to ask include: Is there pain on any movement of the shoulder? Pain on a particular motion of the shoulder? Intermittent pain in the shoulder without relation to movement? Weakness in the shoulder? Limitation of the range of motion of the shoulder? Once the chief com-

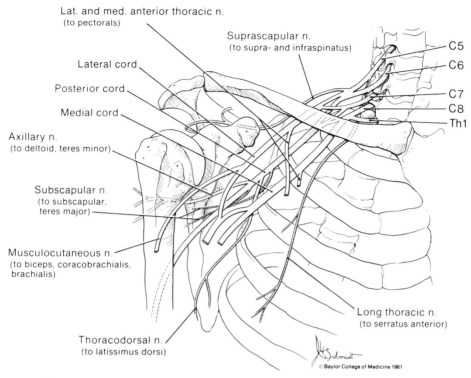

Lat. and med. anterior thoracic n.
(to pectorals)

Suprascapular n.
(to supra- and infraspinatus)

C5
C6
C7
C8
Th1

Lateral cord

Posterior cord

Medial cord

Axillary n.
(to deltoid, teres minor)

Subscapular n.
(to subscapular,
teres major)

Musculocutaneous n.
(to biceps, coracobrachialis,
brachialis)

Long thoracic n.
(to serratus anterior)

Thoracodorsal n.
(to latissimus dorsi)

© Baylor College of Medicine 1981

Figure 6.7. Peripheral nerve supply to the shoulder joint. (From Scott WN, Nisonson B, Nicholas JA (eds): *Principles of Sports Medicine.* Baltimore, Williams & Wilkins, 1984.)

plaint is established, the history then delves into the how, where, and when.

In determining how the problem began, it is important to determine whether it was a traumatic or nontraumatic onset. If traumatic, a description of the trauma (in simple terms) is important. Questions to ask include: Did the patient fall on the point of the shoulder or on an outstretched arm? Was there a blow to a specific part of the shoulder? Was there a specific activity connected with the onset of shoulder pain such as the difficult opening of a stuck window frame or garage door?

In nontraumatic problems one should ask if there was a certain activity that brought about the awareness of the problem, such as repetitive use of the shoulder in an overhead position either at work or at play? Can the patient determine exactly where he/she feels the problem is in the shoulder? Can the patient put one finger on the area of the pain? Is the problem generalized in and about the shoulder? Does pain radiate from

the shoulder upward to the neck or downward to the arm and hand? Does the patient feel something going on inside the shoulder, such as a clicking or a sensation that the shoulder is going out of place? Can the patient demonstrate one particular position where the pain is most acute? Is it reaching overhead at 90° of elevation, in reaching behind the back, in reaching out to the side, or in placing the arm overhead in a throwing position? When did the problem begin? Is it an old recurrent problem or something entirely new? Has it been going on for hours, days, weeks, or months? Does it occur at any particular time of the day or night? Has it been a persistent problem, intermittent, gradually increasing in severity, or changing in severity from time to time? The answers to all of these questions should be recorded precisely and concisely.

Each patient should have a basic past medical history taken and a statement of any present systemic illnesses recorded, as

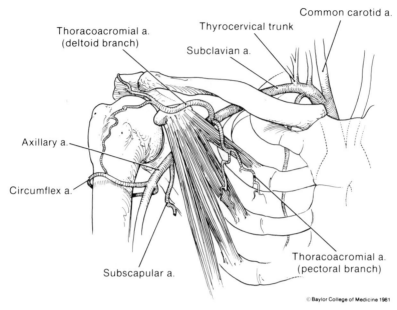

Figure 6.8. Vascular supply to the shoulder joint. (From Scott WN, Nisonson B, Nicholas JA (eds): *Principles of Sports Medicine*. Baltimore, Williams & Wilkins, 1984.)

well as the names and dosages of any medications he/she is taking at the time of the examination.

PHYSICAL EXAMINATION

It is most important that the examination of the shoulder joint be made with the patient properly exposed to the examiner. Men must clearly expose their bodies to the waist. Women must remove undergarments and should be gowned, covered from the breasts in front to below the shoulder blades in back. This can be done either with a sheet that is pinned behind the patient or with a standard cloth or paper gown wrapped around the patient (keeping the arms free) and tied in the back.

The patient must be observed from front and back for any significant shoulder asymmetry including the presence of unilateral swelling, skin temperature or color changes, prominence of a particular part of the shoulder, such as the sternoclavicular joint, acromioclavicular joint, or anterior or posterior prominence of the humeral head area. Atrophy or flattening of the deltoid muscles, trapezius muscle, supraspinatus or infraspinatus muscle groups, or pectoral muscles must be noted and recorded. It is also important to observe if winging of the scapula away from the thoracic cage is present (Fig. 6.9).

Prior to initiating any movement of the shoulder, palpation of the shoulder structures is carried out using the fingertips of one hand. This examination begins at the sternoclavicular joint, moves along the subcutaneous border of the clavicle, directly to the acromioclavicular joint, and then to the acromion. Pressure is exerted below the acromion anteriorly, laterally, and posteriorly to detect the presence of any point tenderness. Pressure is exerted on the trapezius muscle from the occiput to the point of the shoulder. The supraspinous and infraspinous portions of the scapula are palpated. Finally, pressure is exerted over the biceps tendon in the bicipital groove of the proximal humerus. Frequently, it is just as easy to examine the nonaffected shoulder with one hand and the symptomatic shoulder with the other hand. The examination is performed in order to elicit tenderness or to feel any abnormalities, such as swelling, muscle spasm,

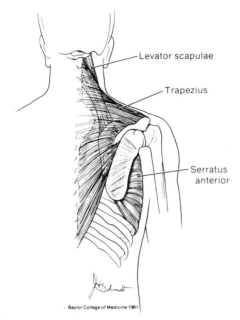

Levator scapulae

Trapezius

Serratus
anterior

Baylor College of Medicine 1981

Figure 6.9. Scapular and muscular attachments. (From Scott WN, Nisonson B, Nicholas JA (eds): *Principles of Sports Medicine.* Baltimore, Williams & Wilkins, 1984.)

or increased mobility of the affected shoulder as compared to the normal shoulder. The examination for range of motion of the shoulder joint is performed both actively and passively. The patient is asked to perform the movements initially, and, if the patient cannot complete a normal range of motion, gentle active assistance is provided by the examiner to determine if the problem is one of restriction by pain or restriction by weakness or actual physical block to movement. The movements of the symptomatic shoulder are compared to the movements of the normal shoulder (Fig. 6.10). The patient is placed with his/her arm at the side, with the palm facing the body. The first movement tested is *flexion* movement or moving the arm forward into the overhead position (a straight overhead position or 180°). The examiner must be sure to record the point in this arc of motion at which the patient complains of any pain. *Extension* of the shoulder begins with the arm at the side. The patient is asked to move the arm directly backward; the normal range is approximately 70°.

Rotation of the shoulder is tested in two positions. The first position is with the arm at the side and the elbow bent to 90° so the thumb points upward. The shoulder is then externally and internally rotated and the range of motion is recorded. A normal range of motion is approximately 70° of external rotation and 70° of internal rotation. Care must be taken to keep the elbow directly against the side of the body. (Testing internal rotation in this position may be difficult in obese patients.) The second position to test shoulder rotation is with the arm abducted to 90°. (This, of course, is impossible if the patient is unable to perform this maneuver because of pain.) The elbow is bent 90° and the palm is facing downward. In this position, normal external rotation is 90° and normal internal rotation is 90°.

Abduction of the shoulder is tested in two positions. In the first position, the arm is at the side with the palm facing the body and the patient is asked to lift the arm away from the side and overhead. This can normally be accomplished to 180°. If the patient resists this movement at some point in the arc of motion, the hand is returned to the side of the body and the palm is turned outward. This maneuver places the greater tuberosity of the shoulder behind the acromion process and therefore reduces any impingement of soft tissues between the greater tuberosity and the acromion. In the second position, the patient is asked to elevate the arm away from the body. If the patient can elevate to 180° with the palm turned outward, but not with the palm turned inward, it is likely that there is a rotator cuff problem.

While the patient is performing these activities, the scapulohumeral rhythm should be observed. Ordinarily, this is a smooth coordination between the motion of the glenohumeral joint and the scapula and thorax. If this rhythm is disturbed so the coordinated motion appears jerky or awkward, this is an indicator of major shoulder dysfunction.

Adduction of the shoulder is carried out with the elbow extended and the arm moved across the chest. This function can also be

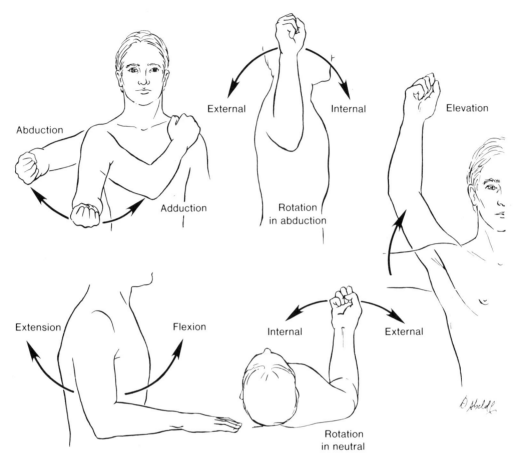

Figure 6.10. Normal shoulder range of motion. (From Burnside JW, McGlynn TJ: *Physical Diagnosis*, ed 17. Baltimore, Williams & Wilkins, 1987.)

tested from the position of 90° of elevation with the arm directly in front of the patient then moved across the chest in this fashion. Adduction normally goes to approximately 45°.

A general sense of strength of these major muscle groups can be obtained by the examiner resisting the specific movements as the patient performs the range of motion maneuvers and comparing how well the patient counters this resistance on the affected side as compared to the normal side. In testing the strength of the abductor muscles, it is important to apply resistance immediately as the arm leaves the side of the body, rather than in the overhead position. Specific testing of the strength of the shoulder elevators is accomplished by asking the patient to shrug while the examiner gently

but firmly resists the shrug with the palms on the top of each shoulder. A specific test for the serratus anterior muscle can be carried out by asking the patient to push forward against the examiner's hand with the elbow at 90°. Winging of the scapula frequently can be detected by this maneuver.

A sense of the stability of the glenohumeral joint can be obtained by grasping the humeral head with the examining hand and moving it forward and backward to detect any unusual laxity. This may be difficult to perform or assess in a markedly obese or very muscular individual. Another test for joint instability may be performed with the patient in a relaxed position on the examining table, lying on the back with the arm elevated directly overhead. Pressure is then exerted on the back of the humeral head thereby pushing it forward. Often the patient with instability in the shoulder joint will resist this movement, stating that it feels as if the shoulder is about to go out of place. Additional physical tests are described with specific pathological entities in the following sections.

There are no motor reflexes about the shoulder joint. However, a sensory examination should be carried out over the entire shoulder, including the area of the anterior and posterior chest, upper arm, and lateral chest wall; the simplest way to do this is to use a pin or pinwheel type of sensory testing device.

DIAGNOSTIC GUIDELINES

The examiner should obtain an A/P shoulder x-ray at the initial visit to rule out tumor, infection, or arthritis of the glenohumeral and acromioclavicular joints. Additional x-rays should include external and internal views to exclude calcification and, if dislocation is suspected, an axillary view. If neck motion produces shoulder pain the examiner should obtain cervical spine films.

THE ADOLESCENT WITH SHOULDER PAIN

The main difference between the adolescent and the adult shoulder is the presence of growth centers in the former. The three growth centers in the proximal humerus—humeral head, greater tuberosity, and lesser tuberosity—do not fuse until approximately age 20. Therefore, in any traumatic injury to the adolescent shoulder, consideration must be given to fracture or avulsion through these cartilaginous plates; comparative x-ray views of both shoulders are mandatory. Common nontraumatic and traumatic conditions of the shoulder are found in Table 6.1.

Nontraumatic Conditions

Overuse Syndrome (Tendinitis)

Overuse syndrome is seen in sports-minded adolescents, particularly those in

Table 6.1
Shoulder Problems Across the Ages

Shoulder Problems	
Traumatic	Nontraumatic
ADOLESCENTS	
Shoulder separation (acromioclavicular joint)	Overuse syndrome (tendinitis)
Shoulder dislocation (glenohumeral joint)	Infection (septic arthritis and osteomyelitis)
Fracture of clavicle	Monoarticular arthritis (juvenile rheumatoid arthritis)
Fracture of proximal humeral epiphysis	Malignant tumor
ADULTS	
Rotator cuff tear	Impingement syndrome
Avulsion greater tuberosity	Calcific tendinitis
Rupture biceps tendon	Bicipital tendinitis
Comminuted fracture of proximal humerus	Frozen shoulder syndrome
MATURE ADULTS	
Impacted fracture (proximal humerus)	Cervical radiculopathy
Hand-shoulder syndrome	Degenerative arthritis
	Degenerative tendinitis

vigorous training conditions as in high school baseball (pitching), tennis, and swimming. Typically, the shoulder ache or pain is only produced on elevation beyond 90°. Point tenderness is common over the biceps tendon and rotator cuff immediately beneath the acromion anteriorly. Treatment is rest, ice after use, and gradual return to sports participation with observation by a coach or trainer who has been alerted to the adolescent's problem. Resolution of this problem may take several weeks.

Infection

Signs of shoulder infection are severe pain (particularly on any motion of the shoulder joint), increased local temperature, systemic fever, and, occasionally, swelling. Diagnosis is made by physical examination and aspiration of the joint with Gram's stain and culture of the aspirate. If there is suspicion of infection the patient should be immediately referred to an orthopaedic specialist.

The early differentiation between septic arthritis and osteomyelitis of the proximal humerus with a secondary effusion of the shoulder capsule may be impossible. An early sterile shoulder aspirate and, after several days, elevation of the proximal humeral periosteum on x-ray, may help to separate the conditions. Treatment is the use of appropriate antibiotics (determined by culture and usually given intravenously, at least in the early stages of treatment). Drainage of pus from the joint and surgical drainage of pus from the medullary canal are secondary treatment modalities.

Monoarticular arthritis (juvenile rheumatoid arthritis) involving the shoulder presents with less pain and fever than septic arthritis. An elevated sedimentation rate may be the only positive laboratory finding. Referral to a pediatrician or rheumatologist is necessary for long-term treatment.

Malignant Tumor

Malignant tumor (osteosarcoma) is usually considered after a shoulder x-ray reveals either a lytic lesion in the proximal humeral bone or periosteal new bone in a young person who complains of a vague pain for some time (weeks or several months). There may be a history of relative minor trauma. The physical examination may not be revealing or it may find localized swelling and tenderness. Immediate referral to a specialist (orthopaedic surgeon or oncologist) is mandatory. These malignancies spread rapidly and are often fatal.

Traumatic Conditions

Most traumatic injuries in the adolescent are related to sports or recreational activities. Such injuries are usually treated on an emergency basis with x-ray facilities and referral services immediately available.

Shoulder Separation

A shoulder separation is an injury to the acromioclavicular joint produced by a downward force on the point of the shoulder. This injury occurs from a fall or a direct blow to the shoulder. The damage to the joint that results depends upon the force of the blow and ranges from a sprain to a complete dislocation. Physical findings range from moderate point tenderness over the acromioclavicular joint to an elevated unstable distal clavicle. The injuries are classified grades I through IV: grade I is a partial tear of the acromioclavicular ligament; grade II is a complete ligament tear; grade III includes the addition of a coracoclavicular ligament tear (Fig. 6.11); and grade IV is an unstable, irreducible grade III injury. The grade III acromioclavicular joint separation with ligament rupture represents 90 to 95% of all dislocations. X-ray evaluation is performed with and without the patient holding hand weights in the upright position. Both shoulders are examined and compared; the subluxing or dislocated joint will be obvious when compared to the uninjured shoulder. Treatment for all, except the grade IV injury, is conservative: ice, sling immobilization, and mild analgesia. Surgery is rarely necessary for these injuries. The grade IV, or irreducible dislocation, requires surgery in order to avoid skin breakdown over the distal clavicle. In conservative care, immobiliza-

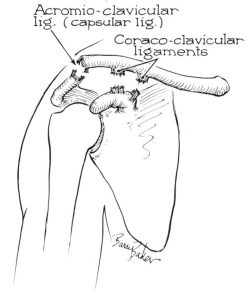

Figure 6.11. Grade 3 acromioclavicular joint separation with ligament rupture. (From Scott WN, Nisonson B, Nicholas JA (eds): *Principles of Sports Medicine.* Baltimore, Williams & Wilkins, 1984.)

tion is necessary for approximately 3 weeks, with an additional 3 weeks of range of motion and strengthening exercises.

Shoulder Dislocation

Anterior shoulder dislocation (glenohumeral joint) represents 90 to 95% of all dislocations that result from a strong blow to the back of the joint with the arm elevated. The humeral head ruptures the anterior capsule and comes to rest anterior and inferior to the glenoid, producing an abnormal anterior prominence and flattening of the posterior shoulder contour. The patient initially is in severe pain, but with the arm at the side the pain is reduced, only to be reactivated by any movement of the shoulder. X-ray evaluation is done primarily to rule out a fracture and confirm the diagnosis. In order to determine if the axillary nerve has been damaged, it is important to perform a sensory test over the shoulder before any attempt at reduction. Stimson's reduction maneuver may be attempted with relative safety. The patient is placed prone on an examining table with the affected limb hanging over the side with 5 to 10 lb of weights strapped to the involved hand. Reduction should occur within 15 to 20 minutes. If reduction cannot be achieved even with light analgesia or muscle relaxation, the arm should be replaced in a sling and immediate consultation obtained with an orthopaedic surgeon for possible reduction and general anesthesia. If reduction is successful, the arm may be immobilized in a sling or shoulder immobilizer for 3 weeks with an additional 3 weeks for protected use of the arm and range of motion exercises.

Clavicle Fracture

A fracture of the clavicle may result from a direct blow to, or a fall on, the shoulder. Often the injury is sustained by "piling on" in athletic endeavors such as football and rugby. The physical findings are local pain, swelling, and painful shoulder motion. X-rays confirm the injury and determine the degree of displacement, angulation, and possible comminution. If the fracture occurs distal to the coracoid process and the coracoclavicular ligament, the fracture is unstable and orthopaedic consultation should be obtained immediately. Cyanosis of the upper extremity indicates vascular compromise and demonstrates the necessity for emergency reduction, possibly by open means.

Treatment of the simple fracture is by means of the figure-of-eight clavicular strap that maintains the shoulder in extension for 6 to 8 weeks. Frequent adjustment of the strap must be made during the treatment period in order to avoid skin breakdown and to maintain reduction (Fig. 6.12).

Proximal Humeral Fracture

A fracture of the proximal humerus in an adolescent may result from a fall on the outstretched arm (either forward or behind the body axis) or on the point of the elbow. It often causes injury to, or displacement through, the epiphyseal growth plate at the base of the humeral head. Pain, swelling, and limitation of motion are the physical findings. X-ray evaluation of both shoulders should be performed to determine any change in the position of the ossified bone on either side of the growth plate. If no fracture is identified but the pain is severe, a crush injury to the growth plate should be considered and the limb should be immobilized in a sling for 3 to 4 weeks. Follow-up x-rays may reveal callus about the growth plate injury.

Displaced epiphyseal injuries require re-

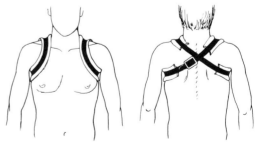

© Baylor College of Medicine 1981

Figure 6.12. Figure-of-eight harness. (From Scott WN, Nisonson B, Nicholas JA (eds): *Principles of Sports Medicine.* Baltimore, Williams & Wilkins, 1984.)

duction only if they are severe. Closed reduction with moderate prolonged downward traction may be successful in restoring satisfactory alignment. Rarely are open reduction and internal fixation necessary.

THE ADULT WITH SHOULDER PAIN

Nontraumatic Conditions

Impingement Syndrome

The impingement syndrome presents as tenderness over the anterior shoulder, beneath the acromion on elevation of the shoulder beyond 90°. The patient usually seeks help only after the condition has been present for several weeks. X-rays are negative. The patient usually describes some repetitive work or sports activity that aggravates the condition (Fig. 6.13).

The etiopathology of the condition may be complex, containing elements of one or more local inflammatory or degenerative conditions within the confined space beneath the acromioclavicular arch. Bicipital and rotator cuff tendinitis and acromioclavicular joint synovitis may be present in varying degrees causing local swelling and painful compression of inflamed tissues on reaching overhead. The treatment is rest

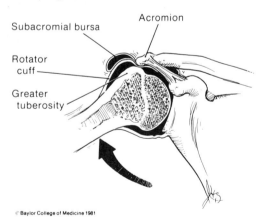

Subacromial bursa
Acromion
Rotator cuff
Greater tuberosity

© Baylor College of Medicine 1981

Figure 6.13. Impingement syndrome between acromion and greater tuberosity. (From Scott WN, Nisonson B, Nicholas JA (eds): *Principles of Sports Medicine*. Baltimore, Williams & Wilkins, 1984.)

and sling immobilization with the use of salicylates or nonsteroidal anti-inflammatory agents. If these measures do not alleviate the problem, referral is indicated for possible steroid injection. A single injection of corticosteroids into the anterior subacromial space may be helpful. Gradual rehabilitation over several weeks, including gentle stretching and strengthening exercises and instructions in avoiding frequent repetitive overhead activities, is usually efficacious in preventing a recurrence. Athletes should be instructed to warm up before overhead sports.

Calcific Tendinitis

Calcific tendinitis is a degenerative condition in which a "calcium boil" develops acutely in the rotator cuff (with a preexisting asymptomatic degenerative calcified tendinitis). The symptoms are severe, localized pain occurring with virtually any movement of the shoulder. X-rays show a radio-dense deposit, usually several millimeters in diameter, just above the humeral head. Treatment is rest, sling immobilization, and anti-inflammatory drugs. Often the use of a large bore needle to puncture the boil and at times to aspirate some of the calcium-containing material with the concomitant injection of a local anesthetic and corticosteroid compound immediately relieves the patient.

Bicipital Tendinitis

Bicipital tendinitis is a local synovitis about the proximal portion of the long head of the biceps tendon in the bicipital groove of the humerus immediately proximal to the point where the tendon enters the glenohumeral joint beneath the rotator cuff tendons. The clinical findings consist of local tenderness in the bicipital groove, pain in the shoulder on resisted elbow flexion and forearm supination, and pain on shoulder elevation.

Pathologic changes include degenerative tears of the tendon and overlying rotator cuff and at times an overly mobile tendon that easily subluxes in and out of the bicipital groove. Rest and anti-inflammatory drugs are the mainstays of treatment. A single injection of a steroid compound and a local anesthetic into the bicipital groove may give immediate and long-lasting relief.

Frozen Shoulder

The "frozen shoulder syndrome" is a complex phenomenon in which capsular thickening and adhesive capsulitis develop in response to a painful stimulus that causes the patient to limit shoulder motion for a prolonged period of time. Conditions such as cervical radiculopathy, diabetes mellitus, and angina pectoris may be associated with the onset of the problem. The patient presents with a history of gradually increasing pain and limitation of motion of the shoulder joint. Clinical findings include generalized shoulder pain on movement with restricted passive motion in several or all directions compared to the opposite shoulder.

Pathological changes include a collagenous proliferation of the shoulder capsule, causing it to become thickened, adherent to the humeral head, and reduced in its intraarticular volume.

In most cases, the syndrome is self-limiting; with rest and gradual gentle rehabilitation, the condition will go through the phases of "freezing, frozen, and thawing" so that a normal, painless range of motion is restored within a period of weeks or perhaps a few months. Often, however, the problem is of several months' duration when the patient presents and the continuing painful stimulus persists. In this case a full range of motion cannot be restored, even after careful rehabilitation. Under these circumstances, the patient should be referred to an orthopaedic surgeon for an "infiltration brisement" under general anesthesia. This procedure involves stretching the capsule with hydrostatic pressure from an intraarticular injection of saline, local anesthetic, and steroid compound, and gently placing the shoulder through a full range of motion to restore capsular length. The procedure may be done on an outpatient basis.

Traumatic Conditions

Rotator Cuff Rupture

Rupture of the rotator cuff is more likely to occur in an adult secondary to the early degenerative changes that may be found—just proximal to the tendinous insertion to the greater tuberosity. The injury is produced during a fall if the patient puts out the hand to break the fall and the weight of the body causes the arm to collapse while the tendon is under tension. The tear may be incomplete through the tendon, complete but small (a few millimeters in length), or large (several centimeters in length). The supraspinatus tendon is frequently involved. The immediate symptoms are pain that may get worse as swelling occurs and an inability to raise the arm, particularly away from the side of the body (abduction).

X-rays may be negative or may show a humeral head resting lower in the glenoid than in the opposite shoulder. Pain on motion and point tenderness over the anterolateral humeral head are the early physical findings. Several days or weeks later, loss of scapulohumeral rhythm, pain on elevation beyond 45°, and weakness in abduction against resistance are prominent findings. Usually the patient's arm can be elevated passively to 180°, but upon lowering the arm to 90° the patient loses control and the arm falls painfully to the side (Fig. 6.14).

If the tear is small, treatment with rest, immobilization, and anti-inflammatory agents, with gradual rehabilitation to full functional use over a period of several weeks to several months, can be prescribed. Larger tears result in permanent pain and weakness. The extent of the tear may be determined by several diagnostic procedures, some noninvasive, some invasive. When properly done, ultrasonography can compare the normal and injured shoulder and can often diagnose a tear and give some idea as to its size. Computerized axial tomography (CAT) and magnetic resonance imaging (MRI) are two additional noninvasive diagnostic studies. Invasive studies include shoulder arthrography and arthroscopy. Arthrography is performed by a radiologist and involves injecting dye into the shoulder joint. The leakage of the radiopaque dye into the subdeltoid bursa is demonstrated on an x-ray and is diagnostic of a tear. Arthroscopy is performed by an

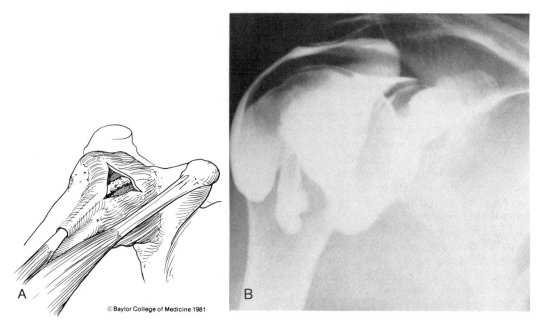

© Baylor College of Medicine 1981

Figure 6.14. **A**, Complete rotator cuff tear. **B**, Arthrogram of rotator cuff tear. (From Scott WN, Nisonson B, Nicholas JA (eds): *Principles of Sports Medicine*. Baltimore, Williams & Wilkins, 1984.)

orthopaedic surgeon under general anesthesia and allows for direct observation and surgical débridement of the tear. Surgical repair of larger tears requires an open operation, followed by several months of rehabilitation.

Greater Tuberosity Avulsion Injury

An avulsion injury to the greater tuberosity occurs through the same mechanism as the rotator cuff tear. Instead of the tendon giving way, however, a piece of the bony attachment of the tendon is pulled away. If x-ray shows the avulsed fragment to be large and with minimal displacement, it may be allowed to heal in place. If the fragment is significantly elevated out of its normal bed, or if a small fragment is pulled into an intraarticular position, the fragment will permanently affect shoulder joint function and therefore an open operation for repair is required.

Ruptured Biceps Tendon

Rupture of the long head of the biceps tendon may occur upon rapid overuse of this partially degenerated tendon, such as in the failed attempt to raise a stuck win-

dow or an overhead door. The tendon may rupture intraarticularly or, more typically, extraarticularly, producing immediate pain and swelling. A deformity of the shortened biceps muscle is immediately noticeable. Treatment can be conservative or operative. Conservative care results in almost normal function with a slightly weakened and permanently deformed biceps muscle. Operative repair may produce an excellent result in terms of function but surgical complications may mar the result and the final outcome may be worse than if the injury had been treated nonoperatively.

Comminuted Fracture of the Proximal Humerus

The comminuted fracture, or four-part fracture of the proximal humerus, may be one of the most difficult injuries to treat about the shoulder joint. After x-ray evaluation, this injury must be referred to an orthopaedic surgeon. The problem with this injury is that the fracture line at the base of the humeral head may cut off all vascular supply. Therefore, no matter what the treatment, closed or open, the result may be avascular necrosis of the head of the humerus, requiring prosthetic joint replacement (Fig. 6.15).

Recurrent Shoulder Dislocation or Subluxation

Dislocation of the glenohumeral joint may produce a tear in the glenoid labrum—the so-called Bankart lesion. This lesion causes instability and recurrent anterior dislocation or subluxation, the latter causing a sudden feeling of loss of function ("dead arm syndrome").

The physical examination demonstrates a sudden click or clunk on elevation and external rotation of the shoulder. Even if a click is not significant, the patient develops an "apprehension sign" with the arm overhead, complaining that the shoulder feels like it is about to dislocate.

The x-ray is an important diagnostic feature in the condition. The view of the humeral head in internal rotation often reveals a posterolateral V-shaped or "hatchet" defect, the so-called Hill-Sachs lesion (Fig. 6.16).

Treatment requires strengthening of the shoulder internal rotator muscles, particularly for the subscapularis. This can be accomplished with a simple loop of rubber tubing (Fig. 6.17). The patient should be counseled to avoid overhead activities. If conservative treatment fails, the patient should be referred for operative treatment.

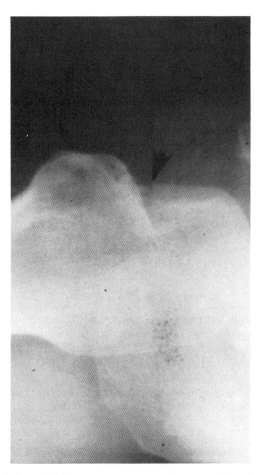

Figure 6.16. Roentgenogram of humeral head defect (Hill-Sachs lesion). (From Scott WN, Nisonson B, Nicholas JA (eds): *Principles of Sports Medicine.* Baltimore, Williams & Wilkins, 1984.)

Posterior Dislocation of the Glenohumeral Joint

A rare (less than 2% of glenohumeral dislocations) and often difficult to diagnose traumatic condition is the posterior glenohumeral dislocation. The most common etiology is a seizure state or the use of electroshock therapy. Occasionally, the patient sustains a strong blow to the front of the shoulder with the humeral head in maximum internal rotation. The humeral head ruptures the posterior joint capsule and dislocates posteriorly.

The physical examination shows a patient in obvious pain holding the arm at the side. External rotation is particularly

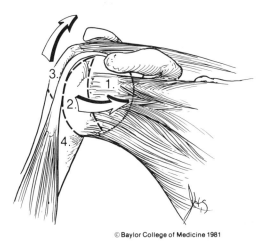

© Baylor College of Medicine 1981

Figure 6.15. Four-part fracture of the humeral head. (From Scott WN, Nisonson B, Nicholas JA (eds): *Principles of Sports Medicine.* Baltimore, Williams & Wilkins, 1984.)

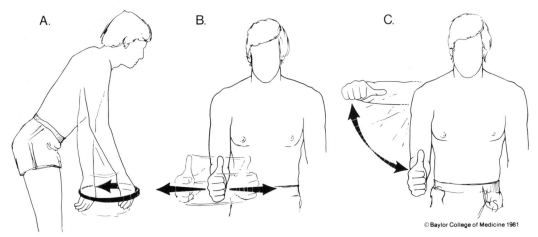

© Baylor College of Medicine 1981

Figure 6.17. Anterior shoulder dislocation/rehabilitation. (From Scott WN, Nisonson B, Nicholas JA (eds): *Principles of Sports Medicine*. Baltimore, Williams & Wilkins, 1984.)

painful. In contrast to the examination in the anterior dislocation, in this examination a bulge (the dislocated humeral head) is palpated posteriorly and a loss of shoulder contour is noted anteriorly.

X-ray evaluation is critical. The anteroposterior view may be interpreted as "normal." Only the axillary view can demonstrate the position of the humeral head posterior to the glenoid. There may also be an impaction fracture of the humeral head as the posterior lip of the glenoid creates a V-shaped defect in the anterior aspect of the head (reverse Hill-Sachs lesion).

Treatment requires traction and an external rotation maneuver (as opposed to internal rotation in the anterior dislocation). This maneuver should be carried out by an orthopaedic surgeon and often requires general anesthesia.

Immobilization and rehabilitation are similar to those required for an anterior dislocation except the arm is immobilized at the side (holster position) and strengthening of the shoulder external rotators is stressed, rather than the internal rotator muscles.

THE MATURE ADULT WITH SHOULDER PAIN

Nontraumatic shoulder problems in the elderly are usually caused by degenerative conditions. Degenerative disc and joint diseases of the cervical spine may refer pain to the shoulder (a manifestation of cervical radiculopathy). Osteoarthritic degeneration of the acromioclavicular and glenohumeral joints and degenerative tendinitis are common ailments that cause shoulder pain.

Shoulder trauma in the elderly may cause an impacted fracture of the proximal humerus or a "hand-shoulder syndrome."

Nontraumatic Shoulder Problems in the Elderly

Chronic shoulder pain in the elderly should bring to mind cervical radiculopathy. Examination of the neck and neurologic examination of the upper and lower extremities should accompany the shoulder examination. X-ray evaluation should include views of the cervical spine as well as the shoulder.

Degenerative shoulder conditions may be present in the face of cervical radiculopathy. Both conditions must be diagnosed and treated for clinical relief of shoulder pain. Pain from tendinitis, acromioclavicular arthritis, and glenohumeral arthritis, responds to rest, heat, anti-inflammatory medication, and gentle rehabilitation to restore a full range of motion.

Rarely, a malignant pulmonary tumor in the apex of the lung (pancoast tumor) is the source of shoulder pain. A normal chest x-ray usually rules out this condition. If any questions concerning the chest film arise, the patient should be immediately referred to a pulmonary specialist or thoracic surgeon.

Traumatic Conditions

Falls on the shoulder or elbow often cause impacted fractures in the osteoporotic bone of the proximal humerus. These injuries, diagnosed by x-ray, cause severe pain and limitation of motion. Treatment requires a brief 10-day immobilization and gradual re-mobilization of the shoulder. If complete immobilization is maintained too long, full range of motion may never be restored.

At times, after an injury to the upper extremity, such as a Colles' fracture, the patient will complain of shoulder pain. In addition, the rehabilitation of the injured part (wrist, hand, or forearm) becomes complicated by pain, stiffness, and persistent swelling. This is the "hand-shoulder syndrome." The etiology of this problem is related to a reflex sympathetic dystrophy involving cervical nerve-root irritation and peripheral autonomic neurovascular responses. Treatment must be gentle, prolonged, and directed at all involved areas—neck, shoulder, and peripheral joints.

REHABILITATION OF THE INJURED SHOULDER

Three words describe the major goal of a rehabilitation program for the injured shoulder: motion, motion, and motion! Only after a full, or nearly full, range of motion is restored should the patient begin to rehabilitate the shoulder musculature for strength.

An appreciation of the capsular structure of the shoulder joint (lax and redundant with the arm at the side, and taut in the overhead position) is pivotal to successful rehabilitation. With injury comes posttraumatic synovitis and capsular fibrosis and shortening. This ruinous triad must be overcome in order to restore shoulder function to normal.

However, the problem is less critical in children and teenagers. The tissues are flexible and heal rapidly, and the patient is well motivated to return shoulder motion to normal in order to rejoin playmates and athletic teams. On the other hand, adults and older individuals have a more difficult recovery. Their tissues are not flexible; they are usually not as well motivated to recover as children, and pain (involved to some extent in all rehabilitation programs) is not well tolerated.

The program to restore normal shoulder motion should begin as soon as possible after the injury (or surgery). The onset of treatment depends upon the stability of the joint tissues (fractures, dislocations, and surgical reconstruction). It also depends upon the motivation of the patient, and factors such as fear and anxiety often need to be overcome by personal contact and encouragement.

In most cases, the injured shoulder, usually supported by a sling, can be moved within 72 hours of the injury. Immediately after the injury, the patient should be instructed to use the hand, wrist, and forearm as a "helping hand" in performing activities of daily living. Early shoulder motion begins in the sling with the so-called Codman exercises. These are performed by having the patient lean forward to allow the arm to hang free (with the elbow bent at 90°). Gravity allows the shoulder to assume a position of 90° of elevation (relative to the trunk of the body). This position eliminates the lax and redundant axillary pouch of the shoulder capsule.

From this relaxed "hung out" position, the patient is asked to begin making increasingly larger circles with the point of the elbow, first in one direction and then in the other. These exercises continue daily, at least temporarily, until the sling can be removed.

Without the sling, motion from 90° to 180° may be restored by two simple maneuvers. The patient is asked to stand at a door frame with both palms at shoulder height resting on the door frame. Then, using the fingertips, the patient climbs up the frame and down the frame, thus allowing the friction between the fingertips and the frame to move the shoulder joint. Gradually, the patient is encouraged to move closer to the door frame and stretch the shoulder structures to 180° overhead. This maneuver must be carried out with both the injured and uninjured extremities in order to prevent the patient from "cheating" by tilting the trunk away from the door frame, thereby reducing effective capsular stretch.

The second maneuver is carried out with the patient lying flat on the back without a pillow. There must be enough overhead room to allow the noninjured limb to be raised 180° to touch the resting surface. The patient then grasps the wrist of the injured limb with the noninjured hand and, using only the power of the noninjured extremity, lifts the injured arm upward. After 90° of elevation is obtained, gravity aids in bringing the arm from 90° to 180°. The arm is *always* brought back to the side by the normal extremity.

After 180° of elevation is achieved and stability of the joint or bone is ensured (at approximately 3 to 4 weeks), more strenuous exercises may begin in order to rehabilitate tendons and muscles. Active, assisted range of motion exercises begin in flexion-extension, internal and external rotation, and adduction-abduction. Strengthening exercises using light (1 to 2 lb) weights, isometric strengthening, and the use of rubber tubing exercises are next in the rehabilitation program. Active stretching of a small (2-foot) loop of rubber tubing is an excellent strengthening exercise. The patient may hold the tubing in front of the body with the opposite hand or in back of the trunk while stretching, thereby strengthening the shoulder rotators. Attaching the loop to a hook or a doorknob, or looping it around the foot allows the patient to control strengthening of most of the shoulder muscles.

The patient should use weighted or hydraulic gymnastic equipment in the final stage of strengthening and rehabilitation.

As long as the program proceeds gradually and progressively, there is no time limit. Some patients may be completely rehabilitated in 3 to 6 weeks. Others, due to the complexity of the injury or surgical reconstruction or due to patient factors (low pain threshold, high anxiety level, or poor motivation) may require 3 to 6 months or more. In general, after 1 year of an adequate rehabilitation program, very little further improvement can be expected.

The shoulder conditions described in this chapter constitute the major shoulder problems seen by medical and nursing personnel in an outpatient setting. It is not meant to be an exhaustive discourse on all shoulder conditions. The nurse-practitioner must know when to treat and when to refer the patient; and the information provided in this chapter should aid in making this decision. The interested reader should refer to texts mentioned in the bibliography for further information.

Recommended Reading

Bateman JE: *The Shoulder and Neck.* Philadelphia, WB Saunders, 1987.

Bremms J: Rotator cuff tear: evaluation and treatment. *Orthopedics* 11:69–86, 1988.

Craig EV: Total shoulder replacement: indication and results. *Orthopedics* 11:125–140, 1988.

DePalma AF: *Surgery of the Shoulder.* Philadelphia, JB Lippincott, 1973.

Ellman H: Shoulder arthroscopy: current indications and techniques. *Orthopedics* 11:45–56, 1988.

Gos TP: Anterior glenohumeral instability. *Orthopedics* 11:87–100, 1988.

Heppenstall RB: Fractures and dislocations of the distal clavicle. *Orthop Clin North Am* 6(2):477–486, 1975.

Heppenstall RB: Fractures of the proximal humerus. *Orthop Clin North Am* 6(2):467–476, 1975.

Murnaghan JT: Capsulitis of the shoulder: current concepts and treatment. *Orthopedics* 11:153–162, 1988.

Nixon JE, DiStefano V: Ruptures of the rotator cuff. *Orthop Clin North Am* 6(2):423–448, 1975.

Nixon JE, Schwamm HA: Do not go gentle. *University of Pennsylvania Orthopedic Journal* 3:41–45, 1987.

Rothman RH, Marvel JP Jr, Heppenstall RB: Anatomic considerations in the glenohumeral joint. *Orthop Clin North Am* 6(2):341–352, 1975.

Rothman RH, Marvel JP Jr, Heppenstall RB: Recurrent anterior dislocation of the shoulder. *Orthop Clin North Am* 6(2):415–422, 1975.

Rowe CR: *The Shoulder.* New York, Churchill-Livingstone, 1988.

Sherk HH, Probst C: Fractures of the proximal humeral epiphysis. *Orthop Clin North Am* 6(2):401–414, 1975.

Simon WH: Soft tissue disorders of the shoulder: frozen shoulder, calcific tendinitis, and bicipital tendinitis. *Orthop Clin North Am* 6(2):521–540, 1975.

Tyson RR, Kaplan GF: Modern concepts of diagnosis and treatment of the thoracic outlet syndrome. *Orthop Clin North Am* 6(2):507–520, 1975.

chapter 7

The Elbow, Forearm, Wrist, and Hand

HARRIS GELLMAN, M.D.

ELBOW AND FOREARM

Functional Anatomy

The elbow is a double hinge joint consisting of the humerus, ulna, and radius (Fig. 7.1). The spool-shaped trochlea of the humerus articulates with the trochlear notch of the ulna, and the capitulum of the humerus articulates with the head of the radius, thus allowing flexion and extension of the elbow. The elbow is enclosed by a relatively thin articular capsule.

The main stabilizer of the elbow is the triangular-shaped medial collateral ligament attaching from the medial epicondyle of the humerus to the medial side of the olecranon of the ulna (Fig. 7.2). The lateral collateral ligament is weaker with attachments from the lateral epicondyle of the humerus to the annular ligament. The annular ligament surrounds the proximal radius, stabilizing the proximal radioulnar joint, and allowing pronation and supination of the forearm. There are three elbow bursae that surround the elbow (Fig. 7.3). These bursae allow gliding between tissue planes. The bursa over the olecranon may become infected after a puncture wound or a chronic olecranon bursitis.

Forearm

The brachial artery crosses anterior to the elbow joint between the biceps tendon and the median nerve to supply vascularity to the forearm and hand. After crossing the elbow, the brachial artery divides into the radial artery and, a short distance later, bifurcates into the ulnar artery and the common interosseous artery. The ulnar nerve passes through the cubital tunnel posterior to the medial humeral epicondyle as it enters the flexor carpi ulnaris. It then continues distally into the forearm deep to the flexor carpi ulnaris lying on the flexor digitorum profundus.

The median nerve leaves the upper arm through cubital fossa by passing between the two heads of the pronator teres to lie deep to the flexor digitorum superficialis. This nerve then continues distally between this muscle and the flexor digitorum profundus. In the forearm it innervates the pronator teres, pronator quadratus, and all the finger and wrist flexors, except the flexor carpi ulnaris and the ulnar half of the flexor digitorum profundus, which are innervated by the ulnar nerve (Table 7.1).

The radial nerve divides into superficial and deep branches shortly after entering the cubital fossa. The superficial branch passes distally deep to the brachioradialis to supply sensibility to the dorsum of the hand. The deep branch (posterior interosseous nerve) pierces the supinator to innervate all the extensor muscles within the forearm (Fig. 7.4).

The flexor muscles of the forearm are divided into superficial and deep groups. The superficial group includes the pronator teres, flexor carpi radialis, and palmaris longus innervated by the median nerve, as

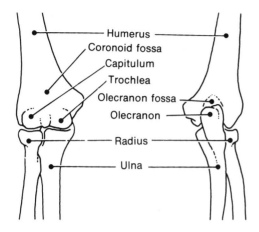

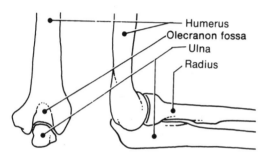

Figure 7.1. The elbow joint. **A**, Anterior view. **B**, Posterior view. **C**, Posterior view, 90° flexion. **D**, Lateral view. (From Ramamurti CP (Tinker RV, ed): *Orthopaedics in Primary Care*. Baltimore, Williams & Wilkins, 1979, p 53.)

well as the flexor carpi ulnaris innervated by the ulnar nerve. The superficial group originates from a common tendon on the medial epicondyle of the humerus. The deep group consists of the flexor pollicis longus, flexor digitorum profundus, and the pronator quadratus, all innervated by the median nerve except the ulnar half of the flexor digitorum profundus (ulnar nerve).

The flexors are separated from the extensors by the interosseous membrane, which passes between the radius and ulna. The extensor compartment (the dorsum of the forearm) contains the brachioradialis, extensor carpi radialis longus, extensor carpi radialis brevis, extensor digitorum communis, extensor digiti minimi, and extensor carpi ulnaris. The deep extensor group is made up of the abductor pollicis longus, the extensor pollicis brevis and longus, and the exten-

sor indicis proprius. All extensor muscles are supplied by the radial nerve.

History and Physical Examination

Taking the patient's history is somewhat analogous to being a reporter obtaining information for a story, particularly when the patient is a teenager or child. A good reporter asks "who, where, what, when, and how?" A good diagnostician needs to know that same information. The who is the patient; where does it hurt—is the pain diffuse or localized, stationary or migratory? What causes the pain and what makes it better? What was the patient doing when the pain started or the injury occurred? When does it hurt? (Tumors typically ache at night, arthritis aches more often in the morning.) Is the pain related to a particular activity such as pitching, or a particular position, or twisting motion? When did the injury occur—at play, at home, or at work? Finally, how did the injury occur—was the patient involved in an unusual or new activity?

Physical examination includes inspection, palpation, active and passive range of motion, vascular and sensory evaluation, and manual muscle testing. With the patient sitting or standing, begin with observation of the carrying angle. The normal arm should have a valgus (lateral) carrying angle of 5 to 15°. More then 15° valgus is called cubitus valgus, and a decrease in the angle to less than 5° is called cubitus varus. Abnormalities in the carrying angle are usually the result of a supracondylar or other elbow fracture in childhood.

Inspection

Inspect the skin for bruises, needle tracks, abrasions, scars, and swelling. Swelling occurs with inflammation, with joint effusions, and following forearm dislocation. A comparison to the opposite arm is useful for subtle cases. With an elbow effusion there is loss of soft tissue contours. Bursae may also be swollen and appear as discrete soft tissue swelling. This is particularly true with the olecranon bursa. Ecchymosis with swelling is suggestive of fracture or dislocation. Loss of symmetry and soft tissue

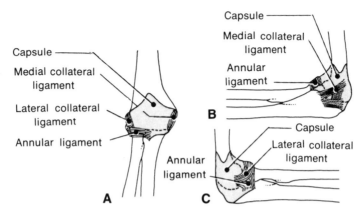

Figure 7.2. Articular capsule of the elbow joint. **A,** Anterior view. **B,** Medial view. **C,** Lateral view. (From Ramamurti CP (Tinker RV, ed): *Orthopaedics in Primary Care.* Baltimore, Williams & Wilkins, 1979, p 54.)

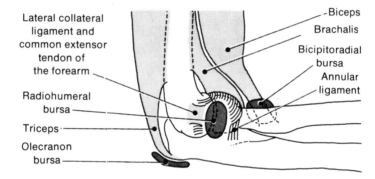

Figure 7.3. Three elbow bursae. The lateral collateral ligament, and common extensor tendon have been reflected away to expose the radiohumeral bursa. (From Ramamurti CP (Tinker RV, ed): *Orthopaedics in Primary Care.* Baltimore, Williams & Wilkins, 1979, p 54.)

contours may be secondary to dislocation. This presents as a deformity with loss of motion.

Palpation

The elbow is moved actively and passively through a normal range of motion. Normal active range of motion of the elbow should be between 0 and 5° extension to 135° flexion, with approximately 90° of pronation and supination (Fig. 7.5).

Synovitis may cause a limitation of normal extension. Assess the supracondylar area (medial aspect of the arm above the elbow) for an enlarged epitrochlear lymph node that would indicate an infection in the arm or hand. Palpate the bony prominences and check for crepitation. With one hand holding the anterior lateral aspect of the arm and with the hand around the biceps, abduct, flex, and extend the arm. Assess the quality of joint gliding, feeling for crepitants indicative of intraarticular pathology, adhesions, fractures, or osteoarthritis. Palpate the elbow for tenderness, warmth, or any changes from normal skin tone. Palpate the medial and lateral epicondyle and the radial head. When the patient's arm is abducted, locate the lateral epicondyle. Palpate along the insertions of the extensor muscles; tenderness here indicates lateral epicondylitis (tennis elbow). Palpate along the medial epicondyle along the insertion of the flexors; tenderness here indicates medial epicondylitis (golfer's elbow). The radial head lies laterally under the skin depression approximately 1 inch below the epicondyle. Tenderness of the

Table 7.1
Summary of Movements of the Forearm, Wrist, and Hand, and Their Chief Controllers[a]

Movement	Muscles	Nerves
Pronation of the forearm	Pronator teres	Median nerve
	Pronator quadratus	Median nerve
Supination of the forearm	Supinator	Radial nerve
	Biceps	Musculocutaneous nerve
Wrist flexion	Flexor carpi radialis	Median nerve
	Flexor carpi ulnaris	Ulnar nerve
	Palmaris longus	Median nerve
Wrist extension	Extensor carpi radialis longus	Radial nerve
	Extensor carpi radialis brevis	Radial nerve
	Extensor carpi ulnaris	Radial nerve
Radial deviation of the wrist	Abductor pollicis longus	Radial nerve
	Extensor pollicis brevis	Radial nerve
	Extensor carpi radialis longus and brevis	Radial nerve
Ulnar deviation of the wrist	Extensor carpi ulnaris	Radial nerve
	Flexor carpi ulnaris	Ulnar nerve
Flexors of the thumb		
Interphalangeal joint	Flexor pollicis longus	Median nerve
Metacarpophalangeal joint	Flexor pollicis brevis	Median nerve
Abduction of the thumb	Abductor pollicis longus	Radial nerve
	Abductor pollicis brevis	Median nerve
Opposition of the thumb	Opponens pollicis	Median nerve
Adduction of the thumb	Adductor pollicis	Ulnar nerve
Extension of the thumb		
Interphalangeal joint	Extensor pollicis longus	Radial nerve
Metacarpophalangeal joint	Extensor pollicis brevis	Radial nerve
Flexion of the fingers		
Distal interphalangeal joints	Flexor digitorum profundus	Median nerve and ulnar nerve
Proximal interphalangeal joints	Flexor digitorum sublimis	Median nerve
Metacarpophalangeal joints	Interosseous muscles	Ulnar nerve
	Lumbricals 1 and 2	Median nerve
	Lumbricals 3 and 4	Ulnar nerve
	Flexor digiti minimi	Ulnar nerve
Abduction of the fingers	Dorsal interosseous muscles	Ulnar nerve
	Abductor digiti minimi	Ulnar nerve
Adduction of the fingers	Palmar interosseous muscles	Ulnar nerve
Opposition of the 5th finger	Opponens digiti minimi	Ulnar nerve
Extension of the fingers	Extensor digitorum	Radial nerve
	Extensor indicis	Radial nerve
	Extensor digiti minimi	Radial nerve
Extension of interphalangeal joint while metacarpophalangeal joint is flexed	Lumbricals and palmar interosseous muscles	Median and ulnar nerves

[a]From Ramamurti CP (Tinker RV, ed): *Orthopaedics in Primary Care*. Baltimore, Williams & Wilkins, 1979, p 91.

radial head suggests a fracture, especially if pain increases with pronation and supination. Place the thumb over the radial head laterally and rotate the forearm. Have the patient slowly pronate and supinate the forearm. The radial head will rotate under your thumb. Pain with this maneuver may indicate inflammatory synovitis, osteoarthritis, or septic arthritis. Palpation continues over the olecranon surface. Tenderness at the insertion of the triceps tendon is seen with tendinitis. Tenderness over the olecranon surface is seen with olecranon bursitis. Palpation of the medial surface includes the ulnar nerve, which lies in a bony groove just below the medial epicondyle. Percussion in this area may produce the sensation of electric shocks or pain ("funny bone"). Next gently roll the ulnar nerve between your middle and index fingers. It should be soft and round. Thickening may indicate scar build-up that may lead to

PALMAR (FLEXOR)   DORSAL (EXTENSOR)

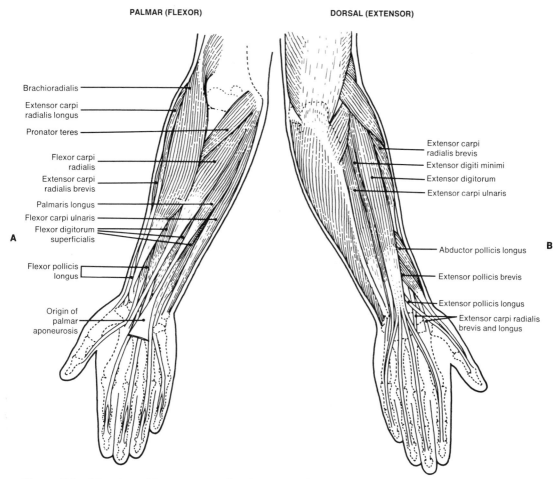

Brachioradialis

Extensor carpi
radialis longus

Pronator teres

Flexor carpi
radialis

Extensor carpi
radialis brevis

Palmaris longus

Flexor carpi ulnaris

Flexor digitorum
superficialis

A

Flexor pollicis
longus

Origin of
palmar
aponeurosis

Extensor carpi
radialis brevis

Extensor digiti minimi

Extensor digitorum

Extensor carpi ulnaris

Abductor pollicis longus

Extensor pollicis brevis

Extensor pollicis longus

Extensor carpi radialis
brevis and longus

B

Figure 7.4. Muscles of forearm; muscles that move fingers. **A**, Anterior. **B**, Posterior. (From Hilt NE, Cogburn SB: *Manual of Orthopaedics*. St. Louis, CV Mosby, 1980.)

compression of the ulnar nerve as it passes through the tunnel and may result in paresthesias that pass along the ulnar distribution. With the elbow fully flexed and fully extended, evaluate the olecranon bursa for swelling and bogginess. Synovitis is palpable as a boggy, or fluctuant, fullness. Evaluate the stability of the medial and lateral collateral ligaments. Cup one hand over the posterior aspect of the patient's elbow and hold the patient's wrist with the other. Instruct the patient to slightly flex the elbow. With the elbow flexed force the forearm laterally. Note any gapping on the medial side. Reverse the direction and force the forearm medially. Note any gapping on the lateral side (Fig. 7.6). Figure 7.7 will

help the examiner with the differential diagnosis.

Muscle Testing

Apply resistance at the wrist as the patient flexes the elbow, and apply resistance on the dorsum as the patient extends the elbow. (Muscle testing of the wrist and hand will be covered in the sections on the wrist and hand.) Evaluation of the radial, median, and ulnar nerves is found in Figure 7.8**A, B,** and **C.**

Vascular Examination

Evaluate the distal pulses, capillary refill, and skin temperature.

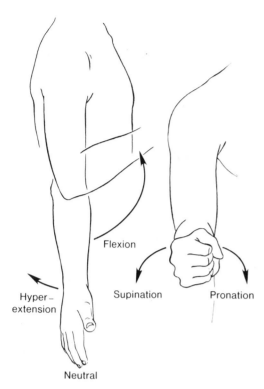

Figure 7.5. Range of motion of the elbow. (From Burnside JW, McGlynn TJ: *Physical Diagnosis*, ed 17. Baltimore, Williams & Wilkins, 1987.)

Special Tests

Tinel's Sign. Tinel's sign is a tenderness or a sensation of electric shocks radiating into the hand when there is tapping over the ulnar nerve where it passes through the groove between the olecranon and the medial epicondyle (cubital tunnel). This may be due to neuroma formation or compression of the ulnar nerve as it passes around the elbow.

Tennis Elbow Test. Stabilize the patient's forearm with one hand. Instruct the patient to make a fist while extending the wrist. Attempt to force the wrist into flexion by applying pressure with your other hand to the dorsum of the fist. If the patient has lateral epicondylitis (tennis elbow) there will be tenderness over the insertion of the wrist extensor muscles of the lateral epicondyle of the humerus.

Diagnostic Guidelines

Radiographic examination should be performed whenever a fracture or dislo-

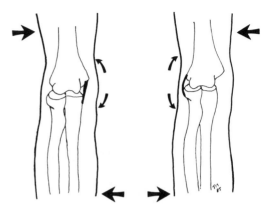

Figure 7.6. Test the integrity of ligaments by exerting medially and laterally directed pressure as shown. If the ligaments are ruptured, abnormal opening of the joint space will occur. (From Burnside JW, McGlynn TJ: *Physical Diagnosis*, ed 17. Baltimore, Williams & Wilkins, 1987.)

cation is suspected. Additionally, radiographs may detect an occult tumor that, although rare, might otherwise be missed.

The Adolescent with Elbow Pain

Pain in the elbow of the throwing arm is a common problem best exemplified by the baseball pitcher. A detailed history includes the precise location of the pain. Referred pain to the forearm may indicate soft tissue inflammation or peripheral nerve irritation. Locking or catching may indicate loose bodies in the anterior or posterior

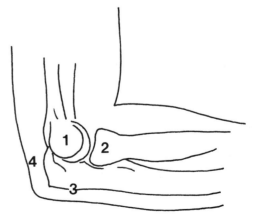

Figure 7.7. Common points of elbow tenderness. *1*, lateral epicondylitis; *2*, radial head fracture; *3*, olecranon bursitis; *4*, triceps tendinitis.

Sensation   Motor function

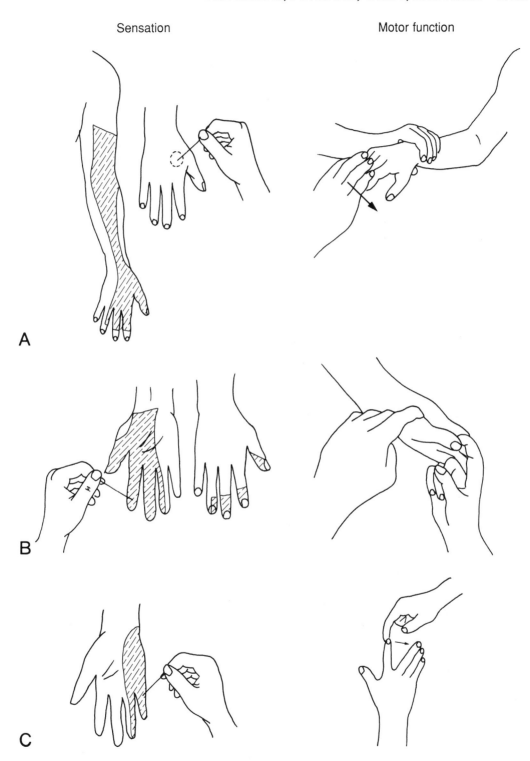

Figure 7.8. Sensation and motor function of radial (**A**), median (**B**), and ulnar (**C**) nerves. **A** from Roy S, Irvin R: *Sports Medicine: Prevention, Evaluation, Management, and Rehabilitation.* Englewood Cliffs, NJ, Prentice-Hall, 1983; **B** and **C** from McRae R: Clinical orthopaedic examination. Churchill Livingstone, Edinburgh, 1976.

compartment of the elbow. Following exercise, recurrent swelling and stiffness of the elbow joint may indicate osteochondritis dissecans. A history of loss of range of motion is common and nonspecific. Examination should be carried out both with the patient sitting and standing. Stability should be checked with the elbow both in full extension and in 45° flexion. Medial stability is tested by applying a valgus stress to the forearm and comparing this to the opposite elbow. An abnormal amount of opening (laxity) of the elbow joint or an increase in pain should make one suspicious of an injury to this area. Lateral stability is tested by repeating the above but applying a varus stress (Fig. 7.6). If instability of the elbow is present, either acute or chronic, a referral should be made for further evaluation and treatment. Even mild instability, if left untreated, can result in the development of premature degenerative arthritis of the elbow joint. If the injury is acute, a long arm posterior splint should be applied and immediate referral made; if the injury is chronic, a splint may not be necessary but the patient should still be referred for further evaluation.

"Little Leaguer's Elbow"

Little leaguer's elbow is a lateral compression injury of the throwing elbow, often resulting in osteonecrosis. Resultant osteochondritis dissecans is the leading cause of permanent elbow disability in pitching athletes. These injuries usually occur in the youngest, least experienced pitchers. Treatment in the skeletally immature patient should consist of rest, immobilization, and anti-inflammatories. Severe flexion contractures and even partial ankylosis may occur as a result of these injuries. Surgery is not usually recommended in the adolescent, as the prognosis after surgery is poor. The basic approach is palliative and many patients will have progression of symptoms at a future date. If a bony injury or loose body is suspected, obtain anteroposterior, lateral, and oblique radiographs of the elbow, and anteroposterior views of the forearm and humerus. If the symptoms persist, an arthrogram or bone scan may be necessary.

The predisposing factors that increase the adolescent's risk for injury are the unfused epiphysis and immature bones. This epiphysis is the last to close.

Prevention of elbow pain is possible if weaknesses found on the preseason examination are corrected. Proper strengthening and flexibility exercises along with aerobic conditioning will decrease fatigue and will build endurance. The young athlete must understand that the best protection for the pitching arm is a 12-month conditioning program. Proper warm-up prior to playing followed by gentle stretching and ice applied directly to the elbow following a game or practice are vital. Coaching techniques now limit the number of throws during practice and the number of curve balls during a game, and these techniques also stress correct throwing mechanics. Instruct the athlete to do the same with pick-up games.

Elbow Dislocation

Dislocations of the elbow are frequent, surpassed in frequency only by shoulder dislocations (Fig. 7.9). As with other types of dislocations, the patient should be referred immediately for further evaluation and the reduction should be done as soon as possible. This is especially important in elbow dislocations as the rapid onset of swelling can result in compression of the neurovascular structures that pass in front of the elbow joint. The immediate danger

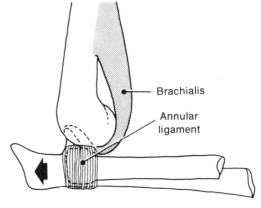

Brachialis

Annular ligament

Figure 7.9. Dislocation of the elbow. (From Ramamurti CP (Tinker RV, ed): *Orthopaedics in Primary Care.* Baltimore, Williams & Wilkins, 1979, p 70.)

with persistent swelling at the elbow joint is that circulation to the forearm is decreased, resulting in a possible Volkmann's ischemic contracture of the forearm and hand. Dislocations are named according to the position of the proximal radius and ulna (olecranon) relative to the distal humerus. Posterior dislocations of the radius and ulna are the most frequent primary elbow dislocations. The deformity is usually obvious; the patient presents with pain and restriction of motion. The most common mechanism is direct trauma from a fall on the outstretched forearm held in extension. Many patients have a concomitant wrist injury and the examiner must look for this. If a wrist injury is suspected obtain AP and lateral radiographs of the forearm and wrist. A significant amount of soft tissue injury, including tearing of one or both collateral ligaments about the elbow, is necessary to allow the elbow to dislocate. Physical examination includes documentation of the neurovascular status including brachial and radial pulses, capillary refill in the fingers, and median, ulnar, and radial nerve function. If this documentation is not performed it will be difficult to tell when a nerve injury noticed only after reduction happened—at the time of dislocation or during the reduction maneuver. Median nerve function is checked by testing sensation to the palmar pulp of the thumb and index finger. Although a pinprick will give a gross indication that median nerve function is present, a two-point discrimination test gives a much better evaluation of the status of the nerve at the time of the test. Normal two-point discrimination should be 6 mm or less. The test can easily be performed by bending the prongs of a small paper clip and setting the distance between the prongs to measure 6 mm. The two points of the paper clip are then lightly applied to the volar pulp of the index finger and thumb to test the median nerve, and then to the small finger to test the ulnar nerve. The autonomous sensory zone of the radial nerve is on the dorsum of the hand in the web space between the thumb and index finger. Sensory testing of the radial nerve is more difficult; pinprick and soft touch are usually sufficient. Muscle function should also be tested: thumb and index finger flexion and thumb opposition test the median nerve; flexion of the tip (DIP joint) of the small finger and the ability to abduct the small finger away from the ring finger tests ulnar nerve function; and the ability to extend the fingers at the MCP joints and extension of the thumb test the posterior (deep) branch of the radial nerve. The ability to extend the wrist, but not the fingers, points to a lesion of the radial nerve after it has crossed the elbow and become the posterior (deep) interosseous branch of the radial nerve. If the radial nerve is injured above the elbow (as with a displaced humeral shaft fracture) then the patient will also be unable to extend the wrist. AP, lateral, and oblique radiographs should be obtained and examined for possible fractures before reduction is attempted. If this is not possible an attempt at mild reduction should be performed due to the danger of impending Volkmann's ischemia from increased swelling in the unreduced elbow. If the elbow is reduced prior to obtaining radiographs, they are essential postreduction to rule out other associated fractures.

Reduction should only be attempted by experienced personnel who have been trained in the evaluation and management of bony injuries, fractures, and dislocations. An attempted reduction of an elbow dislocation by an inexperienced individual can result in accidental fracture of the humerus or ulna or accidental tearing of the brachial artery or one of the nerves crossing the elbow joint. In most cases splinting the patient in a comfortable position and immediate referral are all that is necessary. The technique of reduction, however, is described as follows.

An assistant applies gentle countertraction on the distal humerus by placing his/her hands around the anterior portion of the distal humeral shaft. Following appropriate countertraction, downward traction is applied to the proximal portion of the forearm, which brings the coronoid out of the olecranon fossa. With gentle downward traction continuously applied, the entire forearm is brought into a position of flexion of the elbow. In most instances the elbow will be felt to reduce with this maneuver. If reduction cannot be achieved easily, or if pulses are not present prior to or after reduction the patient should be transported immediately to an emergency facility, as surgical reduction and exploration may be necessary. After reduction, radiographs are again taken to assess the adequacy of reduction. A repeat neurovascular examination should also be performed. The patient is placed into a well padded posterior splint holding the elbow in 100 to 110° of flexion. Stable patients are allowed active flexion after 1 week and may remove the splint for range of motion exercise. The splints remain in place until full extension is achieved. Unstable patients are splinted in flexion for 2 to 3 weeks and then begin an active physical therapy exercise program in a protective hinged elbow orthosis. Radiographs should be taken during this 2 to 3 week period to be sure the elbow remains reduced. All of these patients should be admitted to a hospital overnight to allow monitoring of the neurovascular status of the extremity.

Other Fractures around the Elbow

These other fractures are usually signaled by the patient's complaint of pain and deformity. A long-arm posterior splint should be applied and referral to an appropriate facility should be made. If there is a history of a fall and point tenderness is found on examination, a posterior splint should be applied and referral should be made even if no obvious deformity is observed.

The Adult with Elbow Pain

Tennis Elbow (Lateral Epicondylitis)

By far the most common cause of elbow pain in patients seeking orthopaedic assistance is lateral epicondylitis, frequently referred to as tennis elbow. It is generally believed to be a strain of the common extensor origin. Individuals with occupations that require repetitive work, such as with hammers or screwdrivers, that causes rotation of a pronated forearm are just as likely to develop the problem as the tennis player.

The patient, usually in the 35 to 50 age group, complains of pain radiating from the lateral epicondyle of the humerus along the dorsum of the forearm. The patient may also experience difficulty holding any heavy object at arm's length. A similar syndrome may involve the medial epicondyle (golfer's elbow) but the lateral epicondyle is involved approximately 7 times more frequently. On palpation, the insertion of the extensor musculature into the lateral epicondyle is usually the most painful point (Fig. 7.7). Resisted wrist extension and radial deviation intensify the pain. The radiographic examination should include anteroposterior, lateral, and both medial and lateral oblique views of the elbow. Although radiographic examination is usually negative, occasionally a bony avulsion injury from the medial or lateral epicondyle or a fracture may be seen. The differential diagnosis includes primary pathology of the elbow joint or entrapment syndrome of radial nerve sensory branches at the elbow. This may be the cause in the patient whose tennis elbow is refractory to all attempts at conservative management. Treatment of both lateral and medial epicondylitis is similar and is directed to correction and prevention of reinjury. In the acute phase the extremity should rest to allow healing. Splinting with a removable splint that maintains the wrist in 20° of extension relieves tension on the wrist extensor tendons. Activities that exacerbate the pain should be eliminated and anti-inflammatory medications should be administered. After the 1st week, refer the patient to physical therapy for therapeutic exercise that allows active range of motion of the elbow and active wrist exercises. Wrist exercises are done with the forearm supported on a table and the wrist suspended over the edge to permit wrist extension with radial and ulnar deviation and circumduction. When five repetitions can be done without pain, a 1 lb pound weight is held, and the weight then gradually increased as tolerated (Fig. 7.10). Symptoms usually resolve after 4 to 6 weeks. If treatment is unsuccessful, a steroid injection mixed with lidocaine or surgery may be necessary. Reinjury can be prevented by properly warming up prior

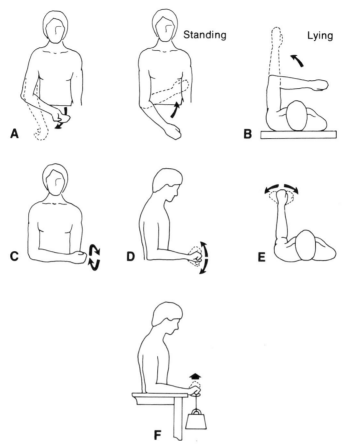

Figure 7.10.   Rehabilitation exercises for disorders of the elbow. **A**, Common extensor tendon stretching for mild tennis elbow. **B**, Acute flexion/extension with and against gravity. **C**, Unopposed forearm rotation. **D** and **E**, Range of motion exercises for the wrist. **F**, Common extensor strengthening exercise. (From Ramamurti CP (Tinker RV, ed): *Orthopaedics in Primary Care*. Baltimore, Williams & Wilkins, 1979, p 56.)

to exercising, particularly for sports activities that require throwing or pitching. For workers it is important to increase the strength of the wrist extensors to the level of the uninvolved extremity prior to returning to the previous level of occupational related activity.

Olecranon Bursitis

Olecranon bursitis is common in carpet layers and others who repeatedly traumatize the posterior aspect of the elbow joint. Swelling of the olecranon bursa is also common in infection, gout, and rheumatoid arthritis. With rheumatoid arthritis there may be associated subcutaneous nodular masses in the proximal part (extensor surface) of the forearm. Acute bursitis is painful; chronic bursitis is usually painless and often resolves spontaneously, unless there is an associated bacterial infection within the bursa. The swelling may be fluctuant and warm. The patient may have decreased elbow flexion and increased pain with flexion beyond 90° and when resting the forearm on a table.

It is essential to distinguish septic from nonseptic bursitis. Refer the patient for aspiration with a 16 or 18 gauge needle. Normally this fluid is clear or straw colored and of serous consistency. Send the aspirated fluid to the microbiology lab for culture, Gram stain, and crystals to rule out infection and gout. If infection is present the patient is treated with antibiotics. Following aspiration the elbow is splinted for 2 to 3 weeks; this usually results in cure. To prevent recurrence local protection such as an elastic band can be applied around the elbow. If the bursitis is recurrent and painful, surgical excision may be necessary.

Ulnar Nerve Entrapment of the Elbow (Cubital Tunnel Syndrome)

Ulnar nerve entrapment, with its frequent accompaniment of small muscle wasting and sensory impairment in the hand, may occur as a complication of local trauma at the elbow or wrist but is most often idiopathic. Inflammation of the ulnar nerve commonly occurs at the elbow where the nerve is abnormally mobile. In these circumstances, the nerve is exposed to frictional damage as it slips repeatedly in front of and behind the medial epicondyle. The nerve is also subject to pressure as it passes between the two heads of the flexor carpi ulnaris below the elbow. This is a common area of compression in weight lifters. Frequent symptoms of ulnar nerve compression at the elbow are paresthesias in the hand, tenderness of the nerve at the elbow, a positive Tinel sign on percussion of the nerve as it passes through the cubital tunnel, and wasting of the small muscles of the hand. The differential diagnosis of ulnar nerve symptoms at the elbow should include metabolic abnormalities such as diabetes or rheumatoid arthritis and infectious diseases such as lepromatous leprosy, which often presents with ulnar nerve palsy. Cubitus valgus at the elbow can result in a tardy ulnar palsy usually appearing between the ages of 30 and 50. Physical examination includes grip strength, sensory testing of the small and ring fingers, motor examination of the ulnar innervated flexors, examination of the small muscles of the hand for wasting, and palpation of the ulnar nerve at the elbow. If on initial presentation there is no evidence of muscle wasting in the hand (compare the involved and uninvolved hands), and the sensory examination of the palmar pulp of the small finger is normal (two point discrimination is less than or equal to 6 mm), then initial treatment is conservative with anti-inflam-

matory medications and splinting of the elbow for 3 weeks to rest the nerve. Occasionally, an injection of l ml of 20 to 40 mg/ml Depo-Medrol or triamcinolone into the cubital tunnel will be necessary, but great care should be taken not to inject into the nerve or too close to the nerve. If conservative management is unsuccessful, or if at the time of initial presentation muscle wasting is present or sensory testing is abnormal, the patient should be referred for evaluation for surgical release of the nerve. Prior to surgical release electromyography and nerve conduction testing is necessary to localize the lesion to the elbow and to be sure there is no pathology at the level of the wrist.

Forearm Injuries

Crush Injuries. A common industrial injury is a crushing injury to the forearm. Usually no serious injury occurs, but affected patients should be observed for the development of a compartment syndrome as a result of swelling, nerve injuries from direct compression, or vascular injuries. Obtain anteroposterior and lateral radiographs of the forearm (elbow to wrist) to rule out fracture or dislocation. Physical examination should focus on the neurovascular examination and signs of impending compartment syndrome. *Pain with passive stretch of the fingers and decreased sensibility of the fingers are the earliest signs of impending compartment syndrome.* Pulselessness is not a reliable sign of compartment syndrome as the pulse is not usually lost. For minor injuries, ice packs to decrease the swelling, along with elevation, splinting, and follow-up by an orthopaedist usually will be all that is required. For severe injuries with open lacerations, a referral to an emergency facility should be made initially. Patients may be hospitalized and compartment pressures monitored with a slit catheter or other compartment pressure monitoring device.

WRIST AND HAND

Anatomy

Joints

The wrist joint includes the distal radius, ulna, and the proximal row of carpal bones (the scaphoid, lunate, and triquetrum) (Fig. 7.11). The distal radius articulates both with the ulna, through a pivot-type joint lying between the head of the ulna and the ulnar notch of the radius, and the carpus through the radiocarpal joint. An articular disc of fibrocartilage is attached to the medial edge of the distal radius and the internal surface of the styloid process of the ulna. This separates the proximal row of carpal bones from the distal ulna. The articular capsule enclosing the joint is strengthened by dorsal and palmar radiocarpal ligaments and the radial and ulnar collateral ligaments. The carpus is made up of eight bones (scaphoid, lunate, triquetrum, pisiform, trapezium, trapezoid, hamate, capitate) aligned in two transverse rows, with dorsal and palmar intercarpal ligaments passing transversely, and interosseous intercarpal ligaments linking the lateral borders of the proximal row to the distal row of bones providing intercarpal stability. The midcarpal joint lies between the proximal and distal rows and allows a considerable range of movement. The hand consists of five metacarpals, five proximal phalanges, four middle phalanges, and five

distal phalanges. The thumb (first) metacarpal articulates with the trapezium in a saddle-shaped joint (trapeziometacarpal joint). The bases of the second through fifth metacarpals are connected to each other and to the distal carpal row by dorsal, palmar, and interosseous ligaments that form the carpometacarpal joints. The deep transverse metacarpal ligaments connect the heads of the metacarpals on the palmar aspect and thereby limit abduction of these bones. The metacarpophalangeal joints are formed by the rounded head of the metacarpals articulating with the concavities of the bases of the proximal phalanges. The joint capsules are reinforced dorsally by the extensor tendons. Palmar ligaments (volar plates) bridge the joints on the palmar aspect of the hand and are continuous with the strong cordlike collateral ligaments that attach proximally to the tubercle of the metacarpal and distally to the lateral aspect of the base of the proximal phalanx. The interphalangeal joints are hinge-type joints that are structurally the same as the metacarpophalangeal articulations with a palmar ligament and two collateral ligaments reinforced dorsally by the extensor expansion.

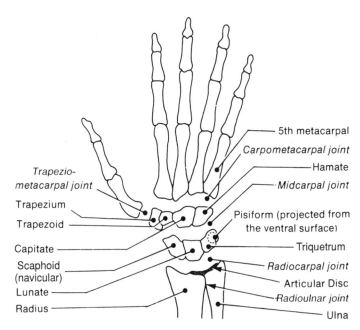

Figure 7.11. Skeletal anatomy of the wrist—dorsal view. (From Ramamurti CP (Tinker RV, ed): *Orthopaedics in Primary Care.* Baltimore, Williams & Wilkins, 1979, p 76.)

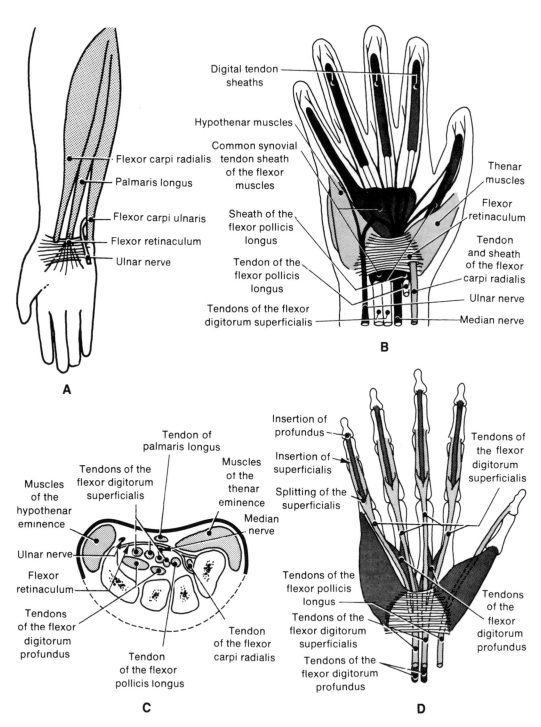

Figure 7.12.   Palmar tendons of the wrist and hand. **A**, superficial tendons. **B**, nerves and tendons deep to the palmaris longus. **C**, transverse section of the carpal tunnel. **D**, relationships of the flexor digitorum in the hand.

Muscles and Tendons

The tendons of the flexor and extensor muscles pass from the forearm to the hand and fingers (Fig. 7.12). The four flexor digitorum sublimus tendons flex the proximal interphalangeal (PIP) joints of the fingers. The four flexor digitorum profundus tendons flex the distal interphalangeal (PIP) joints of the fingers. The thumb interphalangeal joint is flexed by the flexor pollicis longus. The metacarpophalangeal (MCP) joints of the fingers are flexed by the small intrinsic muscles in the hand. The MCP joint of the thumb is flexed by the flexor pollicis brevis.

Extension of the fingers at the MCP joints is achieved by the extensor digitorum communis tendons coming from the forearm (Fig. 7.13). The index and small fingers can also be independently extended by the extensor indicis proprius and extensor digiti minimi, respectively. PIP and DIP joint extension in the fingers is done primarily by the small intrinsic muscles in the hand. Extension of the interphalangeal joint of the thumb is achieved by the extensor pollicis longus; extension at the MCP joint is achieved by the extensor pollicis brevis, and abduction of the thumb is achieved by the abductor pollicis longus. The tendons of the extensor pollicis brevis and the abductor pollicis longus cross from the forearm to the hand through a common sheath in the first dorsal compartment. This is a common area for tenosynovitis (de Quervain's syndrome).

The intrinsic muscles of the hand are divided into three groups: the thenar muscles (abductor pollicis brevis, flexor pollicis brevis, and opponens pollicis) innervated by the median nerve; the hypothenar muscles (abductor digiti minimi, flexor digiti minimi brevis, and opponens digiti minimi) innervated by the ulnar nerve; and the interossei and lumbricals.

Arteries and Nerves

After leaving the forearm the ulnar artery enters the hand by passing to the radial side of the pisiform bone to give muscular branches to the hand. The artery terminates by dividing into a deep branch that joins with a similar branch of the radial

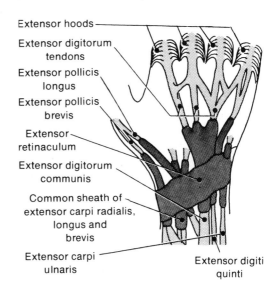

Figure 7.13. Extensor tendons of the wrist and fingers. (From Ramamurti CP (Tinker RV, ed): *Orthopaedics in Primary Care.* Baltimore, Williams & Wilkins, 1979, p 80.)

artery and forms the deep palmar arch as well as a superficial branch that joins with a similar branch of the radial artery and forms the superficial palmar arch. The latter, predominantly from the ulnar artery, lies transverse in the palm immediately under the palmar aponeurosis in line with the fully extended thumb. It gives off the common palmar digital branches, which become the proper digital arteries to supply contiguous sides of the fingers. Passing from the anterior surface of the radius medial to the styloid process, the radial artery enters the hand deep to the tendons of the abductor pollicis longus and the extensor pollicis longus and brevis. Branches of the radial artery include the superficial palmar, which joins the similar branch of the ulnar artery to form the superficial palmar arch. The princeps pollicis and the indicis proprius branches arise as the radial artery pierces the first dorsal interosseous muscle. They supply, respectively, both sides of the thumb and the radial side of the index finger. The deep branch forms the deep palmar arch with the deep branch of the ulnar artery. The deep arch lies on the carpal bones approximately 2 cm proximal to the superficial arch. Branches of the deep arch are the palmar metacarpal arteries. These join the common palmar digital arteries of the superficial arch to supply the fingers.

The circulation of the hand is evaluated by noting the color of the skin and fingernails. The Allen test, which determines the patency of the vessels supplying the hand, is performed as follows:

(1) Compress the radial and ulnar arteries at the wrist.

(2) Have the patient make a tight fist (three or four times to exsanguinate the blood from the hand) and open it into a relaxed position. Avoid forced extension of the fingers; this will maintain blanching.

(3) Release the ulnar artery only while continuing to compress the radial artery. The fingers and palm should fill with blood and the normal pink color should return.

(4) Repeat steps 1 and 2 and repeat the test for the radial artery. This test can also be carried out on a single finger by expressing the blood from the finger and occluding both digital arteries. The test is performed for the radial and then the ulnar digital artery, noting the filling of the finger. This helps to evaluate the patency of each digital vessel to the finger.

The median nerve enters the hand by passing through the carpal tunnel under the flexor retinaculum and transverse carpal ligament along with nine flexor tendons (FDS-4, FDP-4, and FPL). It supplies branches to the thenar muscles as well as the two radial lumbricals. Terminally the nerve supplies cutaneous innervation to the central area of the palm and palmar surface of the thumb, index, middle, and lateral half of the ring fingers, and all of the skin on the distal phalanges of these digits. At the wrist the ulnar nerve divides into a superficial branch that supplies cutaneous innervation to both surfaces of the hand ulnar to a line passing through the midline of the ring finger and a deep branch that supplies all the intrinsic muscles of the hand, except those innervated by the median nerve. The deep branch pierces the opponens digiti minimi muscle and passes around the hook of the hamate to cross the palm with the

deep palmar arch. The radial nerve innervates no muscles in the hand. Its terminal distribution is the cutaneous innervation to a small area on the palmar surface of the thenar eminence and the dorsum of the hand radial to a line passing through the midline of the ring finger, except for the skin over the distal phalanges.

Physical Examination of the Hand and Wrist

Inspect for swelling, erythema, open wounds, or drainage. Note any deformity of the wrist such as radial deviation of the hand that may be seen with Colles' fracture or ulnar deviation as seen in rheumatoid arthritis. Thenar wasting is suggestive of carpal tunnel syndrome or median nerve injury of any etiology. Dorsal swellings are commonly found with ganglions or rheumatoid synovitis. Palmar flexion of the wrist may make a small ganglion more noticeable. Palpate for areas of tenderness or fluctuance. Tenderness in the anatomic snuffbox is common with scaphoid fractures but is also seen with wrist sprains and other minor injuries (Fig. 7.14).

Pain with pronation and supination at the distal radioulnar joint is common with injury to this joint after a Colles' fracture. Diffuse tenderness is common in all inflam-

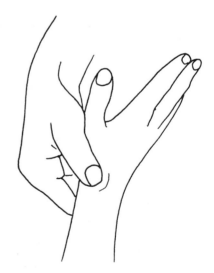

Figure 7.14. Palpation of snuff box. Tenderness suggests a navicular fracture.

matory conditions, whether infections or noninfections. Tenderness and thickening localized to the sheaths of the abductor pollicis longus and extensor pollicis brevis are suggestive of de Quervain's tenosynovitis. Paresthesia with percussion of the median or ulnar nerves at the wrist is suggestive of nerve compression. Observation of active and passive range of motion is a very important part of any examination. Normal wrist motion is 70° dorsiflexion, 75° palmar flexion, 20° radial deviation, and 35° ulnar deviation. Limitations suggest radiocarpal or intercarpal pathology. Pronation of approximately 90° and supination of 90° should be achieved without pain. Limitation suggests a disturbance of the distal radioulnar joint. In the fingers there should be approximately 0 to 90° active motion at the MCP joints; 0 to 100° of motion at the PIP joints, and 0 to 80° motion of the DIP joints. All of the joints of the fingers are involved in grasping and holding, and therefore, when the patient is asked to make a fist, all of the distal phalanges normally will touch the palm at right angles. A loss of motion at any level will result in an inability to touch the injured finger to the palm. The thumb has a slightly different range from that of the fingers, with approximately 55° of flexion at the MCP joint and 20° extension to 80° flexion at the IP joint (100° IP ARC). There should be approximately 60° of abduction of the thumb in a plane at right angles to the palm. Opposition is a composite motion involving abduction of the thumb at right angles to the palm, flexion, and rotation. Normally the thumb should touch the tip of the small finger. Opposition is achieved by the intrinsic muscles of the thumb; loss of opposition occurs with median nerve pathology as with carpal tunnel syndrome. Nerves and muscles are then examined. Sensibility evaluation of the thumb, index, and long fingers tests the median nerve; the small finger and ulnar half of the ring finger test the ulnar nerve; and the web space on the dorsum between the thumb and index finger tests the radial nerve. Flexor tendon function may be abnormal because of tendon, muscle, or nerve injury. The wrist is flexed by the flexor carpi radialis and flexor carpi ulnaris. Flexion of the PIP joints of all fingers is done by the flexor digitorum sublimus (median nerve). The distal interphalangeal joints of the fingers are flexed by the flexor digitorum profundus (FDP). The FDP to the index, long, and part of the ring finger is innervated by the median nerve and the FDP to the small and part of the ring finger is innervated by the ulnar nerve. The long flexor to the thumb (FPL) flexes the IP joint and is median innervated. Extension of the wrist is accomplished by the extensor carpi radialis longus and brevis and extensor carpi ulnaris. Finger extension is done primarily by the extensor digitorum communis, but independent extension of the index and small fingers is performed by the extensor indicis proprius and extensor digiti quinti minimi, respectively. The IP joint of the thumb is extended by the extensor pollicis longus. On the dorsum of the wrist are six compartments for the extensor tendons. The first dorsal compartment contains the EPB and ALP; the second, ECRB and ECRL; the third, EPL; the fourth, EDC and EIP; fifth, EDQM; and sixth, ECU. All extensor musculature is innervated by the deep branch of the radial nerve (posterior interosseous nerve) (Table 7.1).

Special Diagnostic Tests

Allen Test

See Arteries and Nerves.

Tinel Test

This test is performed by having the examiner gently tap the area over the median nerve at the wrist palmarly. While this can be done with a reflex hammer, it is better to use the examiner's long finger bent 90° at the PIP joint as this joint is more sensitive. The test result is considered positive if this produces tingling in the fingers.

Phalen's (Wrist-Flexion) Test

The patient actively places the wrist in complete but unforced flexion. If numbness and tingling are produced or exaggerated in the median nerve distribution of the hand within 60 seconds, the test result is considered positive.

The Painful Hand and Wrist

Colles' (Distal Radius) Fracture

The most common wrist injury in any age group is a fracture of the distal radius. Most distal radius fractures are referred to as Colles' fractures whether or not they are true Colles' fractures. The mechanism of injury is a fall on the outstretched arm with the wrist extended. The classic deformity is described as a "silver fork" deformity with dorsal swelling and displacement of the hand and wrist. A splint should be applied from the fingers to above the elbow, and the extremity should be elevated. Many distal radius fractures are intraarticular and require open reduction and internal fixation. Although cast immobilization is often adequate after reduction, newer techniques of internal and external fixation have greatly improved the results of severely comminuted, displaced fractures. After distal radius fractures, patients usually require 6 weeks in a cast, after cast removal many patients require therapy to regain strength and wrist motion. It is important to be sure that active finger flexion and extension exercises are performed while the patient is in the cast. It may require 3 to 6 months after the fracture before the patient is able to return to full activity. Most patients can return to work after 8 to 10 weeks.

Scaphoid Fracture

The scaphoid fracture is one of the most troublesome of the wrist injuries. The scaphoid is one of the light carpal bones in the wrist and is the one most often fractured. A fracture usually occurs as a result of a fall on the extended wrist with a pronation of the forearm on the fixed hand. Because the scaphoid bone is completely intraarticular in the wrist, it is surrounded by cartilage and has a sparse blood supply. The combination of these factors with the lack of stability of the bone after fracture and the surrounding of the scaphoid by synovial fluid in the wrist joint results in a high rate of nonunion. Patients complain of wrist pain and tenderness in the snuff box (Fig. 7.14). Many times patients (as well as many physicians) ascribe the pain to the sprain and, without an x-ray, the fracture will be missed. Radiographs should include AP, lateral, and oblique views in the wrist. For additional definition of the scaphoid, AP radiographs should be taken with the wrist positioned in radial and ulnar deviation. Treatment of nondisplaced fractures differs from fractures with an element of displacement. If the fracture is nondisplaced initial treatment is by application of a long arm thumb spica cast and referral to an orthopaedist for follow-up. Radiographs should be taken initially at 2 to 3 week intervals to be sure that no displacement of the fracture occurs. Displaced fractures should only be treated surgically, otherwise malunion of the fracture may result and lead to early onset of degenerative arthritis of the wrist.

If the patient has tenderness of the snuff-box at the wrist, but no radiographic findings of a fracture, a thumb spica cast should be applied and the patient re-examined 2 weeks later. Many times a fracture may not be visible on the initial radiographs but becomes visible 2 weeks after injury. After the fracture heals, it usually takes from 3 to 6 months for wrist motion and grip strength to return to near normal.

Wrist Sprains

After what seems a relatively trivial injury, many patients will complain of wrist pain with range of motion of the wrist, especially extension or gripping activities. Most wrist sprains occur as the result of a hyperextension injury to the wrist, either after a fall or catching a heavy object. The diagnosis of wrist sprain should be reserved as one of exclusion when all other possible diagnoses have been ruled out. If one is not carefully looking, it is not uncommon to miss a serious ligamentous injury to the radiocarpal or intercarpal ligaments, or a scaphoid fracture. Physical examination may reveal a decreased active and passive range of motion. There may be diffuse tenderness dorsally over the wrist capsule or an area of point tenderness may be identified. AP, lateral, and oblique radiographs of the wrist should always be obtained. If all studies are negative, it is advisable to place the patient in a short arm cast or a splint for 2 weeks and then re-examine and re-x-ray the patient again.

Many times all symptoms will resolve and the patient can return to work, but occasionally an occult fracture will become obvious at the time of repeat x-rays. If pain is severe, referral should be made initially. If there is moderate or mild pain with a negative examination it is not unreasonable to wait until the repeat examination at 2 weeks or until the referral is made to the hand surgeon.

Wrist Dislocations

Dislocations of the wrist are usually the result of high-energy trauma such as a motorcycle accident. The dislocation is often accompanied by other injuries to the hand and forearm or it may be only one injury in a multiply injured patient. This is one of the most commonly missed injuries by those relatively inexperienced at reading wrist radiographs; dorsal perilunate dislocation is the most frequent. Radiographs demonstrate a loss of the normal articulation of the lunate and the capitate. On the AP view the lunate is often a triangular shape and overlaps the capitate by more than one-third of its height. On the lateral view the capitate is seen to be displaced posterior to the lunate; the lunate may be facing palmar. This is commonly referred to as the "spilled teacup" sign. There may also be a fracture of the scaphoid that is best seen on an AP or oblique view. Median nerve compression occurs as a result of tenting of the nerve over the palmarly displaced lunate by the dorsally displaced carpus and hand. Patients should be splinted and referred to a facility where radiographic examination can be performed and more definitive care provided.

After a wrist dislocation patients rarely get complete recovery. Wrist range of motion exercises (flexion, extension, and radial and ulnar deviation) as well as grip strengthening will help regain function sooner. It often takes 6 months to 1 year for the patient to reach a plateau in wrist motion and grip strength.

Dislocations in the Hand

Metacarpophalangeal Joint. Dislocation of the MCP joint of the fingers and thumb is usually the result of a hyperextension injury. The index finger is most commonly involved, followed by the thumb and small fingers. On physical examination the proximal phalanx is held in extension or hyperextension and there may be dimpling of the palmar skin over the protruding metacarpal head. In the lateral radiograph the base of the proximal phalanx is dorsal to the metacarpal head. On the AP view there is obliteration of the normal joint space because of the overlap of the bones. Reduction can be attempted by hyperextending the finger at the MCP joint followed by traction, distraction, and flexion of the finger. Reduction is frequently unsuccessful because the volar plate is trapped in the joint, lying over the metacarpal head, and often can only be extricated surgically. In the thumb and index finger there is a sesamoid bone in the volar plate that acts as a further block to reduction. If reduction is accomplished a posterior splint should be applied as a block to extension with the MCP joint flexed 70°. Motion (flexion and extension of the MCP joint) should be started in the splint at about 1 week, and the splint can be discontinued after 3 to 4 weeks. It is important to check the range of flexion and extension of the MCP joint after reduction and before applying the splint to be certain there is no obstruction to motion (particularly extension). As always postreduction radiographs should be taken (AP, lateral, and oblique views of the MCP joint). Occasionally a fracture that previously was not well visualized will become obvious.

Proximal Interphalangeal Joint. This is probably the most common dislocation in the body. Dorsal dislocation of the middle phalanx on the proximal phalanx is the type most commonly seen. These occur by hyperextension or a "jamming" injury, often while playing basketball or baseball. The finger appears swollen and malformed with limitation of flexion. There is obliteration of the joint space on AP radiographs and dorsal dislocation of the middle phalanx on the lateral view. Occasionally a fracture will be seen from the volar margin of the middle phalanx. If there is a fracture dislocation surgical reattachment of the fragment is often necessary. Reduction is usually easily accomplished by direct longitudinal traction. Anesthesia should be administered by blocking the digital nerves in the palm at the level of the metacarpal neck rather than in the finger. Instillation of anesthesia into the base of the finger can cause compression of the digital arteries and ischemia to an already injured digit. Lidocaine (0.5 or 1%) *without epinephrine* should be used. After reduction a dorsal extension block splint should be applied blocking the last 15° of extension. Motion can be started in the splint after the 1st week and the splint removed at 3 weeks. "Buddy" taping the fingers after splint removal will help regain motion and overcome stiffness. Stiffness of the PIP joint (usually loss of range of flexion and extension) may be present for 3 to 6 months. Patients often require treatment by a therapist with specialized flexion and extension splints to regain motion.

Volar dislocation of the finger PIP joint occurs by a hyperextension injury at the PIP joint in the extended finger. AP and lateral radiographs should be taken of the finger. Lateral x-rays will show that the base of the middle phalanx is palmar to the head of the proximal phalanx. Volar dislocation of the middle phalanx is much less common and after reduction should be splinted in full extension of the PIP joint. The splint should be applied on the volar side and left in place for 4 to 6 weeks. Volar dislocations often cause traumatic rupture of the central extensor tendon insertion into the base of the middle phalanx. If these are not recognized and treated appropriately a traumatic boutonnière will result and the patient will be unable to extend the PIP joint. AP and lateral radiographs should be checked postreduction to look for any fractures that may have been missed. Flexion and extension of the PIP joint should be started at 4 to 6 weeks postinjury.

Fractures in the Hand

Pain or swelling of the hand or fingers after a twisting or contact injury to the hand should make one suspicious of a fracture in the hand. Physical examination should include palpation along tender areas seeking a point of maximal tenderness. This will usually correspond to the area of the fracture. AP, lateral, and oblique radiographs should be taken. The acute care of most fractures in the hand should include splinting for comfort, elevation of the injured limb, and referral to an orthopaedist or hand specialist. Many of these injuries occur in children and adolescents at school. As most schools do not have access to x-rays or a plaster splint, packing with ice, and referral to an emergency facility for radiographs should be done initially.

Most fractures of the phalanges and metacarpals can be treated conservatively by splinting, casting, or "buddy" taping the fingers if they are nondisplaced and not intraarticular. Intraarticular and displaced fractures should be referred to the appropriate facility where a decision can be made regarding surgical management. Special fractures requiring surgical treatment include:
(1) Displaced intraarticular fractures at the base of the thumb metacarpal (Bennett's fracture),
(2) Fracture dislocations of the MCP or PIP joints in the fingers,
(3) Fracture dislocations of the base of the fifth metacarpal (Baby Bennett's fracture).

Metacarpal Neck Fractures (Boxer's Fracture). Fracture of the metacarpal neck of the fifth finger is the most frequent metacarpal fracture and is commonly referred to as a "boxer's fracture" because these often result from a fight. Patients have tenderness and pain just proximal to the MCP joint of the fifth finger over the neck of the fifth metacarpal. Physical examination reveals a loss of the normal prominence of the fifth knuckle. AP and lateral radiographs should be taken. The angulation of the fracture in a palmar direction is best seen on the lateral radiograph. While this is a displaced fracture, angulation of up to 40° in a volar direction can be accepted. Angulation of other metacarpal neck fractures greater than 10 to 20° is unacceptable and should be treated surgically. If a puncture wound is found over the dorsum of any MCP joint, either alone or in association with a fracture, suspicion should be high that this is due to tooth penetration from a punch to an opponent's mouth. Many of these result in laceration of the extensor tendon over the MCP joint and may communicate with the MCP joint. Infection of the MCP joint can result; prevention consists of treatment with incision and drainage and antibiotics. Joint infection results in cartilage destruction and painful loss of motion. Human bites should be treated with both penicillin (to cover *Eikenella corrodens*, which is an organism specific to the human mouth) and a semisynthetic penicillin or cephalosporin to protect against *Staphylococcus aureus*. The mouths of cats and dogs carry the organism *Pasteurella multocida*, which is also sensitive to penicillin.

Gamekeeper's Thumb. This term is commonly used to describe a tear of the ulnar collateral ligament of the thumb. Disruption occurs after acute radial deviation of the thumb at the MCP joint. Although this is often called "gamekeepers thumb," it is commonly caused when the thumb is forcefully radially deviated by a ski pole or strap when the hand hits the ground after a fall while skiing. Physical examination usually reveals tenderness over the ulnar side of the thumb MCP joint or at the head of the thumb metacarpal. Swelling or ecchymosis is also frequently seen along the ulnar side of the thumb MCP joint. It is important to compare the joint stability of the injured thumb with the patient's uninjured thumb. If there is radial deviation of the injured thumb of 15° greater than the uninjured thumb, or 45° radial deviation is possible, then the collateral ligament is probably disrupted. AP and lateral radiographs should be taken. While radiographs are usually negative, occasionally a bony avulsion will be seen where the collateral ligament inserts into the base of the proximal phalanx. For acute injuries with bony avulsion on the AP radiograph a short arm thumb spica cast is applied and the x-rays repeated. If the bone fragment is reduced, then 4 to 6 weeks in the cast should be adequate. If there is no fracture or avulsion seen on the x-ray the optimum treat-

ment should be either primary surgical exploration and repair or immobilization in a thumb spica cast for 4 to 6 weeks (author's preference is surgical repair).

Nontraumatic Conditions

Ganglions. Ganglions are extremely common about the wrist and hands and often present as painless swellings. They vary in size between the tiny ganglions found in the fingers to the often large, fluctuant ganglions found on the dorsum of the wrist. In most cases the dorsal wrist ganglions communicate with the radiocarpal joint and the ganglions in the fingers communicate with the tendon sheath. Diagnosis is not usually difficult unless the swelling is slight. AP and lateral radiographs of the hand and wrist are usually negative but should be taken in an attempt to rule out any other cause of pain or wrist swelling. Dorsal swelling and tenderness may only be obvious when the wrist is palmar flexed. This type of ganglion is often the cause of persistent wrist pain in young women. Their symptoms are often labeled as functional when the difficulty in examination has not been appreciated. Dorsal ganglions can be aspirated with a large bore needle (16 or 18 gauge) and splinted for 2 to 3 weeks. Up to 50% will respond to this form of treatment. Volar wrist ganglions are usually deep to the radial artery, arising from the volar wrist capsule. Aspiration of these is more difficult as the radial artery is often compressed over the top of the ganglion and aspiration may result in accidental puncture of the artery. Excision is recommended for volar ganglions and those ganglions resistant to conservative treatment.

De Quervain's Syndrome. Tenosynovitis involving the abductor pollicis longus and extensor pollicis brevis is known as de Quervain's disease. It occurs most often in middle-aged females. The walls of the fibrous tendon sheaths on the lateral aspect of the radius are greatly thickened, and there is often marked underlying swelling. The patients often complain of pain with thumb flexion and extension, as well as grip. This is a very common occupational injury as a complication of repetitive movement of the thumb. Treatment is injection of a combination of 1% lidocaine and 40 mg methylprednisolone (Depo-Medrol) into the inflamed tendon sheath, followed by splinting in a radial gutter splint with the thumb immobilized for 3 weeks. For cases resistant to immobilization, surgical release of the lateral wall of the tendon sheath is necessary.

Extensor Tenosynovitis. Acute frictional tenosynovitis occurs most frequently in those 20 to 40 years, generally following a period of excess activity. Any or all of the extensor tendons may be involved. The condition has a benign course and is usually resolved if the wrist is immobilized in neutral to 20° extension for 3 weeks. If the pain has resolved after this period of immobilization the patient can return to the previous level of activity at work or sports.

Osteoarthritis of the Wrist. Osteoarthritis of the wrist is surprisingly rare considering the frequency with which the wrist joint is involved in fractures. It is seen after comminuted fractures involving the articular surface of the radius, nonunion of fractures of the scaphoid, and avascular necrosis of the scaphoid or lunate. Patients commonly present with symptoms of increasing pain with gradual loss of motion, principally in extension. Initial treatment is with anti-inflammatory medications and splinting with a volar wrist splint, such as those available commercially, during particularly painful periods. When symptoms are severe, fusion of the wrist (radiocarpal joint) may be necessary.

Rheumatoid Arthritis of the Wrist. Involvement of the wrist is common in rheumatoid arthritis, and extensive synovial thickening of the joint and related tendon sheaths leads to gross swelling, increased local heat, pain, and stiffness. Rarely, tuberculosis of the wrist may produce a similar clinical picture, but the multifocal nature of rheumatoid arthritis usually makes differentiation easy. Again, anti-inflammatories and splinting may provide relief during painful periods, but arthrodesis or arthroplasty is often necessary for lasting pain relief.

Carpal Tunnel Syndrome. This condition occurs most commonly in women 30 to 60 years. Compression of the median nerve as it passes through the carpal tunnel under the transverse carpal ligament leads to signs and symptoms in the distribution of the median nerve. In some cases premenstrual fluid retention, early rheumatoid arthritis with synovial tendon sheath thickening, and old carpal fractures may be responsible as they restrict the space left for the nerve in the carpal tunnel. The condition is sometimes seen in association with myxedema, acromegaly, and pregnancy. Often, however, no obvious cause can be found.

People in occupations that require chronic repetitive wrist motion in flexion, extension, and gripping are prone to develop carpal tunnel syndrome. Another factor in the development of carpal tunnel syndrome is any activity, such as that of a jackhammer operator, that results in chronic trauma to the volar side of the wrist. More common occupations that are prone to develop carpal tunnel syndromes are assembly line workers, construction work involving repetitive hammering, carpentry, and electrical work. Many times it is helpful if patients can perform different types of activities during an 8-hour shift (part of time assembly line, part of time another job within same factory).

Patients complain of paresthesias in the hand. Often they claim that all the fingers are involved and, although theoretically the little finger should be spared, approximately 30% of patients also have paresthesias in the ulnar nerve distribution. Pain may radiate proximally to the elbow or shoulder; weakness of grip is also common. The symptoms may become most marked at night, often awakening the patient (nocturnal paresthesias) and causing the patient to shake the hand or hang it over the side of the bed. In many cases the history and clinical examination are unequivocal. In others it may be difficult to differentiate the patient's symptoms from those produced by cervical spondylosis or diabetic peripheral neuropathy; indeed, both conditions may be present at the same time as carpal tunnel syndrome.

Two-point discrimination testing is useful when screening for any of the compression neuropathies such as carpal tunnel syndrome. The test is performed by either bending the prongs of a small paper clip so that there is a 6 mm distance between the tips or by using one of the commercially available two-point discrimination calipers. The tips are placed against the volar pulp of the index finger, long finger, and thumb (all fingers should be tested but these three are innervated by the median nerve) until there is a slight blanching of the skin under the prongs. The patient is then asked if he/she feels (is able to discriminate between) one or two points. Normal two-point discrimination is 6 mm or less. On physical examination two-point discrimination may be abnormal (greater than 6 mm), grip strength may be diminished, and thenar atrophy may be present. Flexion of the involved wrist for 60 seconds (Phalen's test) may reproduce the symptoms, or gentle percussion of the median nerve at the wrist may produce paresthesias radiating into the fingers (Tinel's sign). For patients seen early, before the development of abnormal two-point discrimination or thenar atrophy, splinting of the wrist with or without injection of steroids into the carpal canal may prove successful. If conservative treatment does not relieve the symptoms electrodiagnostic testing (EMG, NCV) may prove useful when contemplating surgery or trying to rule out another etiology. If, at the time of presentation, there is either thenar atrophy or abnormal two-point discrimination in the distribution of the median nerve then surgical release of the transverse carpal ligament is the best treatment.

Postoperatively, patients should be protected in a removable volar, resting wrist, cock-up splint for 2 to 3 weeks. During this time finger motion is encouraged. After the splint is removed wrist range of motion exercises and grip strengthening are started. Most patients will return to their preoperative level of grip strength and wrist motion by 3 months. Not all patients require therapy after surgery but if progress appears slow then referral to an occupational or hand therapist should be made. Patients are usually ready to return to work 8 to 12 weeks postoperatively.

Ulnar (Guyon's) Tunnel Syndrome. The ulnar nerve may be compressed as it passes through the ulnar carpal canal (Guyon's canal) between the pisiform and the hook of the hamate. Although isolated ulnar nerve compression at the wrist is much less common than compression of the median nerve, 30% of patients with median nerve compression have concomitant compression of the ulnar nerve. Both the sensory and motor divisions of the nerve may be affected, but often only one division is involved.

Symptoms therefore may include small muscle wasting and weakness in the hand and/or sensory decrease on the volar aspect of the small finger. Pain is rarely seen with ulnar nerve compression at the wrist. Since the ulnar sensory branch to the dorsum of the hand comes off proximal to the wrist in the forearm, sensory disturbance on the dorsum of the hand and little finger excludes a lesion at the wrist level and points more toward a lesion at the elbow. In all cases every effort should be made to exclude a more proximal cause for the patient's symptoms such as ulnar neuritis at the elbow or cervical spondylosis. Nerve conduction studies are often of particular value in this situation. The most common causes of ulnar nerve involvement at the wrist are compression by a ganglion or thrombosed ulnar artery, occupational trauma, and old carpal or metacarpal fractures. After establishing a diagnosis of a lesion localized to the ulnar tunnel at the wrist, surgical exploration of the nerve and decompression are necessary. These lesions do not respond to conservative, nonoperative management, and should all be referred to a hand surgeon for evaluation and treatment.

Tuberculosis of the Wrist. Although tuberculosis of the wrist is now rare, the diagnosis should be considered when an indolent chronic infection is present. Marked swelling of the joint is followed by muscle wasting in the forearm, erosion, destruction, and anterior subluxation of the carpus. Radiographs show marked osteopenia on both sides of the joint with loss of the normal articular joint space. Diagnosis is confirmed by synovial biopsy and culture for *Mycobacterium tuberculosis.* Differential diagnosis includes monoarticular rheumatoid arthritis.

The AP chest x-ray may be typical for tuberculosis or the diagnosis may not be obvious. If tuberculosis is suspected, consultation should be made to an infectious disease specialist. Treatment should include antituberculosis drugs combined with synovectomy and drainage of the wrist joint. Late presenting cases often need wrist fusion as a result of the long-standing joint destruction and cartilage loss.

Dupuytren's Contracture. In this condition there is nodular thickening and contracture of the palmar fascia. The palm of the hand is affected first; at a later stage the fingers become involved. The ring finger is most frequently affected, followed by the little and middle fingers. The index and even the thumb may be involved. Progression of flexion of the affected fingers interferes with the function of the hand. Flexion may be so severe that the fingernails dig into the palm; hygiene is difficult or impossible. The condition predominantly affects men over age 40. In some cases there may be a hereditary tendency, and an association with epilepsy or alcoholism has been reported. The condition may occur in either sex at an earlier age and may be precipitated by trauma. Indications for surgical treatment are flexion of the metacarpophalangeal (MCP) joint greater than 30° and/or any flexion contracture of the proximal interphalangeal joint. Splinting in an extended position at the MCP joint is rarely successful in either correcting or halting the progression of deformity.

When the flexion contracture of the MCP joint is less than 30° and full extension of the PIP joint is possible, patients should be told that until the contracture progresses surgery will not be necessary. Many patients are concerned with how quickly the deformity will progress. Unfortunately, there is no way of predicting how quickly progression will occur other than by observation and follow-up every 6 months. At surgery the contracted fibrous bands are released and excised, which allows improved extension. Postoperatively a splint should be worn on the palmar side of the hand and forearm; the splint holds the MCP and PIP joints in extension. The splint is worn for 6 weeks (day and night) and then for an additional 3 months (night only). Most patients will need hand therapy after surgery and will not return to work for approximately 3 months.

Tendon and Tendon Sheath Lesions

Mallet Finger. In a mallet finger the distal interphalangeal joint is held in a permanent position of flexion and the patient is unable to extend the distal joint of the finger. The etiology is often a tear of the terminal extensor tendon close to its insertion into the distal phalanx as the result of trauma. Many occur after a "jamming" injury to the extended distal phalanx causing a forced flexion injury. This is why the common name for a mallet finger is a "baseball" finger. Treatment is with a metal or prefabricated splint holding the DIP joint in extension for 6 weeks. The splint should not be removed at all during this period as this will allow the terminal phalanx to drop down into flexion. Untreated mallet fingers may be complicated by a swan neck deformity with hyperextension of the PIP joint. This is usually not problematic and if it occurs, does not usually require treatment.

Mallet Thumb. Delayed rupture of the EPL tendon may occur after Colles' fracture, but is more commonly seen in rheumatoid arthritis. Direct repair is usually not possible in an attritional rupture and transfer of the extensor indicis proprius is usually necessary.

Boutonnière Deformity. Traumatic injuries to the PIP joint of the finger may result in detachment of the central slip of the extensor tendon from its attachment at the base of the middle phalanx. This can be secondary to a "jammed" finger that occurred during sports activity or attrition of the joint capsule in rheumatoid arthritis. The characteristic deformity is flexion of the PIP joint with hyperextension at the DIP joint. On physical examination after a traumatic injury, there is usually tenderness dorsally on the finger at the base of the proximal phalanx where the central slip of the extensor tendon inserts. In the rheumatoid patient the deformity usually develops progressively and is not usually tender. Early lesions can be successfully treated by splinting the PIP joint in extension and leaving the DIP free for 6 weeks. Late deformity with fixed flexion contracture often requires fusion of the PIP joint in a functional position (they rarely respond to splinting).

Extensor Tendon Lacerations. Extensor tendon lacerations on the back of the hand are best treated by primary repair and splinting for approximately 4 weeks. These injuries have an excellent prognosis.

Flexor Tendon Injuries. In the fingers, laceration of either the flexor digitorum profundus (FDP) or sublimus (FDS) can be easily diagnosed by physical examination and history. With isolated laceration of an FDP, patients are unable to flex the distal IP joint. With laceration of both FDS and FDP, neither the proximal IP nor the distal IP joint can be actively flexed. Isolated injury to the FDS occurs with lacerations proximal to the wrist flexion crease or in the forearm. Flexor tendon injuries in the fingers are often accompanied by digital nerve or nerve and artery laceration. Patients should be examined closely to determine the circulatory status. These injuries all require surgical repair and should be referred to a hand surgeon for care.

Trigger Finger and Thumb. This condition results from either a thickening of the fibrous tendon sheath or nodular thickening in a flexor tendon. In young children, the thumb is held flexed at the MCP joint, and a nodular thickening in front of the MCP joint is palpable. Frequently the deformity is incorrectly considered untreatable. In adults, the middle or ring finger is most frequently involved. When the fingers are extended, the affected finger lags behind and then suddenly straightens with a painful snap. There is usually a palpable nodular thickening at the level of the MCP joint. Treatment with steroid injection into the flexor tendon sheath and splinting of the thumb for 3 weeks is usually successful. For unresponsive or recurrent cases division of the tendon sheath at the level of the MCP joint (A1 pulley) gives an immediate and gratifying cure.

Rheumatoid Arthritis

It is well known that patients with rheumatoid arthritis commonly have hand and wrist involvement. As the disease progresses, joints, tendons, muscles, nerves, and arteries are affected, resulting in severe deformities and crippling effects on hand function. In the earliest phases the hands are warm and erythematous, later the joints become swollen and tender. Synovial tendon sheath and joint thickening with effusion, muscle wasting, and deformity then become apparent. Tendon rupture and joint subluxation are the main factors leading to the more severe deformities. Surgery of the rheumatoid hand is highly specialized and requires particular skills and experience in judgment, timing, and technique. In the earliest stages of the disease analgesic and anti-inflammatory drugs are used, along with physiotherapy and splinting to alleviate pain, preserve motion, and minimize deformity. When synovial thickening is present before joint destruction and is unresponsive to medical management, synovectomy is often helpful in alleviating pain and delaying progression of deformity. As joint destruction and deformity progress, reconstructive surgery becomes necessary. It is important to watch for tendon rupture (particularly the common extensors to the ring and small fingers); immediate exploration, synovectomy, and repair are recommended. Once tendon rupture occurs it is usually a sign of impending rupture of additional tendons.

Osteoarthritis of the IP Joints

Nodular swellings over the dorsum and sides of the DIP joints (Heberden's nodes) are a sign of osteoarthritis of the finger joints. They occur most frequently in women after menopause, and are often familial. In most cases they are symptom-free, but they may be associated with progressive joint damage and resultant pain. Analgesics and anti-inflammatory drugs can usually control the pain; if not, joint arthrodesis will alleviate the pain.

Carpometacarpal (Basal) Joint of the Thumb

The joint between the thumb metacarpal and the trapezium is the joint most commonly involved with osteoarthritis in the hand. Involvement often leads to disabling pain and impaired hand function, particularly with pinch and grip. There may be a history of a previous Bennett's fracture or of occupational overuse if the job requires repetitive pinching or picking up small objects. Initial treatment with anti-inflammatory drugs, splinting, and occasional intraarticular steroid injections may provide temporary relief. Once symptoms become severe, however, surgical intervention provides pain relief with minimal loss of function.

Tumors in the Hand

Tumors in the hand are not uncommon. Most involve the soft tissues and are benign, but it must be stressed that whenever the diagnosis is in question, malignant potential must be fully investigated. The most common are *ganglions* which occur in the fingers, most commonly along the volar aspects of the flexor tendon sheath between the A1 and A2 pulleys. They are small, spherical, and tender to the touch and may be particularly painful during gripping activities. They do not respond to conservative management and usually need to be surgically removed. Differential diagnosis should include *inclusion cyst* and foreign body granulomas that also occur along the volar surfaces of the fingers and palms. Hemangiomas are small, tender, bluish swellings also found in fingers. *Glomus tumors* are less common. They are small vascular tumors, presenting with exquisite tenderness under the nail bed. They are benign but respond only to surgical removal. *Enchondromas* are most common in the hands, may be multiple, and are often a cause of pathological fracture. They are benign, but may be expansile. Their presence may not be noted until a radiograph of the hand after fracture is taken, but in other cases there may be gross swelling and deformity.

There is rarely any evidence of an enchondroma on physical examination; it is usually best treated by curettage and bone grafting. If a fracture is present, it should be allowed to heal prior to curetment of the lesion.

Infections in the Hand

Paronychia. This is the most common of all infections in the hand; it occurs between the base of the nail and the cuticle.

Apical Infections. These infections occur between the tip of the nail and the underlying nail bed. Infection usually results from introduction of *Staphylococcus aureus* into the paronychial tissue by a sliver of a nail or a hangnail, a manicure instrument, or a tooth. Continuity of the nail fold around the base of the nail may cause infection to extend from one side of the finger to the other. In the very early stages, this process can be aborted by soaking the finger in warm saline solution, using systemic oral antibiotics, and resting the affected part. If there is no response to soaks and oral antibiotics after 24 to 48 hours, surgical incision and drainage should be performed.

Felons (Pulp Infections). These occur in the fibrofatty tissue of the finger tips and are extremely painful. There is often, but not always, an injury preceding a felon. The pain and swelling usually develop rapidly. If untreated, infection frequently leads to osteomyelitis of the distal phalanx. These three common infections are treated by surgical drainage and antibiotics.

Tendon Sheath Infections (Flexor Tenosynovitis). These lead to rapid swelling of the finger and pressure buildup within the tendon sheath. There is always a serious risk of tendon sloughing or disabling adhesion formation.

On physical examination patients will usually demonstrate Knavel's classic four signs: swollen digit, tenderness along flexor tendon sheath, flexed posture of digit, and pain with passive extension of digit. The finger may also have a palpable area of fluctuance with erythema and increased warmth. These infections are often secondary to a puncture wound but may be idiopathic with no identifiable etiology. Infection and swelling spread rapidly, and before the common use of antibiotics these infections were associated with a mortality rate as high as 50%. Rapid treatment will decrease the incidence of adhesions and loss of finger function. In the case of the fifth finger there may be retrograde spread to involve the ulnar bursa, and in the thumb, retrograde spread proximally involves the radial bursa. As two bursae communicate proximal to the wrist (Parona's space), infection may develop in the wrist proximal to the flexor retinaculum, or infection may spread between the thumb and the small finger. Flexor sheath infections should all be treated surgically by incision, drainage, and parenteral antibiotics. Post-operatively, patients are usually hospitalized for 3 to 7 days and the wound may take up to 3 weeks to heal. Most patients require therapy after surgery, and 3 months may pass before finger motion returns to near normal.

Web Space Infections. These are usually accompanied by pain as well as swelling and redness in the palm and affected web space. Physical examination reveals exquisite tenderness in the web space along with erythema. The infection may follow a puncture wound or rupture of a blister in the web. Infection may spread along the volar aspects of the related fingers or to adjacent web spaces across the anterior aspect of the palm. If seen early most web space infections respond to antibiotics, splinting, and elevation; however, surgical drainage is usually necessary. Postoperatively most patients do not need therapy and are able to return to work in approximately 4 weeks.

Midpalmar and Thenar Space Infections. Usually, these occur in the two compartments of the hand that lie between the flexor tendons and the metacarpals. In-

fection may spread to these areas from web space or tendon sheath infections; dissemination through the hand is then rapid. In either case there is usually gross swelling and tenderness of the hand. Unless there is a rapid response (24 hours) to antibiotics, elevation, and splinting, early drainage should be performed and these patients should be referred to a hand surgeon.

Human Bites. A human bite should be suspected if the patient presents with puncture wounds over the MCP joints. These probably originated from a human tooth during a fight. Some patients will, however, admit that they were bitten. The flora of the human mouth include *Eikenella corrodens*, a facultative anaerobe that is sensitive to penicillin, in addition to *Staphylococcus aureus*. Patients should be treated with incision and drainage and penicillin as well as an antibiotic (cephalosporin, or synthetic penicillin) to cover *S. aureus*.

Recommended Readings

Burton RI, Eaton RG: Common hand injuries in the athlete. *Orthop Clin North Am* 4:809–838, 1973.

Conrad RW, Hooper WR: Tennis elbow: its course, natural history, conservative and surgical management. *J Bone Joint Surg* 55A:1177, 1973.

DeHaven KE, Evarts CM: Throwing injuries of the elbow in athletes. *Orthop Clin North Am* 4:301, 1973.

Duncan BF: Rehabilitation of the tennis elbow syndrome. *Contemp Orthop* 7:61–65, 1983.

Gellman H, Gelberman RH, Tan AM, Botte MJ: Carpal tunnel syndrome. An evaluation of the provocative diagnostic tests. *J Bone Joint Surg* 68A:735, 1986.

Green DP, O'Brien ET: Classification and management of carpal dislocations. *Clin Orthop* 148:55–72, 1980.

Nelson CL, Sawmiller S, Phalen GS: Ganglions of the wrist and hand. *J Bone Joint Surg* 54A:1459, 1972.

Phalen GS: The carpal tunnel syndrome: clinical evaluation of 598 hands. *Clin Orthop* 83:29, 1972.

Wehbe MA, Schneider LH: Mallet fractures. *J Bone Joint Surg* 66A:658–669, 1984.

chapter 8

The Hip and Pelvis

PEKKA A. MOOAR, M.D.

ANATOMY AND FUNCTION

The pelvis consists of a complex of bone and ligamentous structures that connects the spine to the hip joint and provides a broad surface for the articulation of the powerful muscles of the lower extremity that are needed for ambulation and to provide a stable attachment of the spine to the lower extremities. The pelvis also protects the abdominal viscera.

The spine is attached to the pelvis through the sacrum. It is secured in all planes by a complex of ligamentous supports and secondary muscle stabilizers (Fig. 8.1).

The pelvis is made up of two paired innominate bones that articulate at the symphysis pubis and the sacroiliac joints. Each innominate has three separate bones: the ilium, ischium, and pubis. The confluence of these three bones is in the acetabulum. In the young, this confluence provides for acetabular growth. This growth area fuses around 16 years of age.

The ilium is the most prominent of the pelvic bones and forms the superior and lateral borders of the pelvis. It also provides for protection of the abdominal viscera and for the broad insertion of the gluteal muscles. It also provides stress transference during standing.

The ischium is posterior and provides for stress transference during sitting. The pubis is the most anterior structure and performs a tie rod mechanism to prevent lateral displacement of the two innominate bones during weight bearing (Fig. 8.2).

The hip joint is a ball and socket type joint composed of the acetabulum (socket) and femoral head (ball). Stability of this joint is produced by capsular ligaments, acetabular labrum, and secondary muscles stabilizers. The forces acting across the hip joint are three times body weight during walking and four times body weight during running. Blood is supplied to the hip through the foveal artery in the acetabulum and by the medial and lateral circumflex arteries. Dislocations and fractures may disrupt the blood supply to the femoral head resulting in avascular necrosis.

The hip moves in four planes and two rotations; flexion, extension, abduction, adduction, and internal and external rotation (Table 8.1).

PHYSICAL EXAMINATION OF THE HIP AND PELVIS

The hip and pelvis are examined in a sequential fashion: inspection and palpation of the bone and soft tissues, evaluation of active and passive range of motion, and assessment of motor strength.

Inspection

Inspection is first performed when the patient enters the examining room. Observe for antalgic gait or Trendelenburg gait (lurching gait). Examine the ease with which the patient stands, walks, sits, and arises from sitting. While the patient is standing, observe for equal weight distribution, symmetry of the pelvis, and height of the pelvis. Look for a tilt of the pelvis that may indicate a leg length discrepancy. Examine the lumbosacral spine for normal contours. Increased lor-

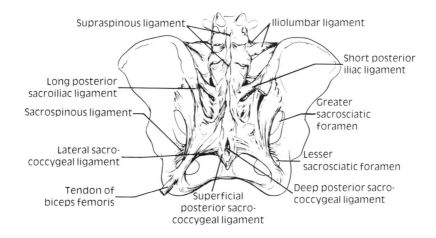

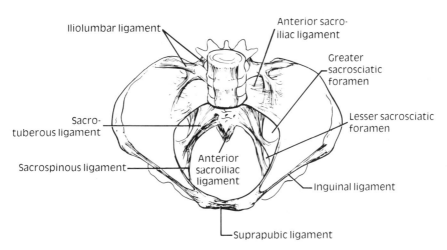

Figure 8.1. Posterior and superior views of pelvis showing bony structures and ligamentous attachments. (From Nicholas JA, Hershman EB (eds): *The Lower Extremity and Spine in Sports Medicine.* St. Louis, CV Mosby, 1981, vols. 1–2.)

dosis is seen with weak abdominal muscles and with hip flexion contractures. Absence of lordosis may be secondary to muscle spasm. The buttocks should be symmetric and the gluteal fold should be at the same level. Observe for ecchymosis, abrasions, draining sinuses, and erythema.

Palpation

Palpation is performed to gauge skin temperature and areas of tenderness. The patient should be in undergarments and may be standing or supine. Beginning an-

terior with the patient directly in front of the examiner, place the examining hands on the patient's waist and slide them down toward the thigh to the bony prominences. This is the iliac crest. With the thumbs palpate inferiorly to locate the most anterior bony prominence. This is the anterior superior iliac spine and the origin of the sartorius. By sliding the thumbs inferiorly the examiner will come upon the pubic ramus (usually just at the line of pubic hair and the prepubic fat). The pubic symphysis is at the level of the greater trochanters laterally. Palpate the trochanters laterally for

LATERAL

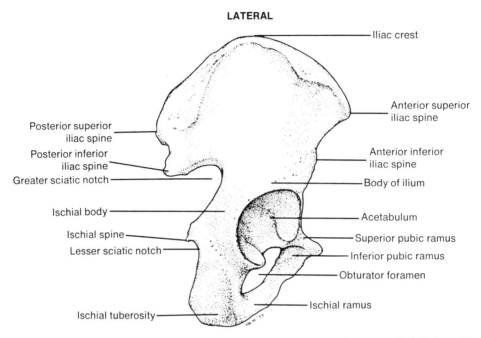

Figure 8.2. Lateral view of the right hip. (From Hilt NE, Cogburn SB: *Manual of Orthopaedics*. St. Louis, CV Mosby, 1980.)

tenderness of the bursa and tenderness of the iliotibial band. The posterior aspect of the pelvis is palpated directly over the posterior brim of the iliac crest (the origin of the gluteus medius). Palpate the iliac crest posteriorly to the iliac tubercle posteriorly. Deep in this most posterior portion of the iliac crest is the sacroiliac joint, which is not directly palpable. Next palpate the ischial tuberosity, the origin of the hamstrings. This is located in the middle of the buttock usually in the gluteus gluteal fold. Flexion of the hip to move the gluteus maximus upward allows for easier palpation of the ischial tuberosity. Perform soft tissue palpation on all muscles to examine for masses, tenderness, and defects. Palpation of the adductors is facilitated by placing the lower extremity in the figure-4-position with the hip flexed and externally rotated, and the foot resting on the contralateral knee. Adductors are now easily palpated at their origin in the groin. Evaluate for range of motion. Range of motion is tested actively and passively and includes flexion, extension, abduction, adduction, and internal and external rotation (Fig. 8.3). Normal hip range

of motion is: flexion, 120°; extension, 30°; internal rotation, 35°; external rotation, 45°; abduction, 45°; and adduction, 25°. Test muscle strength providing resistance in all planes against motion and grade using a scale of 0 to 5 (see Chapter 5 for motor grading scale).

SPECIAL TESTS

Trendelenburg, Gaenslen, Thomas

Trendelenburg Test

This is used to evaluate gluteus medius strength. The patient is observed from posterior and asked to stand on one leg. The pelvis should remain level or slightly elevated. (This assesses the gluteus medius of the weight bearing leg.) If the pelvis drops the gluteus medius is weak (Fig. 8.4).

Gaenslen's Sign

To examine for Gaenslen's sign the patient is supine with both legs drawn to the chest and with one buttock extended over the edge of examining table. The unsup-

Table 8.1
Muscles of the Hip and Pelvis

	Primary	Secondary
Hip extensors	Gluteus maximus ischial portion of adductor magnus	Hamstrings Gluteus medius Piriformis
Hip flexors	Iliopsoas Rectus femoris	Adductors Tensor fasciae lata
Hip abductors	Gluteus medius Gluteus minimus	Tensor fasciae lata
Hip adductors	Adductor magnus Adductor longus Adductor brevis	Gracilis Obturator externus Hamstrings Gluteus maximus
External rotators	Gluteus maximus Piriformis Obturator internus Gemelli Obturator externus Quadratus femoris	Iliopsoas
Hip internal rotators	Tensor fasciae latae Gluteus medius Gluteus minimus	

ported leg is dropped over the edge of the table. This will provoke pain in the SI joint in the presence of sacroiliac disease. An alternative method is pictured (Fig. 8.5). The affected hip is hyperextended against a stabilized pelvis. With the unaffected leg flexed to the chest place one hand on the iliac crest of the affected hip. With the other hand on the knee, move the affected hip into hyperextension. Reproduction of sacroiliac pain indicates a positive test.

Thomas Test

The Thomas test demonstrates hip flexion contractures. The patient is placed supine and both hips are flexed maximally, reversing the normal lumbar lordosis of the spine. While holding one hip maximally flexed, the opposite hip is extended. Lack of complete extension is indicative of a hip flexion contracture (Fig. 8.6).

THE PAINFUL HIP AND PELVIS

Pain in the pelvis and hip region are common complaints and may be due to traumatic or nontraumatic causes (Fig. 8.7).

Referred pain from the spine or viscera must always be included in the differential diagnosis. Trauma is either repetitive persistent microtrauma leading to overuse or "stress" syndromes, or macrooverload resulting in the failure of muscle and bone units (i.e., as in a muscle pull or fracture).

Nontraumatic causes of hip and pelvic pain include: inflammatory conditions, infections, tumors, referred pain, metabolic bone disease, and degenerative arthritis. Inflammatory conditions of the pelvis and hip will usually present in the hip joint or sacroiliac joint. They include rheumatoid arthritis, ankylosing spondylitis, and Reiter's syndrome.

NONTRAUMATIC CONDITIONS OF THE PELVIS AND HIP

Ankylosing Spondylitis

Symptoms. Ankylosing spondylitis presents as low back pain in the buttocks or thighs with protracted morning stiffness that is relieved with activity.

Signs. Localized pain over the sacroiliac joint, and decreased spine motion and chest expansion are two important signs.

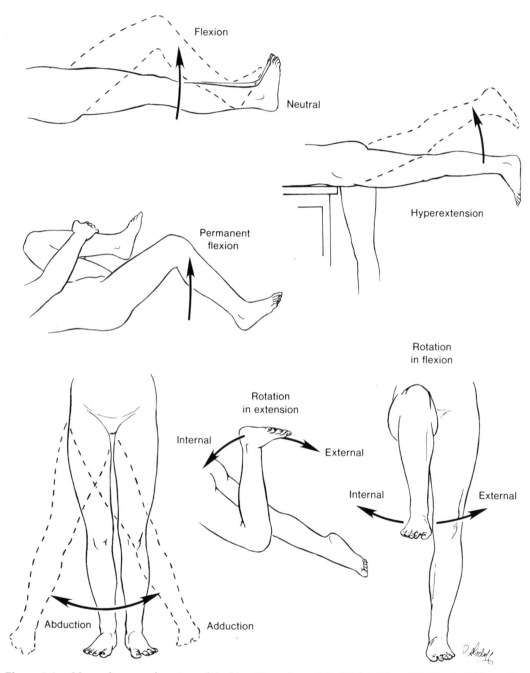

Figure 8.3. Normal range of motion of the hip. (From Burnside JW, McGlynn TJ: *Physical Diagnosis*, ed 17. Baltimore, Williams & Wilkins, 1987.)

Laboratory Evaluation. Collagen vascular screen (RF, ANA, ESR, HLA B-27) is usually negative in these sero-negative spondyloarthropathies.

Radiographic Evaluation. Sclerosis in the SI joints is seen on x-rays. CT scan may diagnose sclerosis earlier. Bone scan is useful when x-rays are negative, showing increased activity in the sacroiliac joint.

Treatment. Indomethacin usually pro-

NEGATIVE TRENDELENBURG TEST

POSITIVE TRENDELENBURG TEST

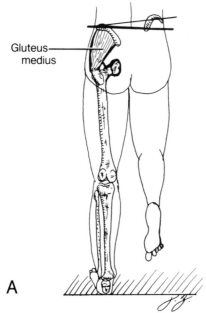

Gluteus medius

A

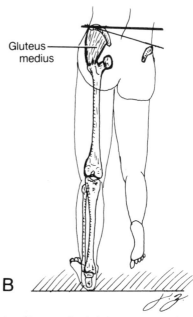

Gluteus medius

B

Figure 8.4. **A,** The Trendelenburg test as performed while standing on the left lower extremity. This person has a negative Trendelenburg test. Note that the right side of the pelvis does rise slightly because the gluteus medius and minimus of the right side act by origin-insertion inversion to straighten the pelvis. **B,** This person is also performing the Trendelenburg test while standing on the left lower extremity. This is a positive Trendelenburg test in that the pelvis tilts to the right side and cannot be recovered to a straight position. This person is suffering from either *(a)* paralysis of the gluteus medius and minimus muscles; *(b)* dislocation of the hip joint, or *(c)* an abnormal angle of femoral inclination. (From Draves DJ: *Anatomy of the Lower Extremity*. Baltimore, Williams & Wilkins, 1986.)

vides prompt relief. Thoracic extension flexibility exercises at least twice each day help to maintain normal spinal curves.

Referral. The patient should be referred to an orthopaedic surgeon or rheumatologist.

Outcome. The outcome can be variable.

Paget's Disease

Symptoms. Paget's disease presents in the adult as pelvic or hip pain. Pain is increased with weight bearing with acetabular involvement, often resulting in degenerative arthritis. Significant acetabular protrusio may be present.

Signs. The signs for Paget's disease are the same as the symptoms.

Laboratory Evaluation. The laboratory evaluation includes increased serum alkaline phosphatase.

Radiographic Evaluation. Mixed areas of sclerosis and osteolysis are the hallmarks of Paget's disease.

Treatment. See Chapter 5.

Inflammatory Arthritis

The hip joint may also be involved in any inflammatory collagen vascular disease.

Symptoms. These diseases present with morning stiffness and painful motion. The stiffness usually decreases with activity. With long standing inflammation joint motion may be lost.

Signs. The signs for inflammatory arthritis are the same as the symptoms.

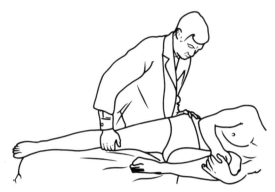

Figure 8.5. *Gaenslen's test.* (From MacNab I: *Backache.* Baltimore, Williams & Wilkins, 1977.)

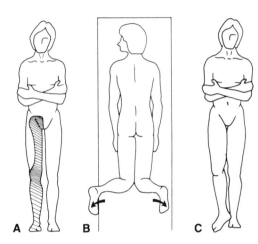

Figure 8.7. Characteristics of hip joint pain. **A,** location of the pain: Initial location over the groin and/or anterior aspect of the knee; referral of pain along the anterior aspect of the thigh, and eventually into the leg as well. **B,** painful manipulation. **C,** posture of the joint. (From Ramamurti CP (Tinker RV, ed): *Orthopaedics in Primary Care.* Baltimore, Williams & Wilkins, 1979, p 184.)

Laboratory Evaluation. A collagen vascular screen should be performed (RF, ANA, ESR).

Radiographic Evaluation. The radiographic evaluation consists of a standing AP with LAT views. These may show joint space narrowing, subchondral cyst formation, and peripheral osteophytes. A bone scan may be useful to demonstrate synovitis.

Treatment. See Chapter 11.

Crystalline Arthritis

Symptoms. Gout and pseudogout usually present with an acutely painful hip. Pain is exacerbated by motion and weight bearing.

Signs. The hip is held in flexion and external rotation. Movement in any plane increases the discomfort. A low grade fever may be present. Pain is increased with weight bearing.

Laboratory Evaluation. Joint aspiration and synovial fluid analysis must be performed to confirm the diagnosis. Crystals will be seen on polarized microscopy. Serum uric acid may be elevated in gout. ESR may be elevated. Cultures should be obtained to exclude infection.

Radiographic Evaluation. In an acute attack the routine radiographs may be normal or show joint space widening consistent with an effusion. With long standing disease joint space narrowing with cyst formation on both sides of the joint may be seen. Calcification in the cartilage (chondrocalcinosis) may be seen in pseudogout.

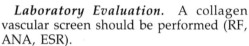

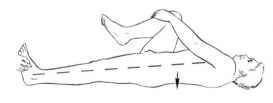

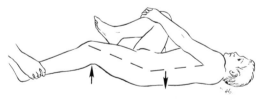

Figure 8.6. Thomas sign. When the patient pulls the knee up on the side without a flexion contracture, the leg on the side with a flexion contracture is pulled up as the normal lumbar lordosis is obliterated. (From Burnside JW, McGlynn TJ: *Physical Diagnosis*, ed 17. Baltimore, Williams & Wilkins, 1987.)

A bone scan will show synovitis in the acute attack.

Treatment. See Chapter 11.

Osteoarthritis

Arthritis is a common finding in the aging patient. It is a result of the gradual loss of articular cartilage secondary to increased stresses (overload), abnormal cartilage metabolism (chondrocalcinosis), or persistent inflammation (crystal-induced arthritis).

Symptoms. Pain is increased with activity. As the disease progresses there is loss of hip rotation and abduction. End stage hip is an uniaxial hip allowing only for flexion and extension.

Signs. These include pain with weight bearing and limited hip motion with an antalgic gait.

Diagnostic Studies. AP and lateral x-rays of the pelvis and hip in weight bearing are necessary. These will demonstrate joint space narrowing, cyst formation, sclerosis, and osteophyte formation.

Treatment. Consists of muscle strengthening, nonsteroidal anti-inflammatories, and use of ambulatory aides, such as a cane in the opposite hand (see Appendix I). Surgery is recommended in those patients who have pain that is unrelieved with conservative measures and in those whose pain interferes with their activities of daily living.

Referral. Referral to an orthopaedic surgeon or rheumatologist is recommended.

Avascular Necrosis

Avascular necrosis is the loss of blood supply to the femoral head and the resultant death to all or part of the femoral head. It may occur in any age group.

Etiology. The etiology may be posttraumatic following hip dislocation or fractures or may be secondary to steroid use or alcohol abuse. The vast majority, however, is idiopathic.

Symptoms. Hip pain occurs with weight bearing.

Signs. Signs include pain on weight bearing and with activity that is relieved with rest, and progressive loss of joint motion as the disease progresses.

Diagnostic Evaluation. X-rays are initially within normal limits with progression seen over time. The weight bearing surfaces of the femoral head collapse with loss of sphericity of the femoral head. Earliest diagnostic imaging is with MRI. Three-phase bone scanning is also a diagnostic tool.

Treatment. Treatment, in the early stages of the disease before collapse, is with protected weight bearing. Conflict exists as to whether or not core decompression of the femoral head is useful in the treatment of this disease. Joint reconstruction for the elderly and hip fusion for the younger patient are the treatments for late disease.

Outcome. This depends upon the stage of the disease when first diagnosed and patient compliance with protected weight bearing.

Referral. An orthopaedic surgeon is recommended for treatment.

Infection

Etiology. The etiology can be drug use, sexually transmitted diseases, and dissemination from other sources.

Symptoms. Severe pain that is increased with any motion and pain that is localized to the groin but may radiate to the thigh or knee are important symptoms. There is also a loss of joint motion, and fever and night sweats are usually present.

Signs. The patient presents with a flexed, abducted, and externally rotated hip as a position of comfort. Fever is usually present. The patient resists any motion, as it increases pain. Inguinal lymphadenopathy may be present.

Laboratory Evaluation. The laboratory evaluation will show an elevated white cell count in the peripheral smear, often with an elevated erythrocyte sedimentation rate. Blood cultures may be useful but are often negative. An aspiration of the hip joint is mandatory and is diagnostic. It will show an elevated white cell count with a predominance of polys. Routine gram stain and cultures of the synovial fluid are mandatory. Cultures for gonorrhea should also be obtained.

Radiographic Evaluation. X-rays may show joint space widening. A bone scan is performed to rule out osteomyelitis.

Treatment. Aspiration for culture followed by surgical drainage for all infections other than gonococcal arthritis is recommended.

Referral. Immediate referral to orthopaedic surgeon if infection is suspected is mandatory.

Outcome. If treated early the outcome should be good. If treated late, chondrolysis from lysosomal enzymes leads to rapid joint degeneration.

Infection Following Total Hip Arthroplasty

Etiology. This infection may be either primary or secondary following a total hip arthroplasty. Primary infections result from infections from innoculum at the time of surgery and occur immediately in the perioperative period. Secondary infections usually are due to a secondary transient bacteremia from dental work, GI or GU instrumentation, or urinary tract infection and are primary gram negative. It is recommended that antibiotic prophylaxis be performed in patients undergoing these procedures.

Symptoms. The patient presents with painful antalgic gait and may present with an acute dislocation.

Signs. Pain with loss of ambulatory range is the primary sign. CBC may show an elevated white count, and the sedimentation rate may be elevated.

Radiographic Evaluation. Radiolucent lines about the prosthesis indicate loosening. Sequential bone scan/gallium scan may be useful in determining septic versus aseptic loosening. Indium white cell scanning is useful. Aspiration is diagnostic only if positive.

Treatment. Treatment includes debridement, irrigation, and antibiotics with immediate or delayed exchange of the prosthesis, dependent upon the organism.

Referral. Refer the patient to an orthopaedic surgeon experienced in the revision of arthroplasty.

Outcome. The outcome is highly variable and depends upon the organism infecting the joint and underlying bone stock.

Tumors

Tumors may either be benign or malignant and either primary or metastatic. Primary bone tumors are primarily a disease of the adolescent. Metastatic disease and multiple myeloma are primarily diseases of the adult and the elderly. Tumors should always be suspected when pain is disproportionate to the physical findings and with the presence of night pain. Visceral tumors should also be considered in the elderly as sources of pelvic and hip pain.

Etiology. The etiology of musculoskeletal tumors is unknown.

Symptoms. Tumors should always be suspected when pain is disproportionate to the physical findings. Tumors characteristically present as night pain. They are often discovered after minor trauma, and often present as persistent discomfort following relatively minor injury exacerbated by activity. Visceral tumors also should be considered in the elderly as sources of pelvic and hip pain.

Signs. Physical examination may reveal localized tenderness, swelling, and loss of normal motion. There may be localized erythema and rubor.

Evaluation should include complete history and physical with abdominal, vaginal, and rectal examination. Laboratory evaluation includes: alkaline phosphatase (elevated), serum calcium (elevated), CBC — hemaglobin is decreased, white count +/−, SPEP (monoclonal spike), UA (proteinuria), and acid phosphatase (increased with prostatic CA).

Radiographic Imaging. Plain films in early lesions are often negative, especially in osteoid osteomas. They may show early areas of sclerosis or periosteal elevation. Tomography is useful to show the nidus of the osteoid osteoma. Bone scanning with tomography is usually diagnostic for malignancies and will localize tumors.

Differential Diagnosis of Tumors.
Adolescent tumors may be either benign or malignant. Benign tumors include osteoid osteoma, osteoblastoma, bone cyst, benign chondroblastoma, and chondromyxoid fibroma. Malignant tumors of the pelvis and hip include periosteal osteosarcoma and chrondrosarcoma. Multiple myeloma is the most common primary malignancy of the bone and it should always be considered in the differential diagnosis in all patients over the age of 60 with pelvic and hip pain. Metastatic tumors are the second most common. Outcome is highly variable depending on the malignancy tissue type and degree of local and distant spread. Excision of benign tumors with curettage and bone grafting is usually curative. Sarcomas may require amputation, although limb salvaging surgery is available for early lesions.

Referral. Referral should be immediate upon the suspicion of any malignancy. The long-term outcome is dependent upon staging.

TRAUMATIC CONDITIONS OF THE PELVIS AND HIP

Contusions (Table 8.2).

Etiology. Contusions result from a direct blow to soft tissue area that have little soft tissue padding; the iliac crest, greater trochanter, and ischial tuberosity are at greater risk for a more painful contusion.

Symptoms. Symptoms include pain, localized tenderness, ecchymosis, and swelling.

Signs. Signs are the same as the symptoms.

Treatment. Ice, compression, and rest will control local bleeding. When pain decreases, therapy is necessary to restore normal flexibility and strength prior to returning to activity. Heat should not be used as it is associated with myositis ossificans.

Bursitis

Etiology. Bursitis usually results from repetitive stress or direct trauma.

Symptoms. Symptoms are characterized by pain that may be aggravated with motion.

Signs. Pain on palpation of the bursa is one sign of bursitis. Erythema and rubor also may be present (Table 8.3).

Treatment. Treatment consists of rest and ice with adjunctive use of nonsteroidal anti-inflammatory medication and the identification of the etiology and correction of the underlying causes. Therapy to restore normal flexibility, range of motion, and strength completes the treatment.

MUSCLE STRAINS

These are the most common injuries encountered in athletes and are a result of stretching the muscle and tendon beyond their normal length. Injury may occur anywhere along the muscle but usually occurs in the muscle tendon junctions. Lack of warm-up or preparation for activity is the common etiology. All muscle groups crossing the hip are at risk for muscle strain (Table 8.4).

Treatment. Treatment consists of rest, ice compression, elevation, and a gradual restoration of activity as symptoms subside and normal painless range of motion and flexibility, endurance, and strength are established.

Table 8.2
Common Contusions

Location	Etiology	Signs
Greater trochanter	Direct blow or fall onto trochanter	Pain with hip abduction, external rotation
Ischial tuberosity	Fall onto buttocks	Pain with straight leg raising Active resisted contraction of hamstring
Pubic ramus	Fall across bar, as in gymnastics	Pain on palpation of pubis
Iliac crest	Direct fall on crest	Difficulty walking, standing upright, pain along the iliac crest

Table 8.3
Bursitis

Location	Etiology	Signs
Trochanteric bursitis	Leg length discrepancy Board pelvis in females Tight tensor fasciality Poor running mechanics Running on banked surfaces	Pain localized to trochanter Increased with abduction, external rotation Positive Ober test
Ischial bursitis	Direct blood Saddle irritation	Pain with sitting, especially increased with legs crossed Direct tenderness on palpation
Iliopectoneal bursitis	Microtrauma	Anterior hip pain and antalgic gait Hip flexion, externally rotated for comfort

Before returning to sports individuals must have:
(1) Full painless range of motion;
(2) Normal flexibility;
(3) Normal strength;
(4) Endurance strength;
(5) The ability to perform the sport without pain.

Sacroiliac Strains

Etiology. Sudden twisting motions of the trunk, pulling while bending forward (weed pulling), or falling on unilateral buttocks can cause sacroiliac strains.

Symptoms. Pain that usually presents a day after injury, with ache and stiffness over the SI joint posteriorly with difficulty bending forward, is a frequent symptom.

Signs. Limited lumbosacral motion and forward flexion as well as pain over the SI joint, a positive Gaenslen's test, and a positive Lasègue sign are frequently noted.

Diagnostic Imaging. This is not needed in sacroiliac strains.

Treatment. Treatment includes rest, ice,

Table 8.4
Muscle Strains

Location	Etiology	Signs/Symptoms
Adductors	Most common usually in the older athlete Forced external rotation of the adducted leg and forced abduction Additional adductor imbalance	Localized tenderness Pain with passive abduction and forced adduction
Hamstrings	Forced flexion of hip with the knee extended	Localized tenderness Pain over muscle and ischial tuberosity with straight leg raising Pain increased with active/resisted hip extension
Iliopsoas	Kicking injury Blocked kick resulting in muscle overload; the thigh fixed or pushed into extension	Deep groin pain May extend into abdomen External rotation of hip in extension increases pain
Rectus femoris	Jumping activities requiring hip flexion and knee extension (i.e., long jump)	Groin pain increased with knee extension while prone; pain increased with passive hip extension and rotation
Gluteus medius	Usually chronic overuse Ice hockey	Pain and attachment to greater trochanter

and analgesics followed by postural education and back rehabilitation programs for both flexion and extension (see Chapter 5 for back exercises).

FRACTURES OF THE HIP AND PELVIS

Apophyseal Avulsion Injuries

Etiology. Apophyseal avulsion injuries usually occur in the adolescent prior to cessation of growth. These injuries are associated with avulsion of the secondary growth centers or apophysis. Injury may occur before the appearance of the secondary ossification centers that develop late in adolescence. A high index of suspicion is needed to diagnose these cases. Diagnosis is confirmed with the development of callous several weeks after injury; this callous formation may be mistaken for tumor (Table 8.5).

Treatment. Treatment is usually conservative and consists of rest, and ice, and resolution in 4 to 6 weeks.

Stress Fractures

Stress fractures are usually the result of overuse and are generally seen after a sudden increase in activity levels. They present as pain with weight bearing and increase with activity. Diagnosis is made with imaging studies. Plain x-rays will show fractures with periosteal reaction. A bone scan provides diagnosis prior to radiographs turning positive. Pain in the groin is the hallmark of a proximal femoral stress fracture and requires prompt intervention to prevent subsequent fracture displacement. If the fracture line progresses across the neck, percutaneous pinning should be performed (Table 8.6).

Pelvic Fractures

Etiology. Pelvic fractures are usually associated with high-energy accidents such as a motor vehicle accident or a fall from a significant height. Injury may occur to a pedestrian struck by a car or to an individual who falls from a horse or scaffolding. These injuries carry associated high morbidity and mortality secondary to associ-

Table 8.5
Apophyseal Injuries

Locations	Etiology	Signs/Symptoms
Iliac crest	Sudden twisting motions Direct trauma	Pain and discomfort over crest Pain with resisted abduction of hip
Anterior superior iliac spine	Forceful contraction of sartorius with running or jumping	Pain over the anterior thigh Pain increased with active hip flexion and passive hip extension
Anterior inferior iliac spine	Kicking activity	Pain and weakness with hip flexion and an antalgic gait
Ischial apophysis	Sudden hamstring contraction with the hip and pelvis flexed and the knee extended. Results in a hamstring avulsion (hurdlers position) Splits during dancing Avulsion–adductor magnus	Pain with antalgic gait Pain with sitting Pain increased with hip flexion when the knee is extended
Lesser trochanter	Rare–sudden contraction of iliopsoas with the thigh flexed and hip extended (i.e., a blocked kick at the point of contact with the ball)	Antalgic gain Pain over trochanter Pain with hip flexion with leg extended Position of comfort, flexed and abducted hip

Table 8.6
Stress Fractures

Location	Etiology	Signs/Symptoms
Pelvic stress fractures	Usually female runners Ischial ramus most common Overuse	Pain over ischial ramus
Pubic ramus	Repetitive trauma Gymnastics	Pain over pubic ramus
Femoral neck	Repetitive jumping activities or running	Pain, antalgic gait Pain with flexion and internal rotation May also present as thigh pain

ated other injuries. The geometry of injury depends upon the direction of the injury and the force that is applied.

Symptoms. Pain, swelling, visible ecchymosis, hematoma, and inability to bear weight are several symptoms. There may be a shift of the iliac crest with vertical or horizontal instability appreciated on palpation. General pressure applied to the iliac wings in compression and distraction may demonstrate this instability.

Signs. The signs are the same as the symptoms. Significant hypotension may be present.

Treatment. The patient must be immediately referred to a trauma center. Vascular support is necessary as bleeding may be life threatening. The use of mast trousers in the acute setting with a comminuted fracture may be beneficial in maintaining vascular volume and controlling pelvic bleeding.

Radiographic Imaging. Imaging consists of AP/LAT, both obliques, and inlet and outlet views to define the planes of displacement. CT scanning is used to define the fracture geometry prior to surgical stabilization.

Definitive Treatment. Stable injuries are treated with protected weight bearing. Unstable injuries require stabilization with either internal or external fixation.

Outcome. The long-term results depend on the severity of the injury. Pelvic fractures associated with sacroiliac joint dislocation and fracture comminution are associated with chronic pain. Fractures involving the acetabulum are associated with late degenerative arthritis.

Hip Dislocation

Etiology. Hip dislocation is usually the result of a motor vehicle accident with direct axial loading of the hip in a flexed position. Posterior dislocations are a result of this position, with the hip in an adducted position. Anterior dislocations are the result of abduction, external rotation, and forced extension of the hip.

Symptoms. Severe pain and inability to walk or stand are two symptoms. Any motion is painful. For *anterior dislocation* the hip is held *abducted, externally rotated,* and slightly flexed. For *posterior dislocation* the hip is held *adducted, internally rotated,* and flexed (Fig. 8.8).

Signs. The signs are the same as the symptoms.

Treatment. This is an orthopaedic emergency requiring immediate referral for closed, possible open, reduction of the hip dislocation. Delays in relocation result in higher incidence of avascular necrosis. Dislocations may occur in conjunction with acetabular or femoral head fractures. Treatment is based upon the position of the fragments' displacement and the degree of displacement. For displaced fractures open reduction internal fixation (ORIF) is the preferred treatment with removal of acetabular loose bodies.

Femoral Neck Fractures

Etiology. In the adolescent and early adult femoral neck fractures occur as a result of high-energy accidents. In the elderly

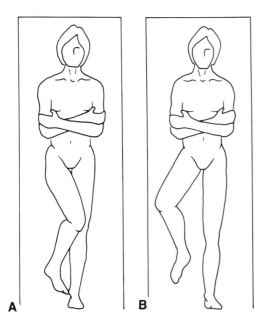

Figure 8.8. Postures of hip dislocation. **A,** posterior dislocation. **B,** anterior dislocation. (From Ramamurti CP (Tinker RV, ed) Orthopaedics in Primary Care. Baltimore, Williams & Wilkins, 1979, p 199.)

they may occur with relatively minor trauma secondary to osteoporosis. Fractures may result from a direct fall on the greater trochanter or from a rotational force along the shaft of the femur.

Symptoms. Symptoms include excruciating groin pain, inability to bear weight, and the extremity held in *external rotation* and *mild adduction*. The pain is exacerbated by motion, particularly internal rotation. In the elderly individual with an impacted fracture, symptoms may consist of pain with ambulation in the groin, thigh, or knee.

Signs. The impacted fracture presents with an antalgic gait. The fracture may be associated with an inability to bear weight and it may have associated swelling and ecchymosis in the thigh.

Diagnostic Imaging. Anteroposterior and lateral x-rays usually confirm the diagnosis. In the elderly with groin pain and osteopenia, tomograms and a bone scan may be necessary to confirm the diagnosis.

Treatment. In the young and in early adults all fractures should be reduced and internally fixed. A high percentage of dis-

placed fractures will undergo avascular necrosis secondary to disruption of the blood supply along the femoral neck. In the elderly, displaced fractures should be treated with hemiarthroplasty or total hip arthroplasty in the presence of acetabular disease. Nondisplaced fractures should be treated with in situ pinning. Failure of fixation may occur secondary to osteopenia. Avascular necrosis is a late sequelae in both displaced and nondisplaced fractures.

Adolescent Slipped Capital Femoral Epiphysis

Etiology. The etiology of adolescent slipped capital femoral epiphysis is uncertain, but it occurs in adolescents who are short and obese or tall and thin. Displacement occurs at the junction of the proliferative cartilage and the provisional zone of calcification. This should be suspected in any adolescent complaining of groin, thigh, or knee pain.

Symptoms. Groin pain often referred to the anterior medial thigh is one symptom. Antalgic gait with external rotation position of the hip and loss of internal rotation are also symptoms. For an acute slip there is usually a history of a fall or direct trauma associated with sudden pain, spasm, or inability to fully bear weight. Chronic slips have a history of mild aching pain in the groin and a limp. An acute slip may occur in the presence of chronic slippage.

Signs. The signs are the same as the symptoms.

Treatment. Early diagnosis before a significant slip occurs is important. Surgical in situ pinning is the treatment of choice.

Diagnostic Imaging. Anteroposterior and lateral radiographs are the appropriate studies.

Intertrochanteric Hip Fractures

Etiology. In the young an intertrochanteric hip fracture is a result of violent trauma. In the elderly it is usually the result of a fall from a standing position and a result of secondary underlying osteopenia.

Symptoms. Pain and an inability to bear weight with ecchymosis are symptoms.

Signs.   A flexed shortened externally rotated hip, thigh swelling, and ecchymosis are several signs.

Treatment.   Immediate referral for surgery with open reduction and internal fixation is necessary.

Diagnostic Imaging.   Anteroposterior and lateral hip radiographs are required.

Outcome.   The outcome is dependent upon the premorbid state of the patient. In a compromised patient the outcome may result in the loss of one level of activity. In an active healthy patient resumption of normal lifestyle after healing usually occurs.

Recommended Reading

Anatomy

Draves DJ: *Anatomy of the Lower Extremity*. Baltimore, Williams & Wilkins, 1986.

Hollingshead WH: *Anatomy for Surgeons: The Back and Limbs*, ed 3. Philadelphia, Harper & Row, vol 3, 1982.

Arthritis

Kelly W, Harris E, Ruddy S, Sledge C: *Textbook of Rheumatology*. vol 1, 2nd ed, Philadelphia, WB Saunders, 1985.

Fractures

Clawson DK, Melcher PJ: Fractures and dislocations of the hip. In Rockwood CA and Green DP, (eds) *Fractures*. Philadelphia, JB Lippincott, 1975, vol 2.

McBride AM: Stress fractures in athletes. *J Sportsmed* 3:212–216, 1975.

Physical Assessment

Hoppenfeld S: *Physical Examination of the Spine and Extremities*. East Norwalk, CT: Appleton-Century-Croft, 1976.

Sports-Related Topics

Scott WN, Nisonson B, Nicholas JA: *Principles of Sports Medicine*. Baltimore, Williams & Wilkins, 1984.

chapter 9

The Thigh, Knee, and Patella

PEKKA A. MOOAR, M.D.

THE KNEE

The Anatomy and Function

The knee joint consists of two joints: the tibial femoral joint and the patella femoral joint. The motion at the knee joint is a complex interaction of flexion, extension, rotation, gliding, and rolling. These complex movements are allowed by the controlled instability of the knee joint. When motions outside of the range of this controlled instability take place, injury occurs. The injury is to the structure or structures that resist the applied force. Knowledge of the anatomy of the stabilizing knee structures is necessary to understand the patterns of injury.

The knee provides motion and stability, allows forces to propel the body forward, and absorbs high loads. Figure 9.1 depicts the structures of the knee. The femur, tibia, and patella are covered on their articulating surfaces with a layer of cartilage. This cartilage derives its nutrition from the synovial fluid and is subjected to the stresses imposed upon it by both normal and abnormal knee motions.

The Meniscus

The menisci (medial and lateral) are crescent-shaped pieces of cartilage interposed between the femur and tibia; they function to absorb energy and to distribute the load across the knee joint. They also provide secondary stability by deepening the tibial plateau. The ligaments of the knee are the medial and lateral collateral ligaments, and the anterior and posterior cruciate ligaments. They function in conjunction with the joint capsule to limit varus (medial), valgus (lateral), and anterior posterior translations of the knee.

The medial stabilizers of the knee are the joint capsule and the medial collateral ligament (Fig. 9.2). These structures resist valgus laxity and medial rotatory instabilities.

These structures have a firm attachment to the medial meniscus that makes it less mobile and therefore at risk for injury during flexion and rotation of the knee. The pes anserine group (sartorius, gracilis, semitendinosus) protects the knee against valgus and rotatory stresses.

The lateral stabilizers (Fig. 9.3) of the knee are the lateral collateral ligament and the lateral joint capsule. Secondary contributions to lateral stability are supplied by the iliotibial band, biceps tendon, and the popliteal arcuate complex in the posterolateral corner of the knee.

The cruciate ligaments are the primary stabilizers for anterior and posterior displacement of the tibia on the femur (Fig. 9.4). The anterior cruciate runs from anterior on the tibia just medial to the anterior tibial spine to the posterior aspect of the lateral femoral condyle in the intercondylar notch.

This ligament prevents anterior displace-

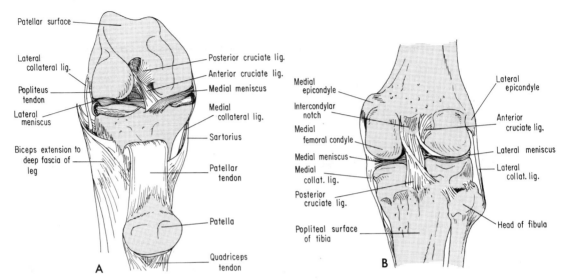

Figure 9.1. *"Internal anatomy" of the knee.* **A,** Anterior view. The knee is flexed, and the patella is "stripped" downward to better illustrate "internal" structure. **B,** Posterior view. (From Reilly BM: *Practical Strategies in Outpatient Medicine.* Philadelphia, WB Saunders, 1984, p 268.)

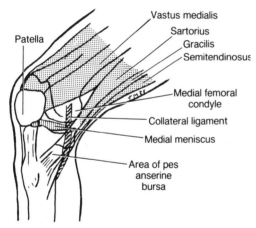

Figure 9.2. Medial stabilizers of the knee. (From Burnside JW, McGlynn TJ: *Physical Diagnosis* ed 17. Baltimore, Williams & Wilkins, 1987, p 271.)

ment of the tibia and helps control rotation and hyperextension of the knee during cutting, twisting, and turning activities.

The posterior cruciate runs from the posterior aspect of the tibial plateau to the anterior aspect of the medial femoral condyle in the intercondylar notch.

This ligament prevents posterior displacement of the tibia on the femur, especially during flexion.

The posterior aspect of the knee contains a hollow space (popliteal fossa) bounded by the biceps femoris laterally and the semimembranosus and semitendinosus medially. Inferiorly it is bounded by the two limbs of the gastrocnemius muscle. Found within the popliteal space are the popliteal artery and vein and the peroneal and tibial nerves (Fig. 9.5).

The Muscles

The muscles about the knee are important to:
(1) Provide locomotion;
(2) Absorb energy;
(3) Provide dynamic stability.

The quadriceps are the anterior thigh muscles and consist of four muscles. These muscles function to extend the knee (Fig. 9.6). They converge to form the quadriceps tendon that inserts on the patella. The patella acts as a pulley across the knee joint and increases the biomechanical advantage of the quadriceps. The patella tendon originates at the inferior pole of the patella and inserts into the tibial tubercle.

The vastus medialis has a secondary function as a dynamic stabilizer of the patella femoral joint. It is also a sensitive indicator of muscle weakness as it is the first

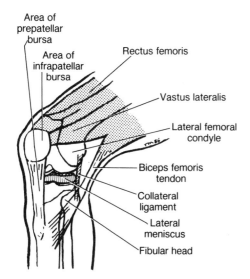

Area of
prepatellar
bursa

Rectus femoris

Area of
infrapatellar
bursa

Vastus lateralis

Lateral femoral
condyle

Biceps femoris
tendon

Collateral
ligament

Lateral
meniscus

Fibular head

Figure 9.3. Lateral stabilizers of the knee. (From Burnside JW, McGlynn TJ: *Physical Diagnosis*, ed 17. Baltimore, Williams & Wilkins, 1987, p 271.)

of the quadriceps muscles to atrophy after injury.

The sartorius, gracilis, and semitendinosus form the pes anserine group that originates from the pelvis and inserts on the medial tibial surface 5 to 7 cm below the joint line. They function as internal rotators and flexors of the knee.

The iliotibial band laterally arises from the iliac crest and inserts on Gerdy's tubercle on the tibia. It functions as both a secondary extensor and flexor of the knee as it shifts anterior to posterior to the axis of the knee motion during flexion and extension.

The popliteus muscle is deep on the posterior lateral corner of the knee with its origin on the femur and insertion on the posterior medial aspect of the tibia. The popliteus helps control external rotation of the femur on a fixed tibia and anterior displacement of the tibia on the femur when the lower extremity is fixed.

The most posterior muscles, the semimembranosus, semitendinosus, and biceps femoris, are collectively called the hamstrings and are the major flexors of the knee. They also function to extend the hip and decelerate the knee during extension.

The semimembranosus dynamically sta-

bilizes the posterior medial corner of the knee and therefore prevents excessive rotation of the tibia on the femur.

The biceps femoris, has two origins. The long head from the ischial tuberosity and the short head from the lateral femur. It inserts on the fibular head posteriorly and has a secondary function of stabilizing the lateral aspect of the knee during flexion. Medially the adductor group of adductor magnus, brevis, longus, and gracilis rise in the pubic ramus and insert along the medial aspect of the distal femur with the gracilis attaching in the pes anserine complex medial on the tibia. These muscles adduct the hip and are hip and knee flexors. The hip abductors are the tensor fascia and the gluteus medius muscles that originate from the crest of the ilium. The gluteus medius inserts on the greater trochanter and the tensor fascia lata travels laterally over the thigh to insert on the lateral aspect of the tibial and femoral condyle. These muscles cover the longest and strongest bone in the body the femur.

Bursae

There are numerous bursae about the knee (Fig. 9.7). These function to reduce friction between structures that glide past one another. They are usually thin but with repeated stress may become thickened and fluid filled secondary to inflammation.

THE PAINFUL THIGH

Physical Examination

Inspection. The patient should be examined appropriately exposed. This usually requires complete removal of clothes to allow exposure of both legs. The patient is inspected in the standing position and is viewed from all directions. This allows the examiner to evaluate alignment of the femur and to look for areas of ecchymosis or swelling. Muscle bulk and symmetry are noted. Attention should be paid to standing postures. If the patient is unable to fully extend the knee there may be a problem with the hamstring or a chronic knee flexion contracture. Observation of the asym-

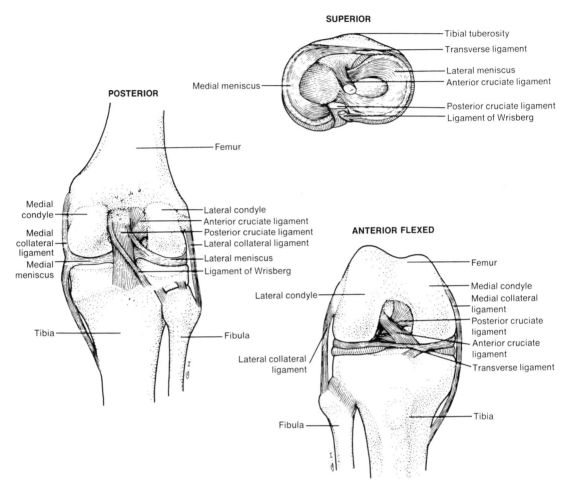

Figure 9.4. Ligamentous stabilizers of the knee. (From Hilt NE, Cogburn SB: *Manual of Orthopaedics.* St. Louis, CV Mosby, 1980, p 25.)

metry of anterior musculature is facilitated by asking the patient to kneel with the buttocks on the heels.

Palpation. The patient is examined with systematic palpation of the origins and insertions of the thigh musculature as well as palpation of the muscles for enlargement, tenderness, or defects. The patient is asked to gently contract his quadriceps and hamstrings to feel for areas of defects or tenderness. With the patient supine, range of motion of the hip and knees is evaluated. Determination of full range of motion is essential. Hamstring tightness is evaluated by lifting the legs off the examining table by the heels with the knees extended. The hips should flex at least 60° before any knee flex-

ion occurs. Early knee flexion is indicative of a hamstring contracture. The patient then is placed in the prone position and the posterior structures of the thigh are examined from the gluteal fold with careful palpation of both the medial and lateral hamstrings. With active knee flexion the hamstring muscles are brought into tension and the examiner may apply resistance to evaluate for muscle defects or tenderness with motion. Palpation in the medial and lateral aspects of the popliteal fossa will allow for palpation of the medial and lateral hamstring tendons. Range of motion is evaluated. Limitation of flexion is indicative of contracture of the anterior thigh musculature. The lateral aspect of the leg is palpated from the iliac crest along

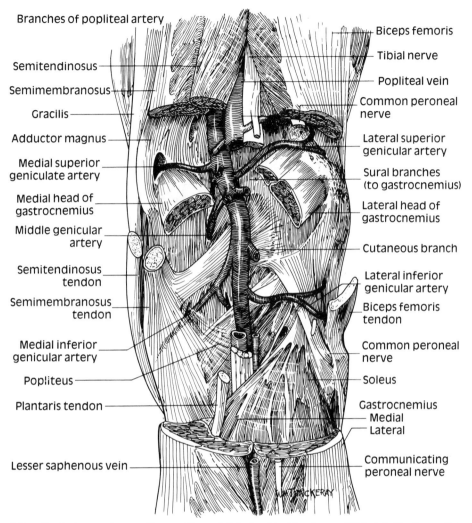

Branches of popliteal artery

Semitendinosus

Semimembranosus

Gracilis

Adductor magnus

Medial superior geniculate artery

Medial head of gastrocnemius

Middle genicular artery

Semitendinosus tendon

Semimembranosus tendon

Medial inferior genicular artery

Popliteus

Plantaris tendon

Lesser saphenous vein

Biceps femoris

Tibial nerve

Popliteal vein

Common peroneal nerve

Lateral superior genicular artery

Sural branches (to gastrocnemius)

Lateral head of gastrocnemius

Cutaneous branch

Lateral inferior genicular artery

Biceps femoris tendon

Common peroneal nerve

Soleus

Gastrocnemius
Medial
Lateral

Communicating peroneal nerve

Figure 9.5.   Posterior anatomy of knee. (From Nicholas JA, Hershman EB (eds): *The Lower Extremity and Spine in Sports Medicine*. St. Louis, CV Mosby, 1980, vols 1 and 2, p 674.)

the fascia lata to its insertion on the tibia. Tenderness over the greater trochanter may be indicative of trochanteric bursitis or snapping iliotibial band (Fig. 9.8). The Ober test is used to test for tightness of the iliotibial band. Most complaints of thigh pain will be the result of direct trauma though sources of referred pain from back, hip, and knee should always be excluded.

Contusions

Contusions as a result of direct trauma are common sequelae of sporting activity. Proper treatment of these injuries is imperative to prevent serious impairment of athletic performance. Following a direct blow to the thigh, there is local damage to blood vessels and muscle. The athlete may continue to play, but as bleeding and swelling continue the thigh begins to get stiff with loss of full knee motion. Treatment consists of ice and compression to control swelling and bleeding. This early therapy is essential to promote painless range of motion. Rehabilitation begins with establishing painless range of motion, followed by flexibility and strengthening exercises.

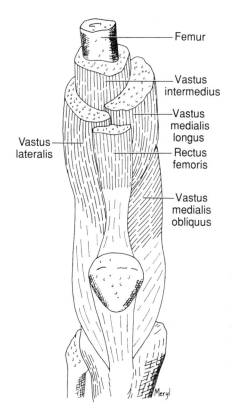

Figure 9.6. Muscles of the knee. (From Scott WN, Nisonson B, Nicholas JA (eds): *Principles of Sports Medicine.* Baltimore, Williams & Wilkins, 1984, p 274.)

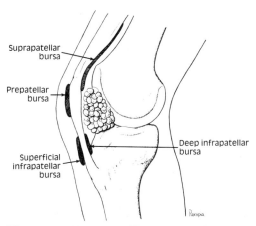

Figure 9.7. Location of bursa in anterior aspect of knee. (From Nicholas JA, Hershman EB (eds): *The Lower Extremity and Spine in Sports Medicine.* St. Louis, CV Mosby, 1986, vols 1 and 2, p 985.)

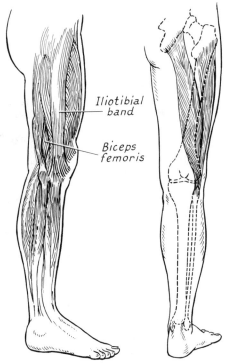

Figure 9.8. The iliotibial band. (From Helfet AJ: *Disorders of the Knee.* Philadelphia, JB Lippincott, 1982, p 6.)

Return to sport is allowed when full painless range of motion and strength equal to the unaffected extremity are obtained. Do not use heat on a contusion.

Myositis ossificans or calcification of muscle at the site of injury is a late sequela of a severe blow to the thigh. Its occurrence is associated with repetitive reinjury before primary healing occurs and when heat is used to treat an acute hematoma. Treatment consists of excision of the mass after it is mature.

Muscle Strains

Quadriceps

Quadriceps strain usually involves the rectus femoris, but may involve the vastus medialis and vastus lateralis. Injury most commonly occurs during rapid acceleration while running, or when a kick is mistimed or blocked. The most common predisposing factor is lack of adequate stretching or warm-up prior to initiation of the activity. Excessively tight quadriceps, short legs, or significant muscle imbalance can also be predisposing factors.

The clinical presentation is usually of pain over the anterior thigh, localized tenderness, and an associated limp. Treatment consists of ice, compression, and rest followed by stretching exercises to restore painless range of motion. The athlete returns to sports when there is equal flexibility in both quadriceps, full painless range of motion, and restoration of strength and endurance strength in the injured muscle.

Hamstring Strain

This injury is the most common of the lower extremity muscle injuries. It is usually a direct result of lack of flexibility in these muscles and lack of appropriate warm-up. Other factors that have been implicated include hamstring/quadriceps imbalance, imbalance between medial and lateral hamstrings, poor running mechanics, overstriding, and too rapid a deceleration during running activities.

This injury presents as sudden onset of pain in the posterior thigh and often the athlete "pulls up lame." Swelling may occur immediately after injury or be delayed. Delayed ecchymosis is common and is often extensive. Treatment consists of ice, compression, and support. Rehabilitation begins after pain subsides with the goal of establishing full painless range of motion prior to strengthening and endurance strengthening exercises.

Iliotibial Band

Lateral thigh pain, especially in a runner, may be due to an irritation of the iliotibial band. This presents as pain over the lateral aspect of the leg and is commonly aggravated by running down hills. Pain may be present over the knee, at 30° of flexion during full weight bearing. This pain pattern is due to a tight iliotibial band and is demonstrated by the positive Ober test and is also associated with inadequate shock absorption in the shoes, poor running mechanics, and with leg length inequality.

THE PAINFUL KNEE

History

When a patient presents with a knee complaint, one should not limit oneself to the knee. A precise review of systems and evaluation of the hip and back will prevent one from overlooking patterns of referred pain from discogenic disease or hip fracture. An assessment of systemic illnesses such as rheumatoid arthritis, systemic lupus, and lyme disease also needs to be considered as well as taking a sexual history to evaluate for gonococcal arthritis.

Determine if the problem is acute or chronic. How, what, when, and where are essential questions. In the acute injury determine the mechanism of injury (how). If it is subacute or chronic, how did the symptoms develop, and were there any changes in the training regimen, activity levels, or work requirements (i.e., did the patient recently increase stair climbing, squatting, or lifting activities) prior to the onset of pain? These activities are often associated with an increase in patella femoral pain, especially in females.

When did symptoms begin? At the time of injury or later? Was the patient able to continue the sport? A tear of the anterior cruciate ligament usually presents with an acute hemarthrosis and inability to continue activity. A meniscus tear may present with an acutely locked knee but may present as a delayed onset of swelling with intermittent catching or giving way episodes associated with joint line pain.

What are the specific complaints? Is there swelling, locking, giving way, pain, weakness, numbness, or sensation of instability? What activities aggravate the symptoms? Walking down stairs and prolonged sitting may bring out symptoms associated with patella femoral disorders. Instability with cutting, twisting, and turning is associated with anterior cruciate lesions and meniscal pathology. Determine the severity of the disability. Are there difficulties with activities of daily living, light sports, or sports requiring vigorous cutting, twisting, and turning activities?

Determine the location of the pain

(where). Meniscus pain will be localized to the joint line but pain of an MCL injury will be diffuse along the medial aspect of the knee along the path of the medial collateral ligament. The pain of patella subluxation or dislocation will be localized to the retinacula structures about the patella.

Physical Examination

Observation. The physical examination begins with observation. Does the patient walk with an antalgic gait? Does the patient sit with the knee extended? If so, there may be a knee effusion.

Inspection. Inspection begins with the patient erect with the legs exposed to mid-thigh. Note the alignment of the knee. Eight to 12° of valgus (knocked knees) is normal. Make note of any excess valgus or varus (bow legs) (Fig. 9.9). Note the location and position of the patella; they should face anteriorly and be at the same level. A medially positioned patella or squinting patella is associated with patella femoral pain syndromes. Inspect the symmetry of the quadriceps; note any muscle atrophy. The vastus medialis oblique is the first muscle to show muscle atrophy. With the knee in full extension, measure the circumference of the thigh at a point 5 cm above the superior pole of the patella. Measure leg lengths, inspect for soft tissue fullness. Loss of soft tissue dimples about the knee is an early indicator of a knee effusion. A knee effu-

sion may give one a false circumferential measurement as the suprapatella pouch may extend significantly proximal to the superior pole of the patella.

Inspection of the bony insertion of the patella tendon may reveal an enlargement that in the adolescent may indicate Osgood-Schlatter disease. Examine the patient's gait. Antalgic gait (avoidance of putting full weight on the painful leg) may represent painful arthropathy. The inability to gain full knee extension at heel strike usually represents intraarticular pathology. An abnormal lateral or medial thrust may indicate ligamentous instability or advanced joint arthritis with joint collapse. Back kneeing, or genu recurvatum, may be an indication of hypermobility syndrome or a posterior cruciate ligament injury. Excessive foot pronation and interior tibial torsion are associated with patella femoral pain syndromes (Fig.9.10). Observation of the inability to duck walk or walking in a squatting position is associated with meniscal injury.

Palpation. Look first for a knee effusion, then gently palpate the knee. A large effusion is seen with a ballottable or floating patella. With the patient's knee extended, depress the patella into the trochlear groove and gently tap; the patella will bounce back with a large effusion. An effusion may also be demonstrated by tapping the lateral retinaculum with a palpable fluid wave appreciated on the medial side. A small effusion may be demonstrated by milking the superior patella pouch inferiorly to force fluid into the knee joint. This will result in a ballottable patella. Palpate the prepatella bursa. If swollen, there may be bursitis; however, the bursa often communicates with the knee joint and may be present with a concomitant knee effusion.

The precise localization of pain in the evaluation of the knee is helpful in defining the pathology (Fig. 9.11). In general it is best to palpate areas of tenderness last as provocation of pain early in the exam may cause anxiety and the patient may become unable to relax and cooperate fully.

Palpate the patella and extensor mechanism; palpate the superior pole. Feel for defects in the muscle attachments over areas

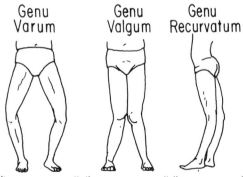

Figure 9.9. Common knee deformities. (From Reilly BM: *Practical Strategies in Outpatient Medicine.* Philadelphia, WB Saunders, 1984, p 221.)

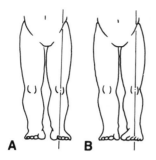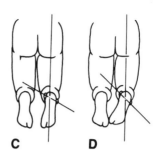

Figure 9.10. Examining for tibial torsion. **A** and **B**, child supine. **A**, normal. **B**, internal tibial torsion. **C** and **D**, child prone, knee-flexed 90°. **C**, normal. **D**, internal tibial torsion. (From Ramamurti CP (Tinker RV, ed): *Orthopaedics in Primary Care*. Baltimore, Williams & Wilkins, 1979, p 258.)

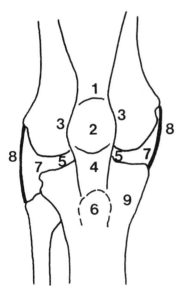

Figure 9.11. Palpation of pain in the knee. *1*, quadriceps tendinitis; *2*, prepatella bursitis, patella pain; *3*, retinacular pain after patella subluxation; *4*, patella tendinitis; *5*, fat pad tenderness; *6*, Osgood-Schlatter disease (tibial tubercle pain); *7*, meniscus pain; *8*, collateral ligament pain; and *9*, pes anserine tendinitis bursitis. (Adapted from Cailliet R: *Soft Tissue Pain and Disability*. Philadelphia, FA Davis, 1977, p 235.)

of pain. This is consistent with rupture or avulsion from the patella. Pain at this location is seen with quadriceps tendinitis. Palpate the anterior patella for warmth, redness, and swelling. Increased warmth, redness, and swelling are found with prepatella bursitis, "house maids," and "brick layers" knee.

Palpate the medial and lateral retinaculum and the medial and lateral facets of the patella. Tenderness over the retinaculum is seen with patella subluxation and dislocation, and facet discomfort is seen with patella femoral pain syndrome. The patella should be gently pushed from medial to lateral to test its intrinsic stability. The patella should not sublux more than 50% of its width. The Q-angle or the angle of the patella tendon with the quadriceps is measured. Increased Q-angles greater than 20° are associated with patella femoral pain syndromes (Fig. 9.12). Palpate the inferior pole of the patella. Pain at this location is seen with jumper's knee or inferior patella tendinitis. The patella tendon is palpated with the accompanying fat pads and bursae. In blunt trauma to the anterior knee these structures may remain painful for many months. Excessive kneeling may also cause infrapatellar bursitis. The insertion of the tendon in the tibial tubercle is palpated next. Pain at this location in an adolescent is the hallmark of Osgood-Schlatter disease. The adult who has had Osgood-Schlatter disease as a child may experience discomfort with repetitive kneeling activities over this bony prominence. Palpate the medial and lateral aspects of the knee.

Examination of the medial aspect of the knee is performed with the knee in extension and in flexion. A repeat examination of the retinacular structures is performed followed by a careful palpation of the femoral condyle and tibial plateau. In the adolescent, pain along the femoral or tibial

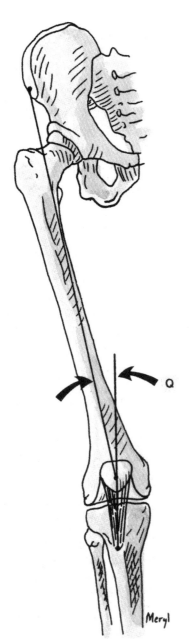

Figure 9.12. "Q" or quadriceps angle is formed by the intersection of lines between the anterior superior iliac spine and the midportion of the patella and the tibial tubercle. It is the angle formed by the quadriceps muscle and the *patellar tendon*. (From Scott WN, Nisonson B, Nicholas JA (eds): *Principles of Sports Medicine.* Baltimore, Williams & Wilkins, 1984, p 302.)

epiphysis after trauma may represent a nondisplaced fracture through the epiphysis. In the adult painful osteophytes of arthritis may be palpated. In the elderly pain over the tibial flair or femoral condyle may be seen with osteonecrosis. In the adult or adolescent with an osteochondritis lesion, pain may be palpated over the involved compartment.

Carefully palpate the joint line. The anterior soft spot between the femoral condyle and the tibial plateau allows us to quickly localize the joint surface. Pain along the joint line is indicative of meniscus pathology. Flex the knee to 90° to allow the pes anserine complex to displace posteriorly. This allows for palpation of the joint line and the medial collateral ligament (MCL). Pain along the course of the MCL from the femur to tibia is seen with injury. Palpation of the medial collateral ligament should include origin, midsubstance, and insertion. Palpate the pes anserine complex and look for tenderness associated with bursitis or tendinitis.

Examine the lateral aspect of the knee from proximal to distal, palpate the lateral femoral condyle, lateral tibial plateau, and lateral joint line. Lateral joint line pain is synonymous with meniscal pathology.

Examine the lateral collateral ligament with the knees crossed or in the figure-4 position. This puts stress on the lateral collateral ligament and allows easier palpation of its origin from the femoral condyle to its insertion on the fibular head. The iliotibial band is palpated along its course over the lateral thigh and knee to its insertion on Gerdy's tubercle on the anterior lateral aspect of the tibia. Pain is often seen in runners with a contracted iliotibial band and is a result of friction as the band is rubbed over the lateral knee structures. This tightness can be demonstrated with the Ober test. Ask the patient to lie on the side with the leg to be tested up. Flex the opposite leg (away from the body) to stabilize the pelvis. Abduct (away from the body) as far as possible and then flex the knee to 90°. The symptomatic leg is allowed to be adducted (toward the body). If the iliotibial band is normal the thigh should drop to the adducted position. If there is a contracture of the iliotibial band the thigh will remain in the abducted position when the leg is released (+ Ober test). If there is inflammation this test will illicit discomfort over the iliotibial band (Fig. 9.13). Next, palpate the posterior aspect of the knee. Fullness may indicate a popliteal cyst. Pain over the medial and lateral heads of the gastrocnemius may represent tendinitis or a muscle injury. Palpate the posterior tibial pulse. In a patient with acute multiplaner instability a knee dislocation should be assumed and an appropriate vascular assessment obtained.

Stability Testing

Stability testing is performed in the anterior/posterior/medial-lateral (varus-valgus) and rotational planes.

The ability to assess the anterior/poste-rior, varus-valgus planes of instability is essential to the basic knee examination. With the knee in full extension and in 30° of flexion, test for medial collateral stability by placing the ankle in one hand, or cradled on your hip, while the other hand is placed over the lateral joint line. Apply a gentle valgus force to the joint line (if the medial collateral ligament is torn); this will open up the medial joint line. If there is instability in full extension then the MCL and secondary stabilizers of the capsule are completely disrupted and this usually represents a surgical problem. Next, examine the knee in 30° of flexion. If instability is only present at 30° of flexion the capsule is intact and there is only a partial injury to the medial collateral or an isolated medial collateral ligament injury.

Reverse the test to evaluate the lateral collateral ligament with a varus force ap-

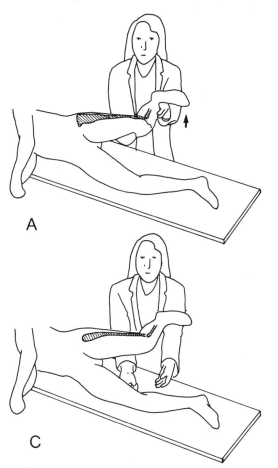

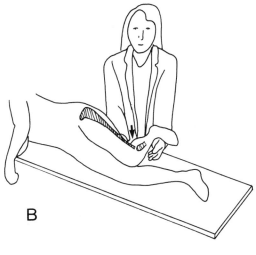

Figure 9.13. Ober test. **A**, Abduct the leg as far as possible and flex the knee to 90 degrees. **B**, Negative Ober test: The leg falls to adducted position when released. **C**, Positive Ober test: The thigh remains abducted when the leg is released.

plied to the medial joint line at both full extension and 30° of flexion.

Anterior posterior displacements evaluate the anterior and posterior cruciate ligaments. The anterior cruciate ligament resists anterior displacement of the tibia on the femur and the posterior cruciate resists posterior displacement.

The anterior and posterior drawer test is performed with the knee flexed to 90°. The foot is kept in neutral rotation to relax the secondary stabilizers of the joint capsule and the collateral ligaments. The test is best performed with the examiner sitting on the neutrally aligned foot. Grasp the knee firmly with both hands as the index fingers palpate the hamstrings for relaxation (Fig. 9.14). The tibia is gently pulled anteriorly for the anterior drawer or pushed posteriorly for the posterior drawer. The degree of displacement from the neutral starting position is assessed as well as the character of the end point (i.e., firm or soft). Comparison is made of the affected and unaffected knees. It is sometimes difficult to assess if the drawer is positive anterior or posterior because of the starting point. This may be evaluated with a drop back test. The test is performed with both knees flexed to 90°, both hips flexed to 90°, and the legs supported only by the ankles and viewed from the side. In a posterior cruciate-deficient knee this will show as a posterior sag or drop back of the tibia on the femur (Fig. 9.15).

Secondary or rotatory instabilities may be assessed with the knee at 90° and the foot rotated internally or externally and the drawer repeated. With internal rotation the lateral structures are tightened. If a drawer is present, anterior lateral rotatory instability is present. Conversely, anterior medial instability is present if the anterior drawer is seen with the foot externally rotated, as this should tighten the secondary medial stabilizers of the knee.

Similar evaluation for posterior rotatory instabilities may be performed (Table 9.1).

Multiplanar instability in the acutely injured knee is a sign of a serious knee injury. All patients with this injury pattern should be presumed to have a knee dislocation. This injury often has associated vascular injury and requires close monitoring and an arteriogram to evaluate the vascularity to the leg.

The patella is examined for stability with the knee in extension and slight flexion. Medial and lateral displacement forces are applied to evaluate stability. "Positive apprehension" may be elicited with existing patella femoral disease. The position of the patella is palpated during passive flexion extension to evaluate its tracking. It is examined to see if it remains centered within the trochlear groove or subluxes laterally. The character of joint motion is also assessed while feeling for crepitus associated with patella femoral pain syndromes (Fig. 9.16).

Provocation testing for patella femoral pain is also performed. The knee is extended and the patella is gently depressed into the trochlear groove as well as slightly inferiorly. The patient is then asked to maximally contract the quadriceps. The location of pain similar to the complaints confirms the diagnosis of patella femoral pain syndrome.

The final provocation testing is for the evaluation of meniscus pathology. The McMurray test is performed with the knee in full internal or full external rotation. The knee is flexed fully and a rotational force applied. The knee is then gently brought out into full extension. The presence of pain localized to the joint line or a palpable joint line click is strongly suggestive of meniscus pathology (Fig. 9.17). The Apley compression test may also be performed. This test is done with the knee flexed 90° while the patient is prone. Axial pressure is applied to the foot during internal and external rotation. The elicitation of pain along the joint line is positive for meniscal pathology (Fig. 9.17).

The inability to gain full extension in conjunction with joint line pain is also highly suggestive of a displaced torn meniscus. An intraarticular loose body also needs to be considered.

Manual muscle testing may be performed but it is difficult to assess subtle differences in strength in the lower extremities. Profound atrophy is usually appreciated on inspection. Diffuse atrophy and weakness seen with muscle degeneration

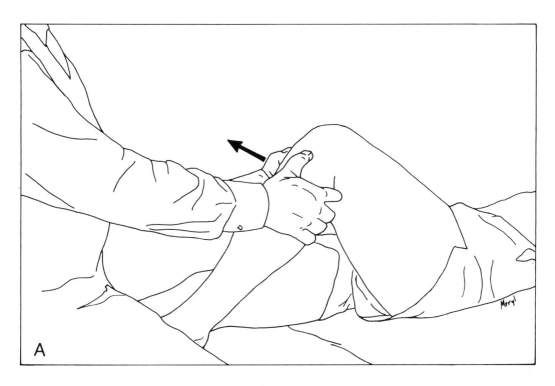

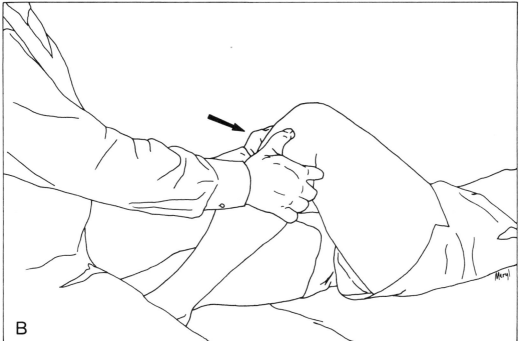

Figure 9.14. **A**, The anterior drawer test. **B**, The posterior drawer test.

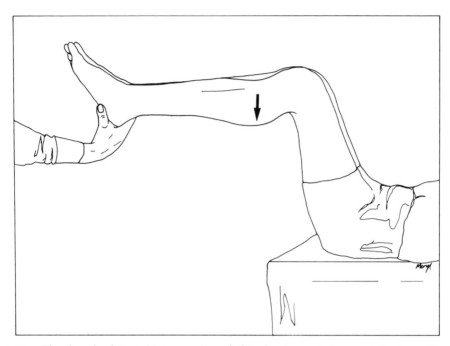

Figure 9.15. The drop back test. Note sagging of tibia due to posterior cruciate disruption. Interpretation may be difficult in patients with previous surgery on the anterior protion of the knee. (From Scott WN, Nisonson B, Nicholas JA (eds): *Principles of Sports Medicine*. Baltimore, Williams & Wilkins, 1984, p 310.)

Table 9.1
Knee Ligament Instabilities[a]

Clinical Instabilities[b]	Laxity Tests
Single plane instabilities	
Medial	Valgus stress at 0° and 30° of flexion
Lateral	Varus stress at 0° and 30° of flexion
Anterior	Anterior drawer at 90° of flexion
	Lachman test
Posterior	Posterior drawer at 90° of flexion
Rotatory instabilities[c]	
Anteromedial	Anterior drawer with foot in external rotation at 90° of flexion
Anterolateral	Anterior drawer with foot in internal rotation at 90° of flexion
	Pivot shift test
Posterolateral	Hyperextension of leg
	Posterior drawer with foot in internal rotation at 90° of flexion
Posteromedial	Posterior drawer with foot in external rotation at 90° of flexion (rare)

[a]*Note*. Classification of instabilities was adapted from the Research and Education Committee of the American Orthopaedic Society of Sports Medicine. From Roy S., Irvin R: *Sports Medicine. Prevention, Evaluation, Management, and Rehabilitation*. Englewood Cliffs, NJ, Prentice-Hall, 1983, p. 310.
[b]Movement of the tibia in relation to the femur. Medial means the tibia is moving away from the femur on the medial side.
[c]Movement of the tibia in relation to the femur. Anteromedial rotatory instability means the tibia is rotating anteriorly and moving away from the femur on the medial side.

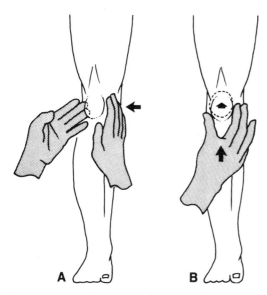

Figure 9.16. Chondromalacia patellae. Examination for characteristic tenderness. **A**, palpation of the lateral margin of the patella. **B**, compression and elevation of the patella. (From Ramamurti CP (Tinker RV, ed): *Orthopaedics in Primary Care.* Baltimore, Williams & Wilkins, 1979, p 222.)

and neurologic disorders will be appreciated on manual muscle testing.

Diagnostic Guidelines

Radiographic Evaluation of the Knee

Radiographs are almost always needed to completely evaluate knee complaints. Obtain AP standing films of both knees on a single cassette with a lateral of the affected knee. This will allow for the determination of most fractures, loose bodies, arthritis, chondrocalcinosis, and osteochondritis dissecans. The presence of joint space narrowing in one compartment is seen with early osteoarthritis. If tricompartmental disease is seen a pansynovial process such as is seen in gout, rheumatoid arthritis, pigmented villonodular synovitis, or chondrocalcinosis should be considered. This finding is also seen in the late stages of osteoarthritis. Obtain a tunnel view to evaluate for flecks of bone off the tibial spine. This is useful to evaluate for acute anterior cruciate injury. Obtain oblique views to evaluate for an avulsion fracture of the lateral tibial attachment of the lateral collateral ligament. This finding, "lateral capsular sign," is strongly suggestive of an anterior cruciate injury with anterior lateral rotatory instability. Calcification in the medial collateral ligament is seen as a late finding following medial collateral ligament injury.

Obtain sunrise views of the patella to evaluate patella femoral tracking and subluxation. Obtain a lateral x-ray to assess the presence of a low-riding or high-riding patella and possible extensor dysfunction. In the skeletally immature adolescent the epiphysis should be examined for evidence of fractures. Stress views are sometimes useful to confirm epiphyseal injury.

Obtain arthrography and MRI to evaluate intraarticular soft tissue injuries of the meniscus, and anterior and posterior cruciate ligaments.

Obtain an arteriogram when multiplanar instability is present in an acutely injuried knee.

Obtain a bone scan to confirm epiphyseal injuries, avascular necrosis lesions, early osteochondritis lesions as well as stress fractures.

Synovial fluid analysis should be performed in all knees with an effusion (Table 9.2). Sterile aspiration is easily performed through medial or lateral patella retinacular portals with a large bore needle 18 gauge. Aspiration of blood is consistent with an anterior cruciate ligament injury and/or other major injury such as osteochondral fracture or retinacular tears or capsular tears. Fat cells may be present with a fracture but are also seen with acute cruciate insufficiency. The fluid should be examined for crystals, looking for both gout and pseudogout. A cell count with differential should be obtained.

Routine cultures should be sent along with cultures for gonococcus, especially in the absence of trauma history.

Arthroscopy allows for direct visualization of the intraarticular structures and anterior cruciate ligament; it may be performed under local anesthesia to complete a diagnostic evaluation of the knee.

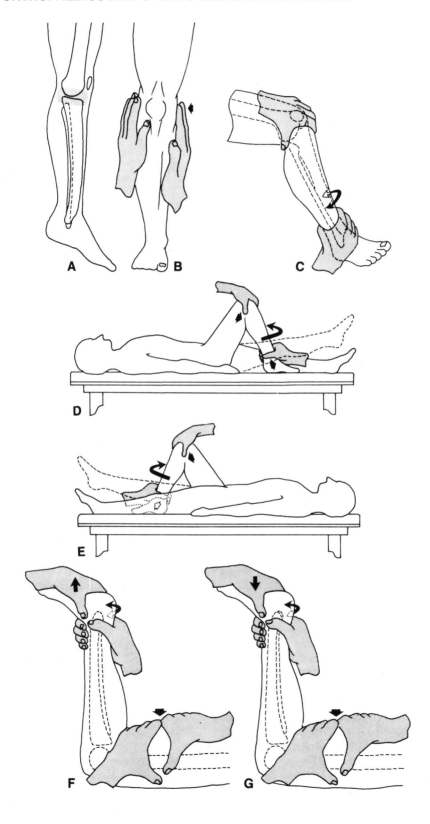

Injuries to the Knee

Meniscus

Etiology. A meniscus injury occurs as an acute injury or as a result of repetitive stresses over a period of time (degenerative tears). Injury to the meniscus is commonly the result of knee rotation on a partially flexed knee (Fig. 9.18). Sports injuries are well documented but simple activities such as getting out of a bucket seat of a car or getting lettuce out of the hydrator of the refrigerator can precipitate an acute meniscus tear. The patient may or may not be able to give a precise mechanism of the injury, especially the older patient with a degenerative meniscus.

Signs and Symptoms. The signs of meniscus pathology are pain at the joint line, swelling, and giving way episodes or a sensation of instability. If the meniscus is displaced it may create a mechanical block to knee motion and may result in a locked knee. The physical examination usually reveals an effusion with joint line tenderness. McMurray's and Apley's provocation testing usually produces pain. Clicking may or may not be present and is nonspecific.

Diagnostic Testing. Diagnostic tests include aspiration and routine x-rays to exclude other causes of symptoms (loose bodies, osteochondritis dissecans). Arthrograms and magnetic resonance imaging are obtained to define the pathology prior to treatment.

Treatment. Initial treatment of the patient with a painful knee that is also suspected of having meniscal pathology should be to control the inflammation with ice and antiinflammatories and to rest the knee with immobilization in a position of comfort. Patients with a locked knee should be referred to an orthopaedic surgeon for immediate evaluation and those presenting with joint line pain and mild meniscal symptoms may have the appropriate tests ordered and be referred to an orthopaedic surgeon for definitive therapy. Arthroscopic repair or resection is the treatment of choice in the symptomatic patient. In the older patient with presumed early degenerative arthritis, care should be taken to preserve the meniscus in its entirety or resect as little as possible. Excision of the entire meniscus leads to an acceleration of the degenerative arthritis in the knee.

Acute Ligamentous Injuries

Ligamentous injuries are always the result of direct trauma and are dependent upon the direction of the applied forces and the position of the knee (Fig. 9.19). A valgus directed force will put the medial collateral, medial meniscus, posterior medial capsule, and anterior cruciate ligament at risk for injury. It is also a commonly encountered injury pattern. Hyperextension results in stresses on the cruciates and may result in anterior cruciate and/or posterior cruciate injury. A varus force (being struck in the medial side of the knee) will put the lateral collateral, posterior oblique ligamentous complex at risk. An injury that results in an immediate effusion is probably due to a hemarthrosis and usually means an anterior cruciate ligament tear or an osteochondral fracture.

Physical examination is best performed acutely before swelling occurs. Localization of the pain and stability testing dictate treatment.

Treatment is based upon the instability patterns that are appreciated (Table 9.3).

Chronic Ligamentous Injury

Often a serious injury is overlooked. The patient experiences a 2- to 3-week disability and resumes a normal lifestyle. Over the next 5 to 10 years the patient develops secondary instability of the knee. This allows

---

Figure 9.17. Examination for meniscus injury. **A,** area of tenderness. **B,** palpation for tenderness. **C,** palpation for "click" during alternate internal and external rotation of the leg. **D** and **E,** McMurray's maneuver. **F,** Apley's maneuver; pain is compatibile with ligament injury. **G,** Apley's maneuver; pain is compatible with meniscus injury. (From Ramamurti CP (Tinker RV, ed): *Orthopaedics in Primary Care.* Baltimore, Williams & Wilkins, 1979, p 236.)

Table 9.2
Examination of the Synovial Fluid[a]

	Normal	Group I Noninflammatory	Group II Inflammatory	Group III Septic
Gross appearance	Transparent, clear	Transparent, yellow	Opaque or translucent, yellow	Opaque, yellow to green
Viscosity	High	High	Low	Variable
White cells/mm³	<200	<200	5,000–75,000	>50,000, often >100,000
Polymorphonuclear leukocytes	<25%	<25%	>50%	>75%
Culture	Negative	Negative	Negative	Often positive
Glucose (mg/dl)	Nearly equal to blood	Nearly equal to blood	>25, lower than blood	>50, lower than blood
Associated conditions		Degenerative joint disease Trauma[b] Neuropathic arthropathy[d] Hypertrophic osteoarthropathy[d] Pigmented villonodular synovitis[b] SLE[d] Acute rheumatic fever[d] Erythema nodosum	Rheumatoid arthritis Connective tissue disease (SLE,[c] PSS, DM/PM) Ankylosing spondylitis Other seronegative spondylarthropathies (psoriatic arthritis, Reiter's syndrome, arthritis of chronic inflammatory bowel disease) Crystal-induced synovitis (gout or pseudogout) Acute rheumatic fever	Bacterial infections Compromised immunity (disease or medication related) Other joint disease

[a]From Rodnan, Schumacher, Zvaifler (eds): *Primer on the Rheumatic Diseases*, ed 8. Atlanta, GA, The Arthritis Foundation, 1983, p 187.
[b]May be hemorrhagic.
[c]SLE, systemic lupus erythematosus; PSS, progressive systemic sclerosis; DM/PM, dermatomyositis/polymyositis.
[d]Group I or II.

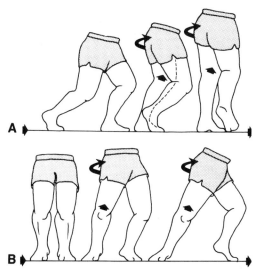

Figure 9.18. The damaging forces acting on the menisci of the knee. **A**, forces which damage the lateral meniscus. **B**, forces which damage the medial meniscus. (From Ramamurti CP (Tinker RV, ed): *Orthopaedics in Primary Care.* Baltimore, Williams & Wilkins, 1979, p 231.)

increased rotation of the femur on the tibia. These abnormal rotational forces result in medial and/or lateral meniscus tears and degenerative changes develop in the knee. Treatment for chronic rotatory instability is based on the functional levels of the patient. Quadriceps and hamstring rehabilitation are the base for conservative treatment and allow many patients to continue sporting activities with a brace. Surgery is the treatment of choice for high-performance athletes and individuals who remain symptomatic during activities of daily living.

Tendon Injuries

Tendinitis

Etiology. Tendinitis is a common complaint and is a result of inflammation secondary to macrotrauma or repetitive microtrauma. Tears in the collagen structure cause inflammation and scar deposition. Persistent tendinitis can lead to weakening of the tendons and ultimate failure. Tendinitis may affect the quadriceps at its insertion into the patella, the

patella tendon, the biceps tendon, the popliteus, or iliotibial band.

Signs and Symptoms. These present as localized pain over the affected tendon. Localized soft tissue swelling may be present. Pain is aggravated by activity and relieved with rest.

Diagnostic Tests. Radiographs are usually normal with persistent inflammation calcific degeneration of the involved tendon may sometimes be seen. Three phase bone scanning may show increased activity in the first two phases of the scan. Blood work to evaluate for an underlying collagen vascular disease may be useful in patients who do not respond to treatment.

Treatment Principles. Primary treatment is rest with treatment of the localized inflammation with ice and antiinflammatory medication. Supportive bracing may be helpful in controlling the acute phase of inflammation and in preventing repetitive episodes.

Quadriceps Tendinitis

Presents as pain localized over the superior pole of the patella. It is seen in patients whose sports or jobs require quick acceleration or quick deceleration movements. Treatment is ice, rest, restoration of flexibility, strength, and endurance and a return to sport. A patella stabilizing brace may be useful in unloading these areas in the rehabilitation phase.

Patella Tendinitis "Jumper's Knee"

The "jumper's knee," or infrapatellar tendinitis, is the most common tendinitis of the knee. It is the result of repetitive microtrauma concentrated at the inferior pole of the patella. Chronic inflammation may result in the rupture of the tendon at its insertion into the patella. It is most commonly found in dancers, basketball players, and athletes who perform jumping activities. The condition may become chronic and not respond to conservative care.

Treatment. If diagnosed early (within the first 3 weeks), rest, ice, antiinflammatory medication coupled with activity modification and progressive return to sports may be all that is needed. If the condition

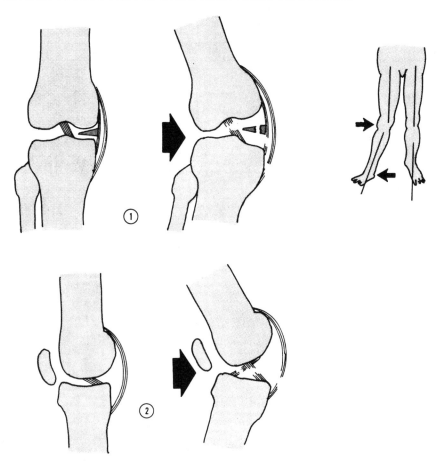

Figure 9.19. *Severe ligamentous sprain* (the unhappy triad). *1*, Lateral (valgus) stress causing disruption of the medial collateral ligament, the medial meniscus, and the anterior cruciate ligament (the unhappy triad). *2*, Lateral view of a severe anterior stress causing hyperextension of the joint and disrupting both anterior and posterior cruciate ligaments and the posterior capsule. Clinically, it has a positive drawer sign. (Modified from Reilly BM: *Practical Strategies in Outpatient Medicine.* Philadelphia, WB Saunders, 1984, p 244.)

has become chronic, complete restriction of activity may be necessary with possible casting. Referral to an orthopaedic surgeon for injection of steroids may be useful in these cases, but great caution should be taken to avoid injection into the tendinous structure itself. Injections of steroids into the tendon significantly weaken the collagen structure and have been associated with tendon rupture. Nonsteroidal antiinflammatory drugs, ice following sports, and compression strapping or bracing of the area may be of benefit in controlling symptoms and allowing for early return to sporting activity. If the knee is completely nonresponsive to rest, surgery may be necessary.

Tendon Rupture

Etiology. Chronic inflammation leading to decrease in collagen strength of the tendon is followed by a load which exceeds the strength of the tendon, resulting in failure.

Signs and Symptoms. Acute loss of the ability to extend the knee against gravity as well as pain and swelling and localized ecchymosis may be present. The patella will be high riding with a complete infrapatellar tendon rupture and low riding with a quadriceps tendon rupture. Partial tears may present as localized pain and swelling with weakness in knee extension. A palpable

Table 9.3
Clinical Diagnosis of Ligament Injuries

	First Degree Sprain	Second Degree Sprain	Third Degree Sprain
Synonym	Mild sprain	Moderate sprain	Severe sprain
Etiology	Direct or indirect trauma to the joint	Direct or indirect trauma to the joint	Direct or indirect trauma to the joint
Symptoms	Pain and mild disability	Pain and moderate disability	Pain and severe disability
Signs and symptoms	Tenderness over the collateral Stable joint exam with no abnormal motions Little or no swelling	Point tenderness over collaterals, swelling, may have localized hemorrhage; loss of normal joint function with laxity tested in 30° flexion; no instability in full extension	Loss of function, marked instability, unstable in full extension
Pathology	Minor tissue tearing Continuity of ligament is intact	Partial tearing with partial loss of ligamentous support	Complete disruption of ligament; no remaining tensile strength
Treatment	Rest, ice, compression, elevation, quadriceps-strengthening exercises	Rest, ice, compression, elevation, immobilization muscle-strengthening activities, protective bracing, fracture brace for 6 to 8 weeks	Rest, ice, compression, elevation, surgery is generally required
Complications	Tendency to recur or be aggravated	Persistent instability, traumatic arthritis	Persistent instability, traumatic arthritis
Prognosis	Normal function, no laxity	Good function, good stability if adequate healing occurs with good bracing	Generally better with primary reconstructive surgery than with casting or fractures bracing

defect in the tendon may be appreciated on physical examination.

Diagnostic Studies. Radiographic evaluation of the knee may show an altered position of the patella. Careful observation for bony avulsion fractures from the patella should be performed. Calcific deposits within the substance of the tendon may be observed and are indicative of chronic inflammation.

Osgood-Schlatter Disease

In the adolescent, Osgood-Schlatter disease presents as pain at the insertion of the tendon into the tibial tubercle. This represents an apophysitis of the tibial tubercle.

Etiology. Robert B. Osgood first described partial avulsion of the tibial tubercle that caused painful swelling in the knee of the adolescent in 1903. Carl Schlatter, some months later, described the same condition and concluded that it was an apophysitis of the tibial tubercle rather than a true avulsion fracture. The argument has never been settled. The condition occurs in the age of rapid growth and is more common in boys than girls. Bilateral involvement is noted in some 20 to 30%.

Signs and Symptoms. The disease is characterized by painful swelling over the tibial tuberosity that is exacerbated by activity, relieved by rest, and usually of several months duration. Tenderness is most marked at the insertion of the patellar tendon. In the adolescent, an acute fracture may occur at this region and present as an acute loss of ability to extend the knee.

Diagnostic Imaging. X-rays may show an irregularity or fragmentation of the tibial apophysis. Fragmentation can also be seen in adolescents with no symptoms. In the occasional acute case, a flake of bone can be detected that suggests an avulsion fracture.

Treatment. The treatment of Osgood-Schlatter disease is purely symptomatic. In persistent or moderately painful knees, one restricts physical activity. When there is a suggestion of a recent acute episode or evidence of a flake fracture, the knee may be immobilized in a plaster cast for 4 to 6 weeks. Knee pads are used to avoid contusions to the prominent tibial tubercle. Symptoms stop after growth ceases. However, the bony prominence will remain throughout life. On occasion, an isolated or separated ossicle may be symptomatic. If it persists in being painful, excision of the ossicle may be necessary. In the case of fracture, if there is significant displacement, open reduction and internal fixation may be required.

Biceps Tendinitis

Biceps tendinitis presents as localized pain over the posterior fibular head. It is most commonly seen in patients with tight hamstrings. Treatment is ice, rest, and nonsteroidal antiinflammatories, as well as stretching and strengthening exercises, with return to sporting activities as symptoms resolve.

Popliteus Tendinitis

Popliteus tendinitis presents as pain in the posterior lateral corner of the knee and is often accentuated by running downhill and descending stairs, as well as prolonged ambulatory activity. The pain is commonly mistaken for a lateral meniscus tear. Treatment is the same as for all inflammatory lesions.

Iliotibial Band Tendinitis

Iliotibial band tendinitis presents as lateral knee pain over the fibular collateral ligament. It is a result of inadequate stretching and results in a tight iliotibial band that then rubs over the posterior lateral corner of the knee, which results in inflammation and pain.

Physical examination reveals localized pain over the posterior lateral corner of the knee and the iliotibial band appears tight (a positive Ober test confirms the diagnosis). The treatment is conservative— stretching, strengthening, and return to sports (Fig. 9.20).

Patella Femoral Pain Syndrome

Anterior knee pain is often vague in its history and common in its presentation. It may result from the sequelae of direct trauma, chronic overuse, or patella femoral malalignment. Patella complaints are more common in women due to the increase in the Q-angle and secondary to increase in the pelvic flair (Fig. 9.12).

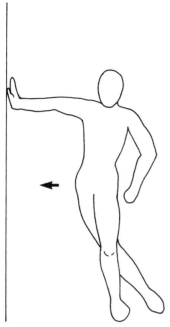

Figure 9.20. Iliotibial band stretching. While standing, place the affected leg toward the wall, crossing this leg over the unaffected leg. Lean your hip into the wall, keeping your body upright. Hold for 10 seconds and repeat 10 times.

Etiology. This increase in Q-angle leads to a tendency for the patella to tilt laterally or sublux laterally during activity. With any injury that limits knee activity, quadriceps strength is lost and the medial dynamic stabilizers of the knee, the vastus medialis obliqus, undergo atrophy. This relative muscle imbalance allows for lateral subluxation of the patella resulting in patella femoral discomfort. Acute dislocations may also result in a lax medial retinaculum and lateral tracking of the patella.

Patella femoral pain may also be a direct result of a repetitive trauma such as long distance running that leads to chronic inflammation. Direct trauma to the patella may result in a chondral fracture with resulting anterior knee pain. This is often seen when the knee strikes the dashboard during a motor vehicle accident or as a sequela of a dislocated patella.

Symptoms. Hallmarks of this problem are pain on rising from sitting, pain on stair climbing, and aches at the end of the day. This pain is often dull and poorly localized

and may be referred to posteriorly in the popliteal recess.

Signs. A sensation of instability with twisting activities may also accompany the syndrome. The diagnosis is made on physical examination with positive patella femoral provocation testing with or without a subluxable patella.

Diagnostic Studies. X-rays to assess patella femoral congruency and tracking are useful. A bone scan with normal x-rays is useful to evaluate whether osteochondral injury has taken place. Arthrograms are not usually useful in this syndrome. Diagnostic arthroscopy may be useful but clinical symptoms do not correlate to the degree of articular softening or chondromalacia found at surgery.

Treatment. Treatment is conservative with quadriceps setting exercises and patella femoral support. If after 6 months symptoms persist and quadriceps are strong, surgical intervention may be considered. Eighty-five percent of patients show improvement with conservative treatment. Surgery is performed to correct the abnormalities of patella-femoral tracking. For severe patella femoral arthritis, tibial tubercle elevation to decrease the patella femoral joint reactive forces may be helpful.

Osteonecrosis

Osteonecrosis is an acute vascular insufficiency of the tibial plateau or femoral condyle. It presents in the 5th to 8th decade as spontaneous onset of severe pain.

Etiology. Unknown.

Signs and Symptoms. It may be accompanied by an effusion and loss of joint motion. The physical examination reveals point tenderness over the involved femoral condyle or tibial compartment.

Diagnostic Studies. X-rays performed at the onset of symptoms are usually normal and the diagnosis is confirmed with technetium-99m bone scanning, with increased activity noted. MRI is also diagnostic of an acute osteonecrosis. The most common sites are the medial femoral condyle and the medial tibial plateau. X-ray changes occur late and appear as collapse of the osteochondral surface.

Treatment is symptomatic with rest and

protected weight bearing, with support, ice, and nonsteroidal antiinflammatories. Core decompression has been reported to relieve pain. If arthritis develops, surgical reconstruction of the knee is the treatment of choice.

Outcome. The outcome is dependent on the percentage of the weight bearing surface involved with the process. Those patients who have more than 50% involvement of the involved compartment usually require some form of reconstructive surgery.

TRAUMATIC CONDITIONS

Fractures

Etiology. Fractures are usually the result of trauma but may occur as a result of bone failure secondary to osteoporosis.

Signs and Symptoms. Fractures usually present with the acute onset of pain and swelling. Ecchymosis develops secondary to the fracture hematoma. Inability to bear weight is often present. Pain is usually increased with weight bearing. Obvious angular deformity of the extremity may be present.

Femur Fractures

Etiology. Femoral shaft fractures are caused by direct blows or by rotary forces.

Signs and Symptoms. Pain and inability to bear weight on the involved extremity. Swelling may be rapid and blood loss may be substantial. Shortening of the extremity with angular deformity is often present.

Diagnostic Evaluation. AP and lateral radiographs of the entire femur are necessary to define the fracture geometry.

Treatment. Primary treatment is to stabilize the extremity in a splint. Definitive treatment will be traction, plate fixation, or intramedullary nailing of the femur. Fracture bracing may be used to facilitate early mobilization of the patient.

Supracondylar Femur Fracture

Etiology. Supracondylar femur fractures are common in the elderly and usually result from direct trauma.

Signs and Symptoms. Pain and swell-

ing immediately above the knee and an inability to bear weight are symptoms. A gross deformity of the knee may be present. With fractures that extend into the joint, a tense hemarthrosis may be present.

Diagnostic Evaluation. Radiographs are needed to define the extent of the fracture and the fracture geometry. AP, lateral, obliques, and tunnel views are usually necessary. Tomography or CT scanning will allow for greater 3-dimensional visualization of the fracture geometry.

Treatment. For a nondisplaced fracture treatment with a fracture brace is the treatment of choice. For a displaced fracture, open reduction internal fixation with restoration of joint congruency is advocated.

Epiphyseal Femur Fractures

Epiphyseal fractures of the distal femur are common in the adolescent.

Etiology. These fractures are the result of varus or valgus stress applied to the knee.

Signs and Symptoms. The adolescent complains of pain over the epiphyseal line and loss of joint motion. Swelling and ecchymosis may be present. Pain is increased with direct palpation of the epiphysis and with stress testing.

Radiographic Evaluation. X-rays are usually negative; stress films may be useful in defining pathology. A bone scan is often diagnostic and reveals increased activity at the epiphyseal line.

Treatment. Treatment is a cast with conversion to a fracture brace to allow for early motion. Epiphyseal injuries have great potential for growth arrest. Patients need to be monitored closely following injury to make sure that growth injury does not occur. For those patients with displacement of the epiphysis, anatomic reduction is required through either closed or open means. Displaced fractures should be closely observed for neurovascular injury.

Tibial Plateau Fractures

Etiology. Plateau fractures are the result of direct trauma and are extremely common. They are secondary to osteoporosis or significant trauma.

Signs and Symptoms. Plateau fractures

present with pain and swelling below the joint line. Ecchymosis usually develops. Bleeding into the fascial compartments of the leg may result in the development of a compartment syndrome and require fasciotomy. Angular deformity may or may not be present depending on the degree of displacement. Pain is increased with weight bearing.

Radiographic Evaluation. AP, lateral, and obliques are necessary to define the injury. Plain radiography tends to underestimate the degree of articular surface depression, and tomography or CT scanning is indicated to define the full extent of the injury.

Treatment. Treatment is restoration of joint congruity with elevation of the articular defects and support with bone grafting and internal fixation. Non-weight-bearing ambulation for 12 to 16 weeks is required. For minimally displaced fractures, treatment with a fracture brace and non-weight-bearing activity are the treatment of choice. Follow-up treatment modalities should be aimed at restoring joint motion as quickly as possible.

Patella Fractures

Etiology. Patella fractures in an adult are usually secondary to a direct trauma or from an avulsion of muscle tendon units. Chondral fractures of the patella are secondary to dislocations.

Signs and Symptoms. Patella fractures present as pain and swelling localized over the patella. Pain is accentuated with active knee extension; the position of comfort is full knee extension. A hemarthrosis of the knee may be present as well as loss of active knee extension.

Radiographic Evaluation. AP, lateral, and sunrise views are usually adequate. The geometry of the fracture and degree of displacement define the treatment modality.

Treatment. If the fracture is nondisplaced, cylinder cast immobilization is the treatment of choice. For displaced fractures, open reduction internal fixation with tension banding technique is preferred. Avulsion fractures of the patella usually require operative stabilization when an extensor lag is present.

Patella Dislocation

Etiology. Patella dislocations are common and may recur as the result of direct trauma or as a result of a contraction of the quadriceps in conjunction with valgus and external rotation of the leg. Dislocations are more common in females secondary to the valgus alignment of the lower extremity.

Signs and Symptoms. The patient often complains that the knee went out of joint. There is usually immediate onset of intense pain and inability to move the knee.

If the patella is still dislocated it will appear as a gross deformity on the lateral aspect of the knee. However, spontaneous reduction often occurs and pain over the medial and lateral retinacular structures may be the only presenting signs in conjunction with a hemarthrosis.

Radiographic Evaluation. AP, lateral, obliques, and sunrise are obtained and evaluated for displacement of the patella as well as for any evidence of a fracture from the patella or the trochlea of the femur or for an osteochondral loose body.

Treatment. Initially, the patella should be gently reduced, iced, and placed in an extension splint. The limb should be held in a cast for 4 to 6 weeks, followed by a full patella rehabilitation program. In a patient with a patella that can easily be dislocated again, consideration for repair of the medial retinaculum is important. Osteochondral fractures should be repaired or excised depending on their size and location.

Patella Subluxation

Etiology. Patella subluxation is a common finding in the female athlete. It is due to a number of causes including increased Q-angle with excessive femoral anteversion, excessive knee valgus, external tibial torsion, and vastus medialis dysplasia or acquired atrophy.

Signs and Symptoms. Usually presents as a sensation of instability associated with cutting, twisting, and turning activities. Discomfort is usually present over the anterior aspect of the knee. It is brought out with flexion, valgus, and external rotation motions on the knee. The patient may complain of sudden giving way or buckling or popping with these activities.

With a subluxing patella there is often a small joint effusion but this may be absent with a relatively normal exam. Physical signs include a lateral squinting patella or lateral tilt, often with a high-riding patella. An increased Q-angle may be present with external tibial torsion and genu valgum often seen.

On physical examination tenderness may be elicited along the medial retinaculum and the medial facet of the patella. The patella should be examined for hypermobility with the knee in full extension and 30° of flexion. Following an acute subluxation this provocation testing may be extremely painful. With provocation testing a positive apprehension may be evident with the patient unwilling to undergo further testing.

Diagnostic Evaluation. X-rays of both knees are useful in the evaluation of this patient. Sunrise views may show the lateral squinting of the patella. Careful observation should be made to look for osteochondral avulsions from the medial facet of the patella or off of the femoral trochlear groove.

Treatment. Should consist initially of ice, compression, and elevation with the knee splinted in full extension. Rehabilitation should then be used to reestablish quadriceps' strength, especially the vastus medialis. A neoprene patella stabilization brace with lateral horseshoe may be useful in providing stability during sporting activities. Surgical intervention is reserved for the patient with functional impairment following adequate rehabilitation.

Tibial Tubercle Avulsion Fracture

Etiology. The adolescent tibial tubercle avulsion fracture occurs as a hyperflexion injury.

Signs and Symptoms. Pain and swelling over the tibial tubercle and loss of active knee extension.

Radiographic Evaluation.. The lateral x-ray is usually diagnostic. Displacement or widening of the apophysis is seen.

Treatment.. Treatment for a nondis-

placed fracture is with a cylinder cast immobilization. A displaced fracture requires open reduction internal fixation with restoration of the epiphysis.

Tibial Spine Avulsion Fractures

Avulsions to the anterior tibial spine occur in early adolescence. The posterior spine injury is less common.

Etiology. Injury is secondary to hyperflexion and hyperextension injury to the knee.

Signs and Symptoms. These fractures usually present as swelling with a hemarthrosis.

Radiographic Evaluation. AP, lateral, and tunnel x-rays show a tibial avulsion.

Treatment. The treatment is to restore the anatomic position, either operatively or nonoperatively.

Osteochondritis Dissecans

Etiology. This injury is believed to be an avascular necrosis of the subchondral plate. It occurs most commonly in the non-weight-bearing portion of the medial femoral condyle. Approximately 70% of patients show bilateral knee involvement.

Signs and Symptoms. Patient presents with pain, limping, and giving way episodes without history of trauma. A knee effusion may be present.

Diagnostic Evaluation. Radiographs are usually diagnostic. The tunnel view x-ray is most useful in showing the pathology. A CT scan or arthrogram is useful to evaluate the integrity of the articular surface. Bone scanning may be useful in picking up the very early lesion.

Treatment. If the epiphyses are open, conservative treatment with protective weight bearing usually results in healing of the lesion. Once the epiphyses are closed the prognosis for healing is guarded. If the fragment is detached, debridement of the bed, drilling, and possible replacement of the osteochondral lesion are preferred, especially if the fragment is in the weight-bearing area. Protected range of motion with non-weight-bearing activity for 6 to 8 weeks is performed. For the patella osteochondritis lesions, debridement and lateral release are the preferred treatments.

Osteoarthritis

Signs and Symptoms. Pain is usually the presenting complaint of the patient and is usually aggravated with activity and relieved at rest; another complaint is morning stiffness that improves as the day progresses only to return later in the day. The pain is often aggravated by activities that require flexion and rotation of the knee, such as stair climbing and squatting. Associated complaints of locking, giving way, or a sensation of instability are often present. A knee effusion or history of knee effusions is usually present. A trauma history may be present. There is often a history of progressive development of bow legs or knock knees.

The clinical exam may reveal a gross angular deformity—either genu valgum or genu varum. A fixed flexion contracture may be present. An antalgic gait with a lateral joint thrust and shortened stride may be present. Pain is usually present at the joint line of the involved compartment. Osteoarthritis may involve one or all of the compartments of the knee.

Diagnostic Imaging. AP weight-bearing x-rays of both knees on a single cassette may demonstrate narrowing of the joint spaces, peripheral osteophyte formation, subchondral sclerosis, and cyst formation; they may also demonstrate the angular deformity of the knee. Lateral and oblique films will demonstrate the presence of peripheral osteophytes and loose bodies. Sunrise views are needed to evaluate the patella femoral joint for osteophytes, sclerosis, and maltracking. Tricompartmental disease suggests a panarticular synovitis process such as crystalline arthritis, rheumatoid arthritis, or chondrocalcinosis. Late presentation of osteoarthritis may also be seen as a tricompartmental phenomenon on x-ray.

Treatment. Initial treatment is rest and nonsteroidal antiinflammatory medication with quadriceps and hamstring strengthening. Ambulatory assistance with a cane or walker is useful, unloading the affected extremity and providing relief of symptoms. Arthroscopic debridement may be useful but menisectomy in the presence of arthritis often leads to an acceleration of the degenerative process.

For varus knees with unicompartmental involvement, high-tibial osteotomy to shift the weight-bearing axis into the lateral compartment is useful in patients less than 65 years of age. For patients older than 65 years hemiarthroplasty or total knee arthroplasty is used to relieve their symptoms. In the presence of tricompartmental disease, total knee arthroplasty gives excellent relief of pain with restoration of ambulatory functions. The young patient with severe tricompartment osteoarthritis, usually secondary to trauma, normally requires a fusion for relief of pain.

Popliteal Cysts

Etiology. Popliteal cysts are usually a symptom rather than an independent process. Popliteal cysts are an outpouching of synovial tissue in the posterior fossa and are a result of increased pressure within the knee secondary to recurrent effusions. This increased pressure results in the distention of a weakened area of the posterior capsule, usually medially with subsequent cyst formation.

Signs and Symptoms. Patients complain of a loss of motion, posterior knee pain, and a sensation of fullness in the popliteal space. There is often a history of knee joint effusions. Rupture of a cyst may mimic deep vein thrombosis with acute calf pain.

Diagnostic Imaging. Confirmation of the popliteal cyst may be done with ultrasonography or arthrography to define the cyst and determine its location and origin. In the older patient it is essential to exclude an aneurysm in the popliteal space. This may be done with ultrasonography or digital subtraction angiography if clinically suspected.

Treatment. Treatment is directed at determining and treating the underlying source of the knee effusion (i.e., crystalline arthropathy or meniscal tear). This will usually result in resolution of the popliteal cyst. Excision is necessary for a cyst that does not resolve. For a cyst that creates venous obstruction, excision needs to be performed. It is important to rule out popliteal aneurysm in the differential diagnosis of a cyst.

Bursitis

Etiology. Bursae are closed, minimally fluid-filled sacks lined with synovium similar to the lining of joint spaces. Their single function is to reduce friction between adjacent tissues. Bursae are subjected to a variety of conditions including trauma, infection, metabolic abnormalities, rheumatic afflictions, and neoplasms.

Signs and Symptoms. Acute bursitis presents as pain and localized swelling. Pain is aggravated by any motion that puts pressure on the bursa. Erythema and localized increased skin warmth may be present.

Diagnostic Evaluation. Radiographic evaluation will show a soft tissue swelling but is usually normal. Aspiration of the bursa should be performed and the fluid evaluated for crystals and signs of infection.

Treatment. In the acute phase, initial treatment should consist of ice and compression, as well as rest. It may be coupled with aspiration and the use of nonsteroidal medication. Padding is used to prevent recurrent trauma. Cortisone may be injected into the bursa once infection has been excluded from the differential diagnosis. It should be used when conservative means of treatment have been unsuccessful. Stretching and strengthening exercises for the knee are needed to reduce the stress on the bursa interposed between moving tissue planes.

Clinically Relevant Bursae (Fig.9.7)

The deep infrapatellar bursa is positioned beneath the patellar tendon below the infrapatellar fat pad on the anterior surface of the tibia. Localized pain and tenderness at this location are frequently due to Osgood-Schlatter disease but can be due to a chronic bursitis. The diagnosis is made by palpation of the bursa.

The superficial infrapatellar bursa rests between the skin and the anterior surface of the infrapatellar tendon. Inflammation of this bursa may be induced by repetitive kneeling or by direct trauma. The pes anserine bursa lies between the pes anserine tendons (sartorius, gracilis, and semitendinosus) and the medial collateral ligament over the medial aspect of the tibia. Bursitis develops because of tendon friction or from direct injury. Pain and tenderness are localized at the anteromedial aspect of the tibia. External rotation and contraction of the pes anserine muscles aggravate the symptoms. Pes bursitis must be distinguished from an injury of the medial collateral ligament. This bursa lies about three cm distal to the medial joint line and pain is localized to this location. Swelling and tenderness may be palpated distal to the semitendinosus tendon.

The lateral aspect of the knee contains many small bursae that are somewhat inconstant. The biceps bursa, however, consistently lies between the lateral collateral ligament and the fibular attachment of the biceps tendon. Inflammation ensues after overactivity. Diagnosis again rests with excluding ligamentous and meniscal injuries. Local swelling is the only real sign, and such swelling includes the differential of cystic degeneration of the meniscus.

Recommended Reading

Draves DJ: *Anatomy of the Lower Extremity*. Baltimore, Williams & Wilkins, 1986.

Ficat RP, Hungerford DS: *Disorders of the Patellofemoral Joint*. Baltimore, Williams & Wilkins, 1977.

Hollingshead WH: *Anatomy for Surgeons, Vol 3*. Philadelphia, Harper & Row, 1958.

Hoppenfeld S: *Physical Examination of the Spine and Extremities*. East Norwalk, CT, Appleton-Century-Croft, 1976.

Kelly W, Harris E, Ruddy S, Sledge C: *Textbook of Rheumatology*, Vol 1, 2nd ed. Philadelphia, WB Saunders, 1985.

Nicholas JA, Hershman EB (eds): *The Lower Extremity and Spine in Sports Medicine*. St. Louis, CV Mosby, 1986.

Noyes F, Basset R: Arthroscopy in acute traumatic hemarthrosis of the knee. *J Bone Joint Surg* 52A, 687–695, 1980.

Rockwood CA, Green DP (eds): *Fractures, vol 2*. Philadelphia, JB Lippincott, 1975.

Schumacker HR, Klippel JH, Robinson DR (eds): *Primer on the Rheumatic Diseases, Ninth Edition*. Atlanta, Arthritis Foundation, 1988.

Scott WN, Nisonson B, Nicholas JE (eds.): *Principles of Sports Medicine*. Baltimore, Williams & Wilkins, 1984.

chapter 10

The Lower Leg, Ankle, and Foot

JAMES E. NIXON, M.D.

Anatomy

The tibia is the second largest bone in the body. It is slightly cup-shaped proximally and is generally cylindrical through most of the shaft. The distal end widens to establish the ankle mortise. Posteriorly and laterally, it is covered by musculature. Anteriorly, the tibia is subcutaneous through most of its length.

The fibula is a slender bone lying laterally to the tibia. It forms an arthrodial joint proximally and a syndesmosis distally with the tibia. It serves primarily for muscle attachment and is the lateral buttress of the ankle joint.

The muscles of the leg are divided into four distinct compartments separated by thick fascial planes (Fig. 10.1). The anterior compartment contains the anterior tibia, extensor hallucis longus, and the extensor muscles to the toes as well as the deep peroneal nerve and anterior tibial artery. The superficial posterior compartment contains the gastrocnemius, soleus, and sural nerve. The deep posterior compartment contains the posterior tibial, flexor digitorum longus, and flexor hallucis muscles. The lateral compartment contains the peroneus longus and brevis muscles, as well as the superficial peroneal nerve. The posterior compartment muscles are innervated by the tibial nerve, while the anterolateral compartments are innervated by the peroneal nerve (Fig. 10.2).

History

The history of the subjective complaint is no more than identification of a temporal period in which the symptoms were initiated, as well as their evolution and modification through time and treatment. That time may be long or short, intermittent or, changing. Nonetheless, if anatomically fixed, there is suggested a continuum and/or relationship. As the present symptoms are of concern, these must be sharply defined.

In the adult, it is a symptom that suggests the patient seeks medical attention. In the child or teenager, it is the concern of the parent to note expressed complaints or observed abnormality. The symptoms may initiate the visit, but they need not be the reason for seeking medical appraisal. Anxiety, not with magnitude, but with chronicity may be the reason. Concern that stress-related symptoms may be harmful may be the reason; or it may be the need to assess the present state to allow continuation of an activity or to obtain advice related to modification, strengthening, or ameliorative routines. In many instances, the patient does not necessarily seek or demand relief, but rather is well treated by assurance or recommendation for modification of activity, or, at times, the presentation of a temporary socioeconomic medical shield. In other words, the history includes finding out what the patient wants.

With disabling symptoms, one works through onset or mechanism of injury if required. One evaluates the duration, frequency, and intermittencey. One ascertains symptomatic modification by treatment, medication, and rest. The examiner seeks to understand restrictions in function, as well as anatomic localization. In a sense, the examiner is attempting to experience what the patient is experiencing.

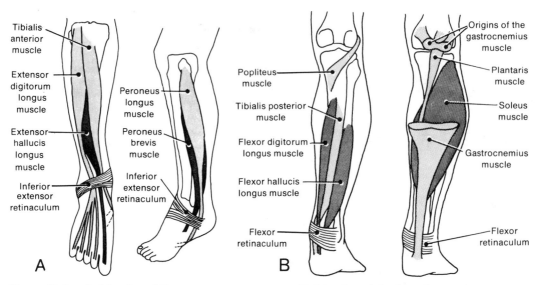

Figure 10.1. **A**, Muscles of the anteror compartment. **B**, Muscles of the lateral compartment. **C**, Muscles of the deep posterior compartment. **D**, Muscles of the superficial posterior compartment. (From Ramamurti CP (Tinker RV, ed): *Orthopaedics in Primary Care*. Baltimore, Williams & Wilkins, 1979, p 249.)

Physical Examination

Examination begins with observation. One cannot observe a clothed lower extremity. One may begin with a screening procedure that includes observation of gait and station. The patient is asked to cross a room. Observe the posture, balance, the swing of the arms, and movement of the legs. If balance is easy, the arms swing at the side, and turns are smoothly accomplished; a "negative" search is appreciated. In examining a reasonably healthy, ambulatory patient, one may ask the patient to hop in place on each foot in turn. The ability to do this indicates an intact motor system for the legs, normal cerebellar function and a good position sense. If one detects abnormal symptoms in the screening of patients, a more specific examination is indicated.

The underlying organization of the assessment is inspection, palpation, assessment of the muscle tone, testing of the muscle strength, and assessment of coordination. One may simply screen the sensory system, especially if there are no neurological symptoms. These symptoms include assessment of vibration in the feet,

brief comparison of light touch over the legs, and assessment of coordination by point-to-point testing. Point-to-point testing consists of placing the patient's foot on the opposite knee and then having the patient run it down the shin to the big toe. If there are tremors or awkwardness, they may suggest cerebellar disease or loss of position sense. Vibration sense is often the first sensation to be lost in peripheral neuropathy. The common cause for peripheral neuropathy is diabetes. The aging process may be associated with a decreased vibratory sense. Loss of position and vibration senses suggests posterior column disease. Obviously, one needs to examine in special detail those areas where (1) there are symptoms such as numbness or pain, (2) there are reflex abnormalities, and (3) where there are atrophic changes, absent or excessive sweating, atrophic skin or cutaneous ulceration.

Leg length discrepancy should be noted in particular as this is frequently associated with overuse syndromes (the longer leg usually being the injured leg). Other subtle anatomic abnormalities that may lead to overuse syndromes are femoral anteversion with excessive internal rotation of the

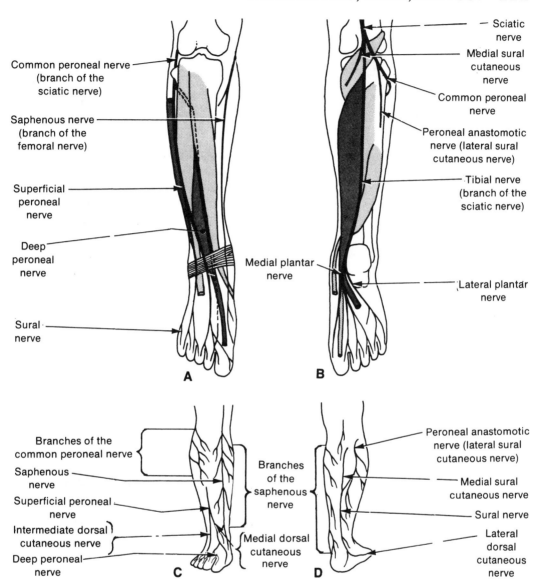

Figure 10.2. Nerves of the leg. **A** and **B**, Major divisions. **A**, Anterior view. **B**, Posterior view. **C** and **D**, Cutaneous nerves of the leg. **C**, Anterior view. **D**, Posterior view. (From Ramamurti CP (Tinker RV, ed): *Orthopaedics in Primary Care*. Baltimore, Williams & Wilkins, 1979, p 249.)

hips, tight hamstrings, genu varum or valgum, excessive Q-angle of the patella, tibial varum (bow legs), functional shortening of the gastrocnemius-soleus, and functionally pronated feet. All can produce distal symptomatology of overuse.

With observation, one may note limping, atrophy, swelling, and bruising as evident objective differences between the limbs.

Vascular Examination

Since venous disease most commonly affects the legs, special attention should be paid to the structure and function of the leg veins. Superficial veins are located subcutaneously where they are supported relatively poorly. Anastomotic channels join the deep and the superficial systems as communicating or perforating veins along the entire course. Deep, superficial, and communicating veins all have thin valves along their course. Aging alone brings relatively few clinically important changes to the peripheral vascular system. Although arterial and venous disorders (especially atherosclerosis) do affect older people more frequently, these disorders cannot be considered part of the aging process. Age may make tortuous or typically stiffen arterial walls, but these changes develop with or without atherosclerosis and therefore are not diagnostically specific. Loss of arterial pulsation is not part of normal aging and demands careful evaluation. The skin may get thin and dry with age. Nails may grow more slowly, and hair on the legs often becomes scant. These are not specific for arterial insufficiency. Diminished or absent posterior tibial, popliteal, or femoral pulse suggests occlusive arterial disease. The dorsalis pedis pulse, however, may be congenitally absent. Its absence is not diagnostic of occlusive arterial disease.

With the patient standing, inspect the saphenous system for varicosities. They may be easily missed when the patient is supine. Look for edema of the legs and check for pitting edema. Look for an increase in the venous patterns of the leg or diffuse red cyanosis of the leg. Feel for increased firmness or tension in the calf muscles. Superficial phlebitis may be characterized by redness or discoloration overlying the saphenous system. Palpate for tenderness or cords. Competency of the venous valves in varicose veins may be assessed by manual compression tests. With the fingertips of one hand, feel the dilated vein. With your other hand, compress the vein firmly at a place at least 20 cm higher in the leg. Then release compression. Feel for an impulse transmitted to your lower hand. Competence of the saphenous valves should block the transmission of any impulse.

If one suspects chronic arterial insufficiency, elevate the patient's leg approximately 12 inches and have the patient move the feet up and down at the ankle for approximately 60 seconds. The maneuver drains the feet of venous blood, unmasking the color produced by arterial supply. Relative pallor is normal. Increased or deathly pallor is ar-

terial insufficiency. Following this, have the patient sit promptly at the edge of the examining table with the legs dangling. The color should return in about 10 seconds, and filling of the veins of the feet and ankle should occur normally in about 15 seconds. If there is delay in color or venous filling return, there is arterial insufficiency (Table 10.1).

Neurological Examination

Peripheral neuropathy is an acute or chronic degenerative condition of either the peripheral nerves, the autonomic nervous system, or the central nervous system. Diabetes mellitus is, by far, the most common cause of peripheral neuropathy. Among other etiologic agents are toxic substances (alcohol, lead, mercury, arsenic, methyl-n-butyl ketone, thallium, and n-hexane, an organic compound in glues), drugs (nitrofurantoin, chloroquine, isoniazid, hydralazine hydrochloride, phenytoin sodium, etc.), systemic disorders (pernicious anemia, vitamin deficiency, etc.) as well as constitutional responses to tetanus anatoxins that may be mentioned.

The toxicity of the work place is increasing. Diagnosis may rest upon an index of suspicions. Symptoms are characterized by complaints located in the distal portions of the limb, particularly the digits, and the symptoms range from paresthesias such as numbness, tingling, and prickling to burning, aching, or sharp intense pain. Frequently tenderness is present along the course of the nerves. The objective findings consist of impairment of touch, vibration, position, and temperature sense. There may be hyperesthesia present. If the condition has progressed to the point of complete functional severance, pain is absent and loss of sensation is complete. Nutritional neuropathy is found most often in the chronic alcoholic as a result of folate and niacin deficiency.

Generalized conditions can produce localized neuropathy. It is found in polyarteritis nodosa, rheumatoid arthritis, Sjögren's syndrome, or in a sense, any condition where the ischemia due to a vasculitis may affect several or more peripheral nerves. The exotoxins of diphtheria, as well as such organic diseases as porphyria, may

Table 10.1
Arterial versus Venous Insufficiency

Clinical Presentation	Arterial	Venous
Edema	Present all the time	Increased at day's end; increased upon walking
Color	Whitish, but when hanging foot down, becomes flame red	Bluish tinge
Ulcers	Often punched out appearance; lateral aspect of leg	Often shaggy; irregular in size/shape, often medial
Pain	Intensity increases with exercise	Aching at rest, aches with exercise
	Foot pain at night	Large muscle pain at night

be typified by a peripheral neuropathy. Trauma or compression of peripheral nerves may lead to a neuropathy.

Peripheral neuropathy must be differentiated from ischemic neuropathy, which is due to a severe degree of ischemia of the peripheral tissues including the mixed nerves. It is produced by chronic occlusive arterial disease, generally arteriosclerotic obliterans of the lower extremity. Although the symptoms of the two conditions are frequently similar (sense of coldness, numbness, or burning in the feet, paresthesia of the toes, and shooting, lancinating pain), the complaints of ischemia appear soon after the patient lies in bed in preparation for sleep and are immediately alleviated by placing the lower limbs over the edge of the bed, sitting up, or standing. This particular posturing may be found in entrapment neuropathies, though in general these positions have no eliciting or controlling effect on the symptoms of peripheral neuropathy.

As one regards the physical findings, ischemic neuropathy is always associated with signs of markedly reduced arterial circulation (absent pulses) that may occur suddenly.

ADOLESCENT WITH LEG PAIN

The adolescent, while not subject to the rigors of the workplace and functioning on youthful tissue, may still present with problems related to the skin, vascular, and musculoskeletal structures.

Common "nontraumatic" problems found in this age group are contact dermatitis from substances used in the manufacture of uniforms and protective equipment. Tincture of benzoin used as a tape adherent is a potential sensitizer. The "neoprene brace" or encasement, when combined with chronic aquatic use, can produce fungal growth, especially in the seam area. The environment itself is a source of contact dermatitis from such elements as poison ivy. Tick-borne disease with both skin and arthralgia complaints are to be considered in this age group.

Some mention should be made of the "history" when the patient is an adolescent. Not infrequently, the adolescent is brought to the provider's office by concerned parents. The condition is fully appreciated by the patient, but is never well verbalized by the teenager. As one seeks specifics of anatomic locations, intensity, duration, frequency, and functional elements that accentuate and relieve the condition, the initial negative attitude is often strongly reinforced. Frequently, it is apparent that the "condition" represents a conflict between the parents, with one parent exaggerating its importance and potential deadliness, and the other denying its existence and allowing a possibly stressful activity to continue.

Contact Dermatitis

The diagnosis of contact dermatitis is found in a history of the recent purchase of an item of clothing or a uniform. Look for localized responses, especially those that follow the outline of the object. It is noted that some of the cream bases used as vehicles for cortisone preparation may be sensitizers. The logical treatment is avoidance of the suspected object. When the dermatitides are secondarily invaded or infected, they present as increasing problems in treatment and diagnosis.

In addition to housing varmints, as well as irritants, the environment is a potential source of nontraumatic consequence upon the lower extremity.

Heat Cramps

This condition is due to excessive salt loss under conditions of high ambient temperature and may be prevented by adequate salt and water intake. Heat exhaustion is due primarily to loss of body water. Peripheral vasodilation and pooling of blood in the lower extremities due to standing may contribute to this condition as well as sustained muscular exercise with no regard for replacing lost water. Psychotropic drugs may have an atropine-like effect. These effects, when combined with high ambient temperatures, may produce symptoms in excess of those expected. Patients complain of painful gastrocnemius and soleus muscle contractions. Attention to the history of drug use in the process of supportive therapy may prove useful. Treatment consists of oral fluid and electrolyte replacement coupled with passive stretching. Instruct athletes to drink water at least every 20 minutes during endurance competition and to stop and stretch periodically.

Frostbite

Prolonged exposure of the body to cold temperatures may produce frostbite that occurs from cooling of the skin and subcutaneous tissues. This cooling can be carried to the point where circulation is closed off. If not rapidly corrected, the skin loses its vascularity. Additionally, frostbite can be found as a consequence of the injudicious use of cooling agents, ethylchloride, and the prolonged use of ice. The clinical presentation consists of pain, loss of sensation, and a cold, white extremity.

The prophylaxis for frostbite is keeping exposed areas of skin covered, reducing local heat loss, and preserving local circulation by avoiding constrictive clothing.

The treatment is rapid warming of the affected part and prevention of re-exposure.

Neuropathies

Neuropathies are usually the result of trauma to the nerve. Adolescents are not good historians. They do not necessarily consider "acceptable" strain as trauma. As a consequence, there may be "nontraumatic" entrapment neuropathy, in which various nerves of the legs may be involved (Fig. 10.3).

Saphenous Nerve

Neuropathy of the saphenous nerve produces pain at or below the level of the knee with radiation downward to the medial side of the foot. The entrapment may be apparent while negotiating stairs, exaggerated with extension of the knee. Adduction of the thigh against resistance reproduces the symptoms by tensing the subsartorial fascia. The area of entrapment is at the site of exit from the subsartorial canal. The point of exit is approximately 4 cm proximal to the medial epicondyle. While palpating the anteromedial muscle (the vastus medialis), one slides the hand posteriorly to the edge of the sartorius. The saphenous opening is beneath this point. Pressure at that point is painful and will cause radiation distally.

Peroneal Nerve

The nontraumatic, noniatrogenic causes for involvement of the peroneal nerve are few. The common mechanism of damage to the peroneal nerve at the head of the fibula is acute compression. Compression is caused by prophylactic braces, stockings and garters, or sitting for a prolonged period, as during a card game with the leg resting against the side of the chair. Squatting or kneeling for extended periods may produce a sudden, painless foot drop. Compression may be produced by ganglia from the proximal tibiofibular joint. Pure entrapment of the fibular tunnel (against the roof of the peroneus longus) is rare.

L-5 radiculopathy may resemble pero-

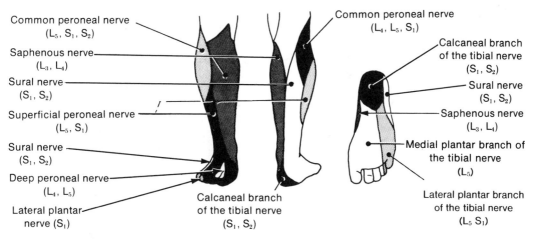

Common peroneal nerve
(L$_5$, S$_1$, S$_2$)

Saphenous nerve
(L$_3$, L$_4$)

Sural nerve
(S$_1$, S$_2$)

Superficial peroneal nerve
(L$_5$, S$_1$)

Sural nerve
(S$_1$, S$_2$)

Deep peroneal nerve
(L$_4$, L$_5$)

Lateral plantar
nerve (S$_1$)

Calcaneal branch
of the tibial nerve
(S$_1$, S$_2$)

Common peroneal nerve
(L$_4$, L$_5$, S$_1$)

Calcaneal branch
of the tibial nerve
(S$_1$, S$_2$)

Sural nerve
(S$_1$, S$_2$)

Saphenous nerve
(L$_3$, L$_4$)

Medial plantar branch of
the tibial nerve
(L$_5$)

Lateral plantar branch
of the tibial nerve
(L$_5$ S$_1$)

Figure 10.3. Distribution of the cutaneous nerves of the leg. (From Ramamurti CP (Tinker RV, ed): *Orthopaedics in Primary Care*. Baltimore, Williams & Wilkins, 1979, p 250.)

neal palsy or entrapment of its branches. In the uncommon individual, there may be no back or thigh pain. Observations that indicate an L-5 radiculopathy should be considered. Some observations include:
(1) Weakness of inversion of the foot. The tibialis is not innervated by the peroneal nerve.
(2) The clear-cut lumbar L-5 lesion sensory loss that is well above the midpart of the calf.
(3) Greater weakness in the extensor hallucis than in the anterior tibial. (The latter muscle receives L-4 innervation.) Complete paralysis of the dorsiflexors of the foot favor a peroneal palsy.

Diagnostic Studies. The electrophysiologic (electromyography (EMG), nerve conduction) assessment of the peroneal nerve has several uses. It may be used in the differential diagnosis as well as to establish prognosis and identify early signs of recovery. Nerve conduction, as well as the electromyographic studies are employed. While the EMG is theoretically useful, clinically, it may not aid in differential diagnosis. Sensory action potentials may identify entrapment of the cutaneous nerves. Prognosis may be suggested by conduction velocity studies. Normal or near normal studies suggest an excellent prognosis. If slowed or undetermined, the prognosis is poor (Berry, 1976).

Treatment. Treatment for the lesions of the common peroneal nerve should consist of bracing. The usual appliance is a plastic orthosis extending from the posterior leg and encasing the plantar surface of the foot as a molded structure. The patient with a slowly progressive disturbance in peroneal nerve function, in which there is pain as well as motor and sensory loss, suggests that an entrapment neuropathy be considered. Ganglion cysts and other tumors should be suspected. In such patients, relatively early exploration is indicated. In entrapment neuropathies, decompression results in rapid and complete recovery in most patients.

The second portion of the superficial peroneal nerve is subjected to entrapment neuropathy in the distal portion of the leg. The usual suggested origin of the neuropathy is forced plantar flexion or an inversion twist of the ankle and foot. The nerve is tethered at the point of derivation at the fibular neck and distally at the subcutaneous exit. The force applied will make a nerve taut against its opening and provide the initiating trauma. Occasionally, repetition of contact over the distal lateral portion of the leg will produce symptom. Injury can occur from a tightly laced boot that ends at the level of the subfascial penetration by the nerve. In general, the pain is burning and superficial.

As the pain distribution strongly resembles that produced by irritation of the L-5 root, the differentiation between the two conditions may present with difficulty. Adding to that difficulty is the fact that the irritated root can cause marked tenderness of the peripheral trunk extension.

ADULTS WITH LEG PAIN

All of the problems found in adolescents, with the exception of overuse and trauma directed against the growth apophysis or epiphysis of growing bone, are found in adults. Musculoskeletal symptoms are not infrequently due to pattern changes. These pattern changes occur because of the change of activities as one ages (attempts to move backward in time at a rapid rate can be somewhat disastrous). One notes these same pattern changes between the sexes because of the difference, overall, of sports and occupation-related differences. Early in life, the more "decelerated" sports, soccer, football, rugby, baseball, and court and field sports with competitors within the same space, produce a greater number of injuries. As many of these do not represent life sports, they are later abandoned because of the team size and playing requirements. The male, as opposed to the female, tends to engage in these activities beyond the school years. Such activity will cross most career fields or may be career field organized.

While the overuse syndromes have been indicated in sports, they have been present in the work place for centuries. These syndromes may be characterized by the external manifestations in the skin. One can see the protective callus in those who kneel, such as a cement finisher, rug and floor layer, as well as tile setters. Beneath the subcutaneous calluses, there are evident chronic bursae formations. The incidental burns of the welder are examples of work-related trauma. The chronic joint and tendon problems related to the repetitive acts of the musician, dancer, factory and clothing worker lead over time to degeneration and disability.

Nontraumatic Problems

The nontraumatic conditions in the adult are those that do not result from specific trauma. A change in the usual or conditioned activities may produce inflammation. If, initially, these traumas are only awareness, stiffness, or temporary aching, there may be little concern. If the symptoms increase and linger, they may be brought to medical attention.

The entrapment syndromes enumerated above may evolve. Laying paving bricks may produce peroneal neuropathy. A change in shoe height, particularly in those with tight heel cords, may produce a peroneal tendinitis. Standing on a ladder or shoveling may produce plantar fasciitis. A garden may be a dangerous as well as a lovesome thing. Gardening not only includes reflection, it may require crouching, squatting, digging with shovels and forks, as well as contact with fertilizers and insecticides, all of which work inroads on the lower extremity.

In evaluating nontraumatic complaints related to the lower extremity, there is a search for a change in pattern that may be the etiologic agent: a holiday, trip, plane flight, household chores induced by weather changes, etc.

Cramps

Lower extremity cramps are common in the gastrocnemius and soleus muscles of the calf. Individuals complain of either a sudden or gradual onset of incapacitating calf pain. This can be related to improper warm-up prior to sports activity, any sustained muscle activity, or salt depletion during an endurance activity. The exact physiology of muscle cramps is unknown.

The treatment consists of proper stretching prior to an activity as well as adequate salt and fluid replacement during athletic competition and passive stretching of the muscle to relieve the painful spasm. Refer to a physician for a trial with quinine those athletes who are refractory to the recommended treatment.

Common Traumatic Problems

Contusions of the Tibia

Contusions over the anterior leg are very common in both sports and the work environment. The nature and severity of the injury depend upon the site of the direct trauma. Much of the tibia is superficial and therefore, has very little protective covering. It acts as a base element of the trauma, entrapping the soft tissue between the bone and the impacting object. As a consequence, rather deep abrasions, lacerations, and involvement of the venous structures are more evident over the anterior leg. The leg is prone to infection. Folliculitis and cellulitis can develop in the more superficial wounds. Lacerations are slow to heal and may be subjected to repeat trauma. Subcutaneous hemorrhage develops from contusion laceration of the superficial veins. This condition may be extensive, and the hematoma may become infected.

Treatment. Cleansing, protection, and repeat observation are demanded by what initially, viewed from a functional standpoint, may be a relatively minor injury. Direct blows to the musculature of the lower leg may result in bleeding. If bleeding or reactive edema in the leg is present to any great degree, the limited expansion allowed within the compartments may cause ischemia. It is extremely important that severe contusions to the muscular areas of the leg be watched closely for increased swelling, changes in skin color and temperature, and loss of peripheral pulses as well as sensation. The presence of any of these signs requires immediate referral to an orthopaedic surgeon. It may be necessary to restore perfusion with an immediate fasciotomy.

Contusions of the Fibula

Contusions over the proximal fibula may injure the peroneal nerve. More distally in the leg, the superficial peroneal nerve in the distal lateral aspect may be injured as it transverses the deep fascia to innervate the distal lateral portion of the leg, the dorsum of the foot, and the dorsum of the first four toes. The sensory alterations of the nerve distribution can range from hyperesthesia to hypoesthesia or analgesia. A complaint following resolution of the trauma can be burning in nature and is generally superficial.

Strains/Sprains

Strains of the muscles and tendons of the leg are frequent in runners and jumpers. The diagnosis of a sprain to the muscle or

tendon is based upon the history of the mechanism, the site of point tenderness, and the degree of disability. Management is directed at reducing the inflammation with the use of rest, ice massage, and the use of oral anti-inflammatory agents. Rehabilitation is directed at increasing muscular endurance. Stretching exercises are begun slowly after resolution of the acute inflammation (Fig. 10.4). Improving strength and endurance is essential before a return to sports. A regimen of stretching before and after running coupled with the avoidance of running on hard surfaces, running downhill, running on uneven surfaces

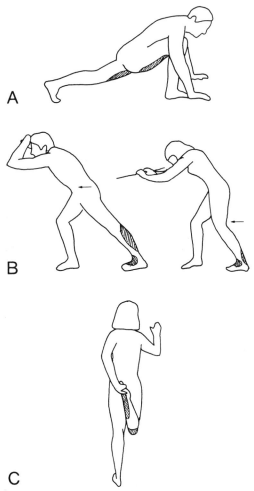

Figure 10.4. Lower leg stretches. Stretch for 10 minutes before and after each exercise session. Stretch gently. Hold the stretch and repeat several times. **A,** Hamstring. **B,** Calf/Achilles tendon. **C,** Quadriceps.

(sand, grass, etc.), and overtraining will decrease the chances of muscle injury.

Instruct runners in the importance of proper foot wear. Shoes should be cushioned, especially at the heel, to absorb shock. Well padded heel counters will support the heel and the Achilles tendon. Mesh uppers will allow the feet to breathe. Padded tongues will prevent irritation of the dorsum. The sole of the shoe should not be stiff as this may lead to lower leg strain. A flexible sole with an arch support that fits is essential. Instruct the athlete in the importance of regularly checking the shoes for wear and replacing worn shoes.

Dislocation of the Head of the Fibula

This injury results from twisting forces applied to the knee that rotate it internally and at the same time direct force is applied to the head of the fibula, levering it out of its shallow pocket. If seen immediately, reduction may be accomplished by closed manipulation. Not infrequently, the injury is missed and later is diagnosed with evidence of a painful luxating phenomenon manifest with traction of the hamstrings. If the joint remains unstable, the ligamentous structures may have to be repaired.

Shin Splints

"Shin splints" is a catch-all term that has been used to include tibialis posterior tendinitis, stress fractures, muscle tears and strains, periosteal strains, and certain vascular disorders (compartment syndromes). The frequent cause is hyperpronation caused by forefoot varus.

While the posterior tibial syndrome and shin splints have become synonymous, characteristic scintigraphic findings do not define the posterior tibial muscle origin. Abnormal tracer accumulation is localized to the middle and distal thirds of the posterior medial aspect of the tibial cortex on delayed images. A high-resolution gamma camera must be used to obtain both lateral and medial views. The pattern suggests that the soleus muscle margin is involved as opposed to the posterior tibial or other muscle tendon complexes of the leg (Holder and Michael, 1984).

The patient presents with aching pain along the medial tibial border, usually after a long run on uneven surfaces and with inadequate foot support.

Treatment. Management focuses on the cause of injury in the given patient. A collapsing medial arch should be supported with orthotics. Symptoms can be treated after the biomechanical cause of the injury is corrected. Strength and flexibility exercises can be instituted after pain subsides. Heel cord stretching is accomplished on an incline board.

Overuse Syndromes

Overuse syndromes generally present as leg pain without a history of specific injury. Their common denominator is that they are all associated with exercise. The overuse syndromes include acute muscle cramps, tenosynovitis of the anterior tibial, flexor hallucis longus, posterior tibial or Achilles tendon, periostitis of the tibia, stress fracture of the fibula or tibia, partial subcutaneous ruptures of the Achilles, tears of the musculotendinous junction of the medial head of the gastrocnemius, chronic and/or acute anterior compartment syndromes.

Compartment Syndrome

Compartment syndromes may develop as the result of an acute injury or may be the result of muscle swelling in the encased compartment. Any of the four compartments of the lower extremity may be involved. Because the compartments are bounded by tight fascial structures, swelling or bleeding within these compartments can raise the intercompartmental pressure, resulting in decreased perfusion and relative anoxia of the muscle compartment. The initial presentation of this ischemia is that of pain. This pain is disproportionate and is not relieved with minor analgesics. Pain is increased with passive stretch of the involved compartment. With progression parethesias and paralysis develop. With the development of paresthesias and paralysis, the muscle compartments have usually undergone irreversible cell damage and death. The standard evaluation for pulses in this condition is not useful. The clinical sign of pain with passive stretching of the involved compartment should trigger automatic compartment pressure monitoring.

This condition is an orthopaedic emergency and requires immediate referral for monitoring of compartment pressure and possible fasciotomies. Crush injuries of the lower extremities and tibial fractures are common etiologies for development of compartment syndrome. In a patient with head trauma or in a polytraumatized patient, indwelling compartment pressure monitoring should be performed, as neurovascular assessment is not possible.

Acute exercise-induced compartment syndromes produce pain in the lower extremity and are due to muscle swelling within these compartments as a consequence of physical exertion. This can be demonstrated by increased compartment pressure after exercise. This syndrome presents predominantly as pain after a period of exercise. This condition may be improved with rest and modification of training programs, but in a high performance athlete this problem may require fasciotomy in order to obtain relief.

With the intensification of interest in running, distances and the training periods have lengthened. As a consequence, there have developed chronic compartment syndromes of the anterior, the posterior superficial, as well as the deep posterior compartments. In general, all of these conditions improve with rest or modification of the running program. Correction in leg length patterns and the use of an orthosis for skeletal deformity of the foot have also been useful. These chronic exercise-induced compartment syndromes can be studied utilizing treadmills and pressure catherization techniques. The energy cycle of muscle action may be studied by magnetic resonance techniques.

Gastrocnemius Tear

The medial head of the gastrocnemius can be ruptured. It occurs at the musculotendinous junction, usually in the older age group, although it can occur in the hypertrophied muscle of the overdeveloped athlete. The postrupture state is characterized by an upward migration of the muscle, tenderness over the medial head, and at the junction of the musculotendinous area evidences of swelling and ecchymosis with distal migration of subcutaneous blood in the more severe cases. Generally, the condition is caused by a sudden eccentric force on the muscle. The individual is now but an intermittent participant in a skilled sports activity. Irregularity, as opposed to regularity of the exercise program, is a definite factor. The condition can be confused with deep thrombophlebitis, but in general the episode itself, the sudden onset, and the sharply defined anatomic location do not cause diagnostic problems.

Treatment. Treatment is directed at control of pain and inflammation, and restoration of normal motion and strength of the lower leg before return to sports. Conservative care generally suffices, although in the occasional case, recurrence can occur. Pressure dressing, elevation, and icing is used early. A heel lift will relieve tension with ambulation. Crutches are used with weight bearing to tolerance. The healing phase requires not less than 6 weeks with subsequent rehabilitation. Early return to sports usually guarantees recurrence.

Achilles Tendinitis

Repetitive overextension or overuse of the Achilles tendon, such as jumping at basketball or distance running may cause the sheath to become inflamed and thickened. This results in chronic pain and tightness over the Achilles tendon. More frequently, it is insidious in onset, peaking in the midthirties. At times, the condition may become chronic and incapacitating, particularly to the competitive athlete. Examination may reveal a diffuse or localized swelling and tenderness to palpation over the tendon. The contour of the tendon should be smooth and even, and there should be no evidence of nodulations or scar formation. In the more chronic tendinitis, nodulation or distortions in contour can occur, and these suggest degeneration within the structure of the tendon itself or partial subcutaneous tears.

Treatment. The initial treatment includes rest, until acute inflammation subsides, ice to the affected area, and oral nonsteroidal anti-inflammatory drugs. A heel lift may be useful to decrease tension on the tendon. Once the condition subsides, active stretching and strengthening of the gastrocnemius soleus complex can begin. If conservative treatment is unavailing and the patient disabled, consideration should be given to surgery.

Achilles Rupture

Acute Achilles tendon rupture occurs, but generally there is a prodromal period of "tendinitis." The occurrence is usually 1 or 2 inches above the insertion of the tendon on the calcaneus. A palpable gap is apparent. There is a distinct history of a sudden, lancinating (knife-like) pain with loss of function and inability to stand on the toes.

Physical examination of the complete tear reveals swelling and ecchymosis over the posterior aspect of the leg and heel. This can be confused with an "ankle sprain." Generally, there is a palpable gap and the absence of active plantar flexion with good strength. Thompson's test is performed by squeezing the calf musculature (Fig. 10. 5). If there is no continuity between the gastroc soleus muscles and the Achilles tendon, the transmitted squeeze ("shortening" the muscle) will not produce plantar flexion of the foot. Splinting and compression dressings with the foot in a relaxed plantar flexion mode with advised elevation and early icing can be useful in reducing the reaction about the area. In the young, active individual surgical repair is advised; additionally the condition can be treated in an equinus cast.

Stress Fracture

The tibia and fibula frequently sustain stress fractures as a result of overuse. While one tends to identify these strains with distance runners, they can be found in teens with "normal activity." It is well identified in dancers, as well as basketball players, soccer players, and lacrosse players. The condition frequently occurs in the preseason training period. These fractures do not occur at any particular time, but rather are the end product of an adaptive process in which a bone attempts rapidly to remodel itself along the lines of increased stress. The bone becomes partially or completely disrupted by rhythmic, repeated sub-threshhold stress. Symptoms usually begin with a mild discomfort in the long shaft of the tibia or fibula after activity. Simple rest relieves the symptoms. With continued activity, the pain becomes more persistent, lasting from day to day. Ultimately, the pain is severe enough to prohibit activity.

Clinical examination may demonstrate localized tenderness to palpation directly over the fracture sites. There may be evident subcutaneous swelling. Early x-ray films may be negative but reveal periosteal reactions or cortical thickening 2 to 4 weeks after the onset of symptoms. A bone scan (Fig. 10.6) will be positive before x-ray changes. Bone pain may precede scintigraphic evidence of stress fracture and repeat scanning may be necessary in highly motivated individuals whose bone pain increases with continued activity. Such positive scans might be included under stress reaction of bone as opposed to the fracture. Stress fractures are generally found in the lower one-third of each bone, and may be single or multiple (Fig. 10.7). Management of these fractures is rest from sports. Generally no cast is required, and ordinary walking is allowed providing it is not excessive. In some instances a tibial Aircast fracture brace maybe useful in decreasing symptoms and allowing earlier return to sports. It is to be noted that some patients require a cast primarily to induce rest. If the advice is ignored, the bone may completely fracture.

Fracture

Isolated fracture of the tibia and fibula occur but are not overly common in sports. Fractures of the neck of the fibula can occur with sudden turns in skiing as well as "cutting" in basketball. There may be secondary associated injuries due to bleeding that involve the peroneal nerve.

Frequently, high fractures of the fibula can occur with sprains about the ankle as well as the associated injuries involving the interosseous membrane as well as the ligamentous structures of the medial ankle joint (Fig. 10.8). While the ankle itself may not be fractured, the evidences of trauma

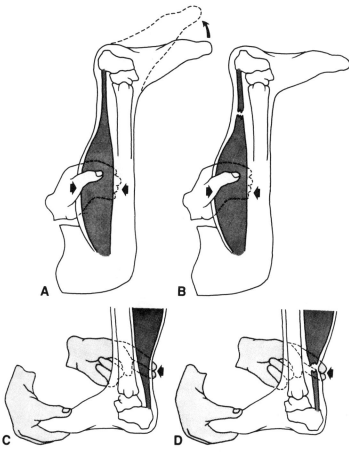

Figure 10.5. Diagnosis of the ruptured achilles tendon. **A**, Normal. **B**, Ruptured. **C**, Normal. **D**, ruptured. (From Ramamurti CP (Tinker RV, ed): *Orthopaedics in Primary Care*. Baltimore, Williams & Wilkins, 1979, p 279.)

about the ankle, as well as the high fibular fracture, strongly suggest a transmitted disruption through the interosseous membrane across the front of the ankle and through the deltoid ligamentous structures. Thus the high isolated fracture may be associated with serious injuries.

With fractures of the leg, the primary concern is restoring integrity of the tibia. The immediate management should be application of a splint and transportation to a facility where x-ray examination can be performed and more definitive care extended. Splinting, gentle compression, and external application of cold packs where feasible, as well as medication for relief of pain should be routine. Definitive treatment requires res-

toration of length, alignment, and joint congruity by either closed or open means.

THE ANKLE

Anatomy

The ankle joint is formed by three bones: tibia, fibula, and talus. (Fig. 10.9).

The dome of the talus fits into the mortise (concavity) formed by the tibia and fibula. The medial and lateral malleoli project downward to articulate with the side of the talus. The ankle joint essentially moves in one plane upward and downward with a central axis of rotation. As the ankle goes into plantar flexion, the more narrow posterior positions of the talus are brought into

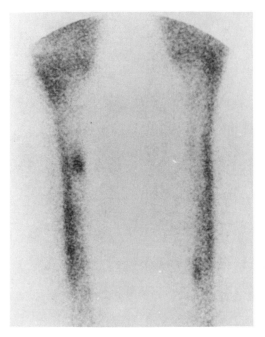

Figure 10.6. Stress reaction of bone in both tibias.

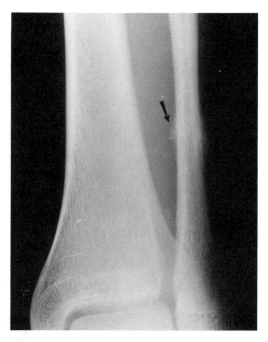

Figure 10.7. Healing stress fracture.

contact with the wider anterior portions of the tibia. This permits a small amount of free play in the ankle joint which, in dorsiflexion, is lost. On the other hand, as the tibia is driven forward on the plantar flexed talus, the narrower portions of the tibia impinge on the wider anterior portions of the talus, blocking dislocation of the tibia on the talus.

The relationship of these three bones is maintained by three groups of ligaments: the deltoid ligament medially, the lateral collateral ligaments, and the anterior tibiofibular ligament and syndesmosis. The deltoid, the strongest of the three ligaments, has a broad triangular shape and is defined by the bony insertions on the navicular, the talus, and the calcaneus as it fans from the medial malleolus. The lateral collateral ligament of the ankle is T-shaped and consists of three distinct parts. The posterior talofibular ligament arises from the posterior portion of the tip of the fibular and runs backward and slightly downward to attach to the lateral tubercle of the posterior process of the talus. This is essentially an interarticular ligament. It is the strongest of the three ligamentous elements

and helps to resist posterior dislocation of the foot. The calcaneofibular ligament is the largest of the three and passes inferiorly in a posterior direction to insert on the lateral surface of the calcaneus. The ligament is extrascapular, but may be associated with the peroneal tendon sheaths. This ligament is completely relaxed when the foot is in a normal standing position. The anterior talofibular ligament arises from the anterior border of the lateral malleolus and passes forward somewhat medially to attach to the neck of the talus. Its direction corresponds to the longitudinal axis of the foot and is taut in all positions of flexion. The anterior talofibular ligament is the primary stabilizer of the ankle joint and is most commonly injured. The ligaments of the tibiofibular syndesmosis maintain the relationship of the distal tibia and fibula. The ligaments hold the fibula snug in the groove on the tibia where the fibula rotates around its longitudinal axis, as well as rising and falling with dorsi and plantar flexion of the ankle. The anterior tibiofibular and posterior tibiofibular ligaments blend into the interosseous membrane approximately 2 to 3 cm above the ankle joint.

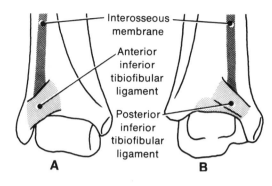

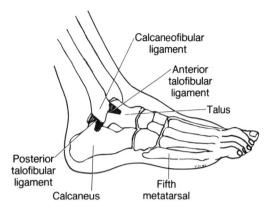

Figure 10.9. The ankle joint. (From Burnside JW, McGlynn TJ: *Physical Diagnosis*, ed 17. Baltimore, Williams & Wilkins, 1987, p 275.)

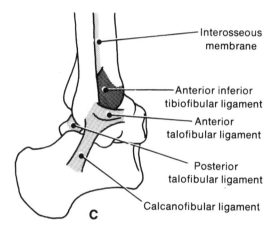

Figure 10.8. Distal tibiofibular joint and tibiotalar joint. **A**, Anterior view. **B**, Posterior view. **C**, Lateral view. (From Ramamurti CP (Tinker RV, ed): *Orthopaedics in Primary Care*. Baltimore, Williams & Wilkins, 1979, p 245.)

Ankle Sprains

The best time for accurate assessment of the degree of damage is immediately following the injury when muscle spasm is absent, pain is not as severe, and swelling and hemarthrosis have not developed. Unfortunately, the reaction about the ankle, as it relates to swelling and hemarthrosis, is extremely rapid. It is estimated that ankle injuries account for 20 to 25% of all lost time injuries in running and jumping sports.

There are frequent corollaries in the work place that are sustained on insecure footing secondary to slips or falls, dismounting from vehicles, and encounters with unexpected potholes.

Mechanisms of Injury. Injuries to the ankle must be considered in relationship to the magnitude and direction of forces applied to the ankle. Once inversion is initiated, the ankle loses the bony stability of its neutral position. As inversion increases, the medial malleolus may lose its stabilizing function and begin to act as a fulcrum for further inversion. Since inversion injuries are the most frequent, sprains to the lateral collateral ligament are by far the most common ankle injury. The same mechanism of inversion and supination can lead to a fracture, usually an oblique fracture of the fibula with or without a fracture of the medial malleolus.

The other important mechanism of ankle injury is pronation and external rotation. This is rarely a pure ligamentous injury, and when it does occur the deltoid and anterior tibiofibular ligaments are torn. Usually, the deltoid ligament ruptures with the fracture of the fibula.

Physical Examination. With serious ankle injuries, there may be a history of immediate pain and difficulty in bearing weight. Often the patient will describe a "pop," or a "snap," or a sense of giving way.

Initial evaluation reveals localized tenderness over the involved ligaments (Fig. 10.10).

Motion may or may not be restricted (Fig.

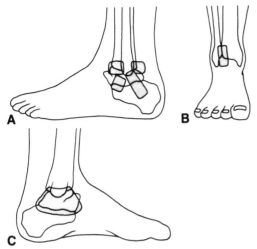

Figure 10.10. Examination of the ankle—zones of tenderness of the individual ligaments. **A,** The lateral ligaments. **B,** The anterior-inferior tibiofibular ligaments. **C,** The deltoid ligament. (From Ramamurti CP (Tinker RV, ed): *Orthopaedics in Primary Care.* Baltimore, Williams & Wilkins, 1979, p 290.)

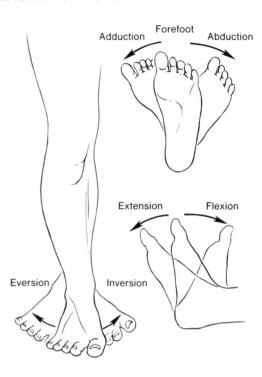

10.11). In general, the more difficulty an individual has in weight bearing, the more serious the injury.

The initial evaluation of acute injury includes the neurological and vascular functions of the extremity. If these are intact, attention is turned to the other elements. Initially a fracture must be differentiated from a sprain (Fig. 10.12). This may be difficult with the undisplaced spiral fracture of the fibula or the avulsion fracture of the tip of the fibula. Fibular pain with compression away from the area of trauma or with tapping the heel often indicate a fracture if there is a specific referral area. Fracture at the base of the fifth metatarsal must be considered. Careful palpation of the anatomic structures generally locates the maximized area of pathology.

Diagnostic Guidelines. Routine x-ray films (AP, lateral and mortise) of the ankle, including oblique views, identify fractures. The very specific indication of an ankle x-ray may exclude the base of the fifth metatarsal; if this is suspect, obtain additional films of the foot.

Sprains are classified as first, second, or third degree. The classification is to deter-

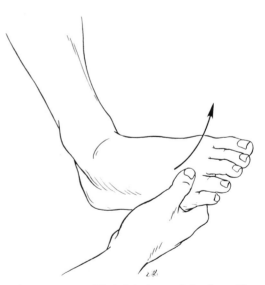

Figure 10.11. (*Top*). Motions of the foot. (*Bottom*). Inversion of the foot. Note that the entire foot is inverted, not just the digits. (From Burnside JW, McGlynn TJ: *Physical Diagnosis*, ed 17. Baltimore, Williams & Wilkins, p 276.)

mine treatment and prognosis. In essence, the mild stable injury with minimal disability can be treated quite conservatively with

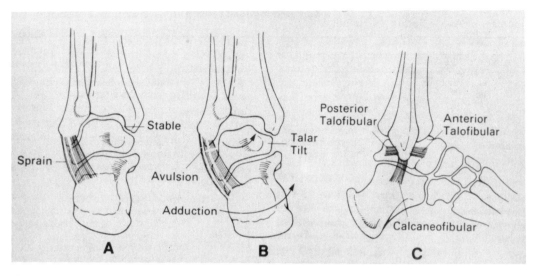

Figure 10.12. Lateral ligamentous sprain and avulsion. **A,** Simple sprain in which the ligaments remain intact and the talus remains stable within the mortise. **B,** Avulsion of the lateral ligaments; the talus becomes unstable and tilts within the mortise when the calcaneus is adducted. **C,** Lateral ligaments of the ankle. The anterior talofibular and the calcaneofibular ligaments are the ligaments most frequently involved in inversion injuries. (From Goroll AH, May LA, Molley A: *Primary Care Medicine*, ed 2, p. 684, Philadelphia, JB Lippincott, 1987.) (Redrawn from Cailliet R: *Foot and Ankle Pain.* Philadelphia, FA Davis, 1968)

prompt return to ambulation and afforded support. The moderate injury is of greater symptomatic distress to the patient. The treatment emphasis is in controlling the process of inflammation, maintaining muscle tone and range of motion with protective ambulation. The more severe and/or unstable ankle joint present with ligamentous injuries and instability (Table 10.2).

The most common injury to the anterior talofibular ligament results in anterior instability. This is demonstrated by a positive anterior drawer test (Fig. 10.13) or x-ray of the ankle. To evaluate laxity of the anterior talofibular ligament the patient must be relaxed and facing the examiner while seated on the examining room table with the knee flexed over the edge. The examiner should grasp the patient's heel in one hand and manipulate it in the sagittal plane back and forth. To the examining hand, there is a sense of instability or "opening" of one joint compared to the other. Ligamentous structures have an end point, but further, the talus is controlled, and the recoil slap of the unstable ankle is not appreciated (positive talar slap

test). Gross laxity on inversion indicates tears of both the calcaneofibular ligament and the anterior talofibular ligaments.

If instability is suspected on clinical examination (Fig. 10.14), refer the patient to an orthopaedic surgeon for stress testing under x-ray. Local anesthesia is used in the acute injury as muscle spasm secondary to the painful injury can hide instability. If, on a stress AP x-ray film, the talus opens 15 to 30° laterally, the diagnosis is rupture of the anterior talofibular and calcaneofibular ligaments. In the lateral view, if the foot is forced forward, the talus will sublux anteriorly and be documented on the lateral x-ray film.

One always suspects an injury to the deltoid ligament with any fracture of the fibula or any pronation mechanism of injury. Stress testing can be diagnostic by revealing widening of the medial joint space on x-ray. Avulsion at the very tip of the lateral malleolus is diagnostic of a major injury to the lateral collateral ligaments. Osteochondral fractures of the dome of the talus may accompany any injury resulting in instability. Anteroposterior x-rays with the foot in

Table 10.2
Summary of Ankle Sprain Treatment

Ankle Sprain		
Classification	Characteristics	Treatment
First degree (stretching of the ligaments)	No pain Swelling Tenderness on palpation over the joint Normal range of motion Normal talar tilt sign Negative anterior draw	Ice to the affected area for 20 minutes every hour for 24 hours, then PRN, elevation of the affected ankle, elastic wrap Weight bearing Active ROM exercise Encourage swimming Return to sports 1 to 3 weeks
Second degree (tearing of some part of the ligamentous fibers, anterior talo fibular ligament)	Pain Swelling Pain on range of motion Inability to bear weight Positive anterior draw Normal talar tilt sign	Ice for 24 hours, elevation, elastic wrap 1 to 2 weeks Partial weight bearing as tolerated until pain subsides Partial weight bearing exercise 2 to 3 days after injury (active plantar, dorsi, toe flexion, inversion, eversion) Full weight bearing after swelling resolved, with sprain brace (protects against inversion and eversion while permitting plantar and dorsiflexion) No sports 4 to 8 weeks Tape ankle prior to athletic activity
Third degree (complete tearing of entire ligamentous fibers)	Severe pain (exam difficult) Pain with passive inversion Swelling anterior lateral malleolus Positive anterior draw Talar tilt >20 degrees Positive talar slap	Prompt referral Cast immobilization 4 to 6 weeks or surgery Return to sports after rehabilitation

equinus (ankle joint plantar flexed) may be helpful to show this lesion and osteochondral loose bodies. While arthrograms of the ankle are interesting, they offer little information that impacts upon treatment and prognosis. With classification based on an evaluation of stability, treatment is directed toward protective support and early rehabilitation. In essence, the moderate or second degree sprain is treated the same as the minor injury. It simply takes a longer period of time to heal. Immobilization or splinting with such devices as an Aircast is more frequently employed.

Treatment. The treatment of the unstable or third degree sprain of the lateral collateral ligament is still controversial. The choices are (1) short leg plaster for 4 to 6 weeks, (2) cast, bracing, and/or an Aircast, and (3) surgical repair.

Surgery is considered in displaced interarticular fractures involving the weight bearing surface of the joint. It may be considered in the unstable ankle joint in young competitive athletes. There are also many individuals who work on extremely unstable surfaces and a consideration of joint use may condition surgical judgment for nonathletes. In the very unstable ankle, where there is rupture of the anterior talofibular and calcaneofibular ligaments, the conservative versus open repair controversy continues without an absolute position established. In addition to the interarticular fractures, ankle luxation may be accompanied by peroneal tendon dislocations; this may prompt the consideration of surgery. A combination of surgical repair and cast bracing may speed the process of rehabilitation.

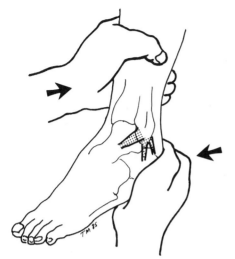

Figure 10.13. The anterior drawer sign. To test the stability of ankle ligaments, cup the heal in the palm of one hand and exert anteriorly directed pressure while you grasp the ankle with the other hand; this exerts posteriorly directed force. With both hands cupping the ankle, it is also easy to stabilize the foot and ankle and medially and laterally rotate the foot through motion within the ankle mortise. You can palpate the ligamentous areas with your fingers or thumb at the same time and identify abnormal opening of the joint space and tenderness over the talofibular and calcaneofibular ligaments. (From Burnside JW, McGlynn TJ: *Physical Diagnosis*, ed 17. Baltimore, Williams & Wilkins, 1987.)

Rehabilitation. Rehabilitation in ankle sprains begins at the onset of treatment. Strengthening of the medial and lateral stabilizers of the ankle may begin as soon as a pain-free exercise program is made possible. Although there are arguments about full weight bearing before the pain has cleared, there are very definite benefits to progressive partial weight bearing. Exercises for dorsiflexion, plantar flexion, inversion, and eversion involve the four major muscle groups of the lower leg (Fig. 10.15).

Walking is followed by jogging, running, figures of eight, and other exercises to re-establish neuromuscular integration disturbed by the injury. External support such as taping or an Aircast is extremely useful when an individual with a second or third degree sprain is returned to running activities.

Definite emphasis on regaining proprioception should be made, and this is done on tilt boards and similar apparatus. This not only aids in neuromuscular recovery, but improves the subtalar motion. The rehabilitation following fractures is similar to that of sprains, but prolonged because of the injury and the required immobilization.

Subtalar Joint Sprain

Overlooked in the ankle sprain is the not infrequent concomitant sprain of the subtalar joint. It is not unusual following conservative treatment of sprains in a plaster cast that the subtalar joint motion is markedly restricted. This may become a chronic problem. An "ankle sprain" that continues to be disabling beyond a 6-week period of rehabilitation should be evaluated for involvement of the subtalar joint. The joint is painful on testing of the motion. The involvement can be defined by a CT scan as well as a bone scan. It may not be defined with conventional x-ray. Such studies may disclose ill-defined, small fractures as well as arthritis of the subtalar joint (Fig. 10.16).

Fractures

Fractures of the ankle are clinically quite different from sprains in that they will require cast or cast brace immobilization and may require surgical stabilizations. Rehabilitation is more difficult and prolonged due to the severity of the injury, and there is evident muscle atrophy that results from immobilization. Rigid internal fixation of these fractures may reduce the rehabilitation time and lead to a faster recovery. Presuming anatomic reduction, the ultimate prognosis in ankle fractures is related to the damage to the articular surface, which may not be evident for some period of time after the injury.

Osteochondral fractures of the ankle usually involve the superior surface of the talus, either medially or laterally, and may occasionally involve the inner surface of the fibula. Surgical removal of the bone and cartilage fragments is usually necessary to affect cure. These fractures may be missed if oblique views are not obtained on x-ray examination of the injured ankle. Tomograms and CT scans may prove useful in

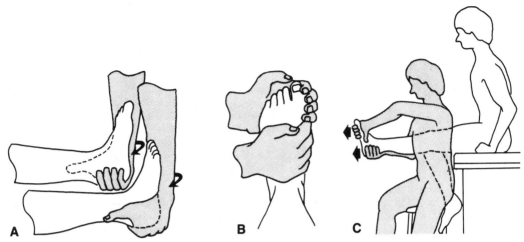

Figure 10.14. Examination of the ankle—manipulation of the ankle. **A,** Manipulation for instability of the tibiotalar joint. The injured ankle may be compared to the normal ankle by simultaneous manipulation. **B,** Gentle manipulation in dorsal and plantar flexion. **C,** Application of rhythmic traction to the ankle. (From Ramamurti CP (Tinker RV, ed): *Orthopaedics in Primary Care.* Baltimore, Williams & Wilkins, 1979, p 291.)

defining the condition, as well as extent of placement. Arthroscopic techniques may be employed to treat these very specific fractures of the joint surface. The overall principles of management of ankle fractures are concerned with the stability of the ankle joint and maintenance of the mortise. Internal fixation with screws and plates and repair of ruptured ligaments is frequently indicated to restore the integrity of the joint.

Peroneal Tendon Dislocation

These primary lateral stabilizers are the ankle's protection against an inversion injury. Injury results when the individual's foot is fixed in a position of maximal dorsiflexion, such as occurs in cross-country skiing, down-hill skiing, and wrestling. Patients complain of a sudden giving way sensation. Physical examination reveals swelling and tenderness behind the lateral malleolus that extends proximally over the peroneal tendon. Active manipulation will dislocate the tendon when the ankle is dorsiflexed. With dislocation of the peroneal tendon, there is a strong possibility of recurrence. Therefore, it is best treated initially by repair of the retinaculum, despite the fact that such treatment may lengthen the recovery phase.

THE FOOT

Anatomy

The bony skeleton of the foot is composed of 26 bones (Fig. 10.17). The inferior surface of the talus articulates with the calcaneus making up the subtalar joint that contributes greatly to inversion and eversion movement of the foot. The combination movement of these three articulations, talocalcaneal, talonavicular, and calcaneocuboid, result in the complex foot movement of eversion and inversion, pronation and supination. The midtarsal joints, navicular cuneiform, and cuneiform metatarsals are very stable and produce very little movement. Metatarsals and proximal phalanges make up the metatarsophalangeal joints. They are important for push off, particularly at the first MP joint. The bones are arranged structurally to form two arches, the longitudinal arch and the transverse arch. The individual bones are mortised together to form the architecture of the arches. The ligaments of the foot provide intrinsic support, and the muscles provide extrinsic support. The longitudinal arch starts at the weight bearing surface of the calcaneus and ends at the metatarsal heads. It is supported intrinsically by the spring ligament. This lig-

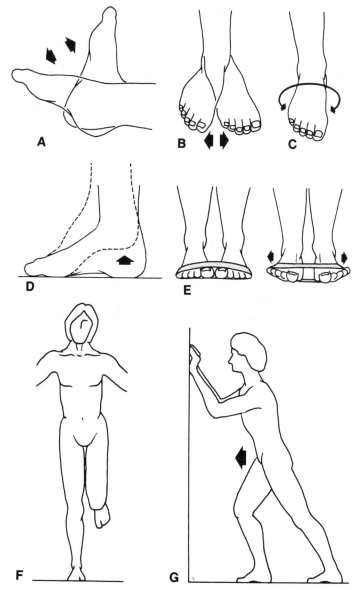

Figure 10.15. Range of motion and strengthening exercises of the foot and ankle. **A,** Active movement of the tibiotalar joint by alternate dorsiflexion and plantarflexion. **B,** Active movement of the subtalar, intertarsal, and tarsometatarsal joints by alternate supination and pronation. **C,** Active movement of the tibiotalar, subtalar, intertarsal, and tarsometatarsal joints by circling the foot. **D,** Repeated elevation onto the toes, standing. **E,** Pronation against elastic resistance. **F,** Balancing on one foot. **G,** Heel cord stretching. (From Ramamurti CP (Tinker RV, ed): *Orthopaedics in Primary Care*. Baltimore, Williams & Wilkins, 1979, p 268.)

ament supports the head of the talus. The arch is also supported by the plantar fascia that runs from the calcaneal tuberosity to the proximal phalanges. The plantar fascia acts as a bowstring for the longitudinal arch and

supports the muscles on the plantar surface of the foot. The extrinsic support for the medial arch comes from the anterior tibial tendon pulling upon its insertion on the first cuneiform and the posterior tibial tendon and

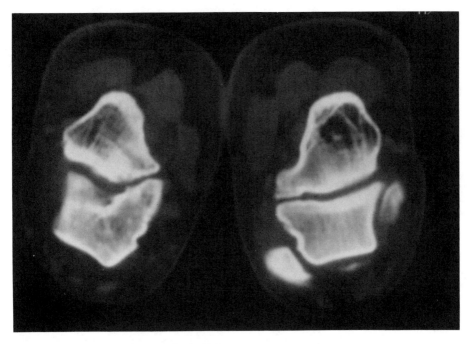

Figure 10.16. CT scan of arthritic subtalar joint.

peroneus longus tendon that pass under the foot and create a dynamic sling supporting the longitudinal arch.

The three main muscle groups of the lower leg all insert on the foot and thus control the action of the foot. The deep portions of the posterior compartment contain the posterior tibial, flexor digitorum longus, and flexor hallucis longus. The posterior tibial muscle supports the longitudinal arch and inverts the foot. The flexor digitorum longus flexes the lateral four toes, and the flexor hallucis longus flexes the great toe. These three muscles enter the foot through a ligamentous tunnel behind the medial malleolus along with the posterior tibial nerve, the artery, and the vein.

The posterior tibial nerve divides into the medial and lateral plantar nerve and supplies sensation to the plantar surface of the foot while innervating the plantar muscles.

The lateral compartment is composed of two muscles, the peroneus longus and brevis. The longus crosses under the longitudinal arch from lateral to medial and inserts on the plantar surface of the first cuneiform and first metatarsal. The peroneus brevis inserts on the base of the fifth metatarsal. These muscles evert and plantar flex the foot.

The anterior compartment consists of the anterior tibial that inserts on the medial cuneiform, the extensor digitorum longus, and the extensor hallucis longus. This group dorsiflexes the foot and toes. The anterior tibial and extensor hallucis longus muscles are invertors, and the extensor digitorum longus is an evertor. The intrinsic muscles of the foot are primarily related to toe function.

The plantar nerves are subjected to entrapment neuropathy as they turn around the medial edge of the foot to enter the plantar region. The posterior tibial nerve passes behind the medial malleolus where it is covered by the lanciniate ligament. This configuration has been called the tarsal tunnel. Near the tunnel, the posterior tibial nerve splits into the medial plantar, lateral plantar, and calcaneal nerves. Some of the calcaneal branches innervate the skin of the heel and pierce the ligament, but some pass completely through the tunnel. This latter group is made up of nerves that innervate the inferior aspect of the calcaneus. The medial plantar nerve carries sensation from the me-

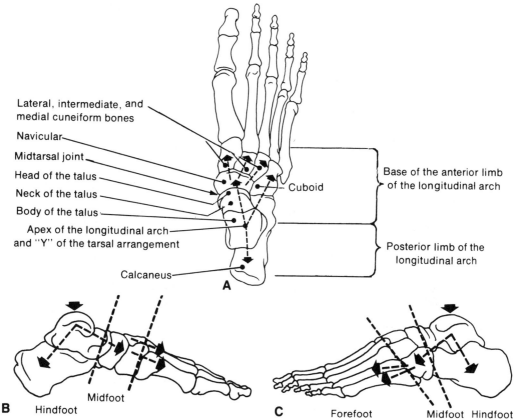

Figure 10.17. The tarsal bones and the dispersion of weight throughout the foot. **A,** Superior view. **B,** Medial view. **C,** Lateral view. (From Ramamurti CP (Tinker RV, ed): *Orthopaedics in Primary Care.* Baltimore, Williams & Wilkins, 1979, p 246.)

dial side of the sole in front of the heel and from the plantar surface of the three and one-half medial toes. The nerve innervates muscles whose chief action is plantar flexion motion of the toes, particularly at the metatarsophalangeal joint of the first toe. The flexor brevis and the abductor hallucis are very important in providing the necessary stability of the first toe phalanges for a final pushoff in walking. The lateral plantar nerve carries sensation from the lateral side of the sole past the heel and from the plantar surface of the lateral one and one-half toe. Motor action of this nerve helps maintain the functional conformity of the foot innervating muscles that cause flexion at the lateral MP joints and adduction and abduction of the toes.

Entrapment of these elements may pro-

duce heel pain, or medial and lateral plantar burning pain, numbness, and changes in sweat patterns of the plantar foot. The diagnosis may be aided or established by nerve conduction and EMG studies. It has been demonstrated that forcing a foot into an overpronated position will stress the posterior tibial nerve against the fibrous edged opening in the abductor hallucis muscle. One may suspect the involvement of the nerves in acute foot strain that presents with marked tenderness at the posteromedial plantar aspect of the foot. Although usually described as a sprained ligament, it may be due to plantar nerve trunk sensitivity. The painful heel, additionally, may be caused by involvement of the calcaneal nerves as they innervate the common origin of the muscles and fascia at the anterior inferior surface of the calcaneus.

The deep peroneal nerve is subject to an entrapment neuropathy in its terminal portions on the dorsum of the foot. Traumatic involvement of the nerve or one of its branches is a frequently unrecognized complication of a direct blow to the dorsum of the foot. As the deep peroneal nerve approaches the foot, it passes deep to the inferior extensor retinaculum. This has been designated as the anterior tarsal tunnel. In the lower portion the nerve divides into medial and lateral branches. The lateral branch innervates the digitorum brevi. The medial branch continues on the bone plane down the dorsum of the foot to reach the junctions of the first and second metatarsal. At this point, it passes immediately under the tendon of the extensor hallucis brevis and then pierces the deep fascia to reach its final innervation of the skin of the cleft between the first and second toes.

Physical Examination

Physical examination should include complete evaluation of the lower extremity. Flat feet (or the pronated foot) is a condition in which the longitudinal arch is flattened (Fig. 10.18). The hindfoot may be in valgus; this should be observed from the rear with the patient standing. Occasionally, there is an associated accessory navicular bone. The navicular tuberosity fails to fuse to the main bone and remains as a bony prominence on the medial side of the foot. This is often locally painful.

Flat feet are classified as flexible or rigid. The flexible flat foot (pronated foot) is the most common and is usually asymptomatic in the milder forms. Moderate to severe deformity may be symptomatic. Proper attention to footwear and longitudinal arch supports are helpful. The rigid flat foot is a much more difficult problem and may prohibit such activities as long, continued running. Rigid flat foot or a peroneal spastic flat foot is often due to congenital tarsal coalition, although symptoms may be delayed until adolescence or later.

Congenital deformity such as metatarsus varus or valgus may be present. Metatarsus varus (adductus) is a deformity of the forefoot in which the forefoot is angulated and rotated medially in relation to the hindfoot.

Metatarsus valgus (abductus) is the opposite deformity of the forefoot. With extensive use, these deformities may place abnormal stress on the foot resulting in painful callosities. Proper footwear and orthoses may prevent problems.

The hindfoot may also be angulated either medially or laterally. Deformities are usually associated with a cavus (varus) angulated medially, or flat foot (valgus) angulated laterally. Deformities of the toes are common. Hallux valgus with or without a bunion is associated with widened angle between the first and second metatarsals. Clawing of the toes is hyperextension of the MP joint and flexion of the interphalangeal joint. This usually results from some subtle muscle imbalance of the foot. Painful callosities can develop over the dorsum of the interphalangeal joint, as well as under the metatarsal heads. Hammertoe is a deformity in flexion of the distal interphalangeal joint that puts pressure on the nail and end of the toe with contact against the sole of the shoe.

Common Problems of the Foot

Blisters

Friction produces blisters. In sports, the premonitory sign of a blister on the sole of the foot is the appearance of redness and tenderness. If this is treated promptly with application of ice and covering with adhesive tape, the formation of the blister is prevented. Once the blister has formed on the foot, premature removal of the roof only prolongs pain and disability. One may aspirate and preserve the roof by taping. The aspiration should be performed with a fine gauge needle through intact skin beyond the blistered area. If a blister ruptures spontaneously, the space between the roof and skin has been contaminated, and care must be exercised not to seal infection within or below the blistered skin. There should be a fairly wide area of excision. The prevention of blisters depends on minimizing the unfavorable effects of friction. Instruct the patient on the importance of properly fitting shoes, socks that fit properly, stay up and avoid wrinkles, the use of insoles, shoes that do not bind the sole to the foot with rotary

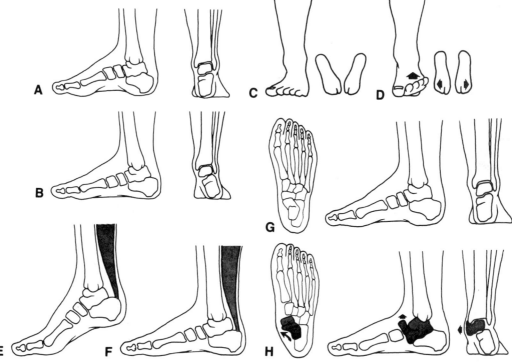

Figure 10.18. Pronated foot. **A** and **B**, Hypermobile flatfoot. **A**, Non-weightbearing. **B**, Weightbearing. **C** and **D**, Correction of internal tibial torsion by intentional pronation. **C**, Pigeon-toed stance of internal tibial torsion. **D**, Straight stance at expense of pronation. **E** and **F**, Adaptation to short heel cord by intentional pronation. **E**, Non-weightbearing. **F**, Weightbearing. **G** and **H**, A form of rigid flatfoot. The talus is angulated medially and plantarward. The navicular is dislocated and lies dorsal to the head of the talus. **G**, Normal. **H**, The rigid flatfoot. (From Ramamurti CP (Tinker RV, ed): *Orthopaedics in Primary Care.* Baltimore, Williams & Wilkins, 1979, p 259.)

movements, and consideration of lubrication of the sole before use.

Contact Allergy

On the feet, contact dermatitis is commonly caused by four major groups of materials: (1) components of shoes and stockings, (2) applied medicaments, (3) appliances used on the feet, and (4) substances encountered in occupational exposures. In the classic case, shoe dermatitis presents as an eczematous dermatitis beginning on the dorsal aspect of the big toe with eventual extension to other toes, sparing the toe webs and soles. Climatic and environmental factors play a role in the development of some occupational skin diseases. Chemical agents are the predominant causes of industrial dermatitis from leakage of chemical agents that spill on the shoes and feet.

Cement, for instance, can cause contact dermatitis through the corrosive action of the cement and/or allergic reaction from the chromates in the cement. Another type of exposure may arise from the components of specially designed work shoes or rubber boots worn in various occupations.

The diagnosis of allergic contact dermatitis depends upon history and eczematous eruption and its localization. Special patch testing is valuable in defining the causative agent.

Athlete's Foot

The concept that athlete's foot is strictly a ringworm infection of the toe webs is no longer accepted. The athlete's foot represents a continuum from a relatively asymptomatic scaling eruption caused by fungi to a symptomatic macerated hyperkeratotic variety that is caused by an overgrowth of bacteria. Thus, symptomatic athlete's foot ranges from mild scaling to a painful, exudative, erosive, inflammatory process. Tinea pedis, the most common of the dermatophytoses is usually due to *Trichophyton rubrum*. The acute clinical manifestations are oozing, macerated vesicular eruption that leads to loss of epidermis, fissuring, pruritus, and occasional secondary bacterial infection. Frequently, the initial area of involvement is a toe web where maceration and fissuring occur. The process may then extend. In marked contrast to the acute vesicular inflammatory tinea pedis, there may be a chronic, scaling, often nonsymptomatic hyperkeratotic type. In this disorder, the involvement is on the soles and often extends onto the sides of the feet in the so-called moccasin distribution. The toe webs are usually spared. This type of tinea pedis is generally due to *Trichophyton rubrum*. Oncomycosis may be the only manifestation of tinea pedis, or it may be present with the cutaneous involvement of the feet.

Treatment. For the chronic or mild infections, powders, tinctures, and solutions are used during the day, and antifungal creams or ointments are prescribed for night use. The proprietary powders and ointments are effective in treatment. The feet are kept thoroughly dry and the socks are changed twice a day. Synthetic materials are avoided. Shoes are changed and the feet powdered. Proper foot care leads to a decrease in the amount of moisture and corresponding clinical improvement. Broad spectrum antifungal agents, such as clotrimazole and miconazole, work against the fungi and also against the bacteria as they control the collaborative infections.

Soft Tissue Injuries

A bursa is a potential soft tissue space that may, with inflammation, fill with synovial fluid. External pressure from ill fitting shoes may cause inflammation or bursitis, which is seen predominantly over the MP joint of the great toe.

The pre-Achilles bursa can suggest a tendinitis. The presenting symptom is localized to the soft tissue area immediately anterior to the Achilles tendon. There may be a definite swelling anterior to the tendon. A bursa, generally related to footwear, may develop between the Achilles tendon and the overlying skin.

A callosity is an area of thickened skin overlying a bony prominence. The presence of a callus usually indicates abnormal pressure between the shoe and the bony projection; this can be noted over the distal medial great toe. The callus can be quite bothersome over the second, third, and fourth metatarsal heads and can often be relieved by padding just proximal to the metatarsal heads. This padding may, in addition, partially correct the toe deformity that, with hyperextension of the MP joint, produces a prominence of the metatarsal head.

Neuropathy

Neuropathy of the interdigital or common digital nerve is a frequent source of foot pain. The classic Morton's neuroma is found between the third and fourth web space. Other interdigital nerves, because of a similarity in anatomic relationship, are subject to the same lesion. There are multiple causes: wearing high-heeled shoes, association with the hallux valgus or bunion formation, fixed hyperextended positions of the MP joint, and positions habitually assumed in the work place or as a result of injury to the bones of the distal foot. The neuropathy is due to pressure and chronic irritation to the nerve with the production of a neuroma, or nerve mass, that sets in place a cycle that leads to disability.

Anterior Tarsal Syndrome

The clinical symptoms of the anterior tarsal syndromes are chiefly sensory. Numbness and paresthesias occur in the first dorsal web space. There may be aching and tightness about the ankle and dorsum of the foot. The complaints may be relieved by posturing of the foot. There may be nocturnal paresthesias that awaken the patient. Upon examination, there may be sensory loss in the web space. A Tinel's sign (reproduction of sensory symptoms by tapping with a reflex hammer over the tarsal tunnel) may be defined at the level of the ankle joint just medially to the dorsalis pedis. The extensor digitorum may be atrophic. Distal motor latency of the peroneal nerve to the extensor digitorum muscle may be useful in diagnosis.

If conservative treatment consisting of rest, night splints, and steroidal injections is unsuccessful, surgical release may be necessary.

Pain in the Hindfoot

Arthritis

Juvenile rheumatoid arthritis may present as a monoarticular arthritis usually seen in the lower extremity, rather than in the upper extremity. The most common site is the ankle and knee; it may occasionally arise in the subtalar joint. The painful, swollen ankle or subtalar joint in a juvenile carries a high index of suspicion for rheumatoid arthritis, especially in the absence of a history of trauma or infection. The differential diagnosis includes a screening for gonorrhea.

Posterior Tibial Tendon Strain

A strain of the posterior tibial or tenosynovitis of the posterior tibial tendon may give rise to a painful flat foot. The pain may persist with swelling and definite tenderness along the course of the posterior tibial tendon, as it passes beneath the medial malleolus.

Treatment. A valgus flat foot support or insole coupled with rest and nonsteroidal drugs will generally suffice. The condition may be associated with an accessory tarsal navicular over the medial foot. In the face of local symptoms, padding may be afforded. If the complaints continue, it may be necessary to excise the navicular prominences of the medial foot.

Posterior Tibial Tendon Rupture

The posterior tibial tendon is subject to rupture. It may be concomitant to an "ankle sprain" or it may occur during sports and because of local swelling, it may be difficult to diagnosis. Chronic "tendinitis" with fluid collection may disguise the condition. Complaints of acquired flat foot and chronic medial pain require exact definition of the condition. To aid diagnosis obtain MRI studies of the soft tissues.

Treatment. With rupture, if foot support and conservative measures do not relieve the complaints, reconstruction may be necessary.

Plantar Fasciitis

The plantar fasciitis is an acute or chronic condition that is characterized by plantar heel pain. Runners with cavus feet or individuals who stand for long periods of time (i.e. waitresses) may be particularly vulnerable. The heel is most painful, especially with the first steps upon arising in the morning. Runners find that pain is severe as they begin to run. Pain is most severe at the calcaneal tuberosity, but may spread along the course of the plantar fascia. Conceptually, it is a tennis elbow equivalent that is found anterior to the heel at the point of attachment of the long plantar fascia and the flexor brevis digitorum. On physical examination there is pain with palpation along the plantar surface of the heel where the calcaneus attaches to the plantar fascia. Anteroposterior, lateral, and oblique foot x-rays may reveal a calcaneus spur (osteophyte) that represents calcification secondary to chronic inflammation.

Treatment. Treatment includes the introduction of an anterior heel pad, rest, and, on occasions, injection of cortisone. In refractory cases, surgical release may be indicated.

Stress Fracture

Stress fracture of the calcaneus in adults occurs at any age and often accounts for a chronic painful heel. The calcaneus has the longest latency period in developing radiologic change. A bone scan will be positive long before the subtle radiologic change. Correct differential diagnosis avoids the overenthusiastic diagnosis of plantar fasciitis (calcaneal spur). Plantar fasciitis is sharply localized to the anterior heel. The stress fracture is much more diffuse about the heel. Gout must be excluded. The treatment is reduced activity, and stress relieving pads or heel cups.

Sever's Disease

Calcaneal apophysitis or "Sever's Disease" is thought to be a strain of the attachment of the tendinoachilles at the apophysis of the calcaneus or an equivalent of Osgood-Schlatter disease of the tibial tubercle. The lateral foot x-ray may demonstrate increased density or fragmentation of the apophysis. This is found on film, as opposed to the symptoms, and is almost always bilateral. There is local tenderness over the apophysis, and the patient demonstrates a limp and complains of pain with running. The condition resolves spontaneously over 3 to 6 months. Frequently, simple rest from activity will promptly reduce the symptoms and an elevated heel pad may be useful. Occasionally, in the severe case, a short leg walking plaster cast may be required for 3 to 6 weeks.

Pain in the Forefoot

Hallux Rigidus

Painful hallux rigidus occurs in the young and may be difficult to treat. It follows stubbing of the big toe. X-rays may show a change that suggests osteochondritis of the first metatarsal head with subsequent changes that progress to degenerative arthritis with a narrow joint line and peripheral osteophytes.

This condition is a limitation of dorsiflexion of the metatarsal phalangeal joint of the big toe. Subsequent flattening of the head and osteophyte formation produce a typical "squared-off" appearance of the metatarsal head. Repeat trauma may be the cause.

Chronic hallux rigidus may be due to gout or rheumatoid arthritis. X-rays may reveal an erosive process at the articular margin as opposed to hypertrophy, as well as osteoporosis and joint line narrowing.

Treatment. Treatment consists of modification of the shoes with a rocker sole. Injections may be used but have no lasting effect. With continued disability, surgery is recommended.

Anterior Flat Foot

Diffuse callosities of the midfoot or the so-called anterior flat foot is an acquired disorder found in the obese middle-aged individual whose occupation requires standing.

Treatment. Treatment consists of foot supports with stress absorptive material in the shoes, as well as soles, and exercises for the foot (Fig. 10.19).

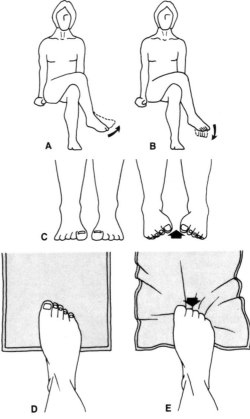

Figure 10.19. Active supination and toe-gripping exercises. **A**, Supination. **B**, Toe gripping. **C**, Standing supination. **D**, Grasping with the toes. (From Ramamurti CP (Tinker RV, ed): *Orthopaedics in Primary Care*, ed 17. Baltimore, Williams & Wilkins, 1989.)

Hallux Valgus (Bunions)

Hallux valgus does occasionally develop in adolescents. Although 90% of the cases that come to surgery are female, the overall incidence is approximately equal for male and females (Johnson, 1956). Discrepancy is probably found in the difference between the sex as related to footwear. The condition may present during adolescence from the age of 12 on, or may present at any age during adult life. Congenital hallux valgus is rare. In the adult, hallux valgus or a bunion is confused in the relevant literature. The condition may be defined by the inclusion of the following conditions:
(1) Rotation of the hallux;
(2) Metatarsus primus varus;

(3) Overriding of the hallux on the second toe;

(4) Metatarsalgia;

(5) Hammer- and clawtoe deformities of the lateral toes.

The condition has multiple origins. They may be (1) hereditary, (2) secondary to metatarsus primus varus, (3) a muscular imbalance, (4) foot pronation, and (5) shoewear.

With hallux valgus, the condition is bilateral with a dominant symptomatic side. A family history is present in approximately 60% of the cases. Conservative care may produce some relief, or may control symptoms once they occur. The "surgical shoe" has a place, more particularly in the rheumatoid form. When all conservative measures fail, surgery becomes necessary for pain relief.

Osteochondritis

Osteochondritis of the second metatarsal is probably an infraction of the metatarsal head. It generally occurs after 13 years of age and is more common in girls than boys. Symptoms may be treated by a metarsal bar, and inner pad; or in adults, surgery may be necessary.

Stress Fractures

There is a gradual onset of pain and swelling in the foot that is aggravated by activity and relieved by rest. On palpation a definite swelling in the dorsum of the foot may be felt. One can detect this swelling along a specific metatarsal shaft. This is particularly evident in the older individual and the fracture presents with very distinct swelling, redness, and heat.

Treatment. Conservative treatment is a reduction in the general level of activity. Referral to an orthopaedic surgeon may be necessary for casting. Extreme care is taken in attempting to cast the elderly osteoporotic foot, as a stress fracture, with beginning ambulation, may evolve in the contiguous metatarsals.

Morton's Metatarsalgia (Morton's Toe)

Morton's metatarsalgia can be found from the ages of 17 to 70. The patient is usually a young or middle-aged woman. Acute neuralgic pain is felt under the middle of the forefoot, with radiation into one or more of the three central toes. In "Morton's toe," the pain is referred to the fourth toe. Pain develops with standing or walking in closed, tight fitting footwear. The patient often takes off the shoe and manipulates the forefoot, prompting a relief of the pain. Pain is produced on physical examination by pressure upward and backward in the web space. The forefoot is alternately compressed with one hand while maintaining the pressure in the web space. Refer the patient to an orthopaedic surgeon for local anesthetic injection; if the symptoms are relieved, this is diagnostic of the condition.

Minor symptoms may be controlled by the low-heeled, open type of footwear. Occasionally, hydrocortisone injection may afford relief. When the symptoms are disabling, the treatment is excision of the interdigital nerve.

References

Berry H, Richardson, PM: Common peroneal palsy: a clinical and electrophysiologic review. *J Neurol Neurosurg Psychiatry*, 39:1162, 1976.

Holder LE, Michael RH: The specific scintigraphic pattern of "shin splints" in the lower leg: Concise Communication. *J Nucl Med*, 25:865–869, 1984.

Johnson O: Further studies of the inheritance of hand and foot anomalies. *Clin. Orthop*, 8:146–159, 1956.

Recommended Readings

Abramson DI, Miller DS: *Vascular Problems in Musculoskeletal Disorders of the Limbs.* New York, Springer-Verlag, 1981.

Bateman JE, Trott AW (eds): *The Foot and Ankle: A Selection of Papers from the American Orthopaedic Foot Society Meeting.* New York, Thieme-Stratton, 1980.

Dawson DM, Hallett M, Millender, LH: *Entrapment Neuropathies.* Boston, Little, Brown & Co., 1983.

Devas M: *Stress Fractures.* New York. Churchill Livingston, 1975.

Kelikian H, Kelikian AS: *Disorders of the Ankle.* Philadelphia, W.B. Saunders, 1985.

Levin ME, O'Neal LW (eds): *The Diabetic Foot.* St. Louis, CV Mosby, 1973.

Samitz MH: *Cutaneous Disorders of the Lower Extremities.* Philadelphia, JB Lippincott, ed 2, 1981.

chapter 11

Arthritis

SALLY PULLMAN-MOOAR, M.D.
WENDY W. McBRAIR, R.N., B.S.N.

Arthritis is the most common disabling disease in the United States. Over 7 million people are disabled by arthritis, and it costs $14 billion annually in lost wages and medical bills. In 1980, the National Health Interview Survey found that 36 million Americans had arthritis. Women are affected more than twice as often as men.

Arthritis is the general term used to describe conditions causing pain in and around joints. The following discussion will outline general principles concerning the approach to a patient with arthritis so the best care plan can be formulated.

The most important step in assuring the best treatment for the patients' condition is discovering the type of arthritis that is present. There are more than 100 hundred types of arthritis, all of which are associated with a different pathogenesis, treatment, and prognosis. Knowledge of the normal anatomy of a joint is essential in understanding different types of arthritis (Fig. 11.1).

ANATOMY OF THE JOINT

The normal joint functions as a hinge mechanism between two adjacent structures. Ideally, there will be very little friction in the joint and very little instability or laxity around the joint so that movement occurs effortlessly and painlessly. The normal diarthrodial joint is lined with smooth cartilage that provides a surface with a low-gliding coefficient of friction. A normally small membrane, called synovium, lines the joint cavity and attaches to the rim of bone

immediately outside the gliding surface. Healthy articular cartilage is not covered by synovium. Tendons, muscles, and ligaments, which act as the mechanical "pulleys" across a joint that cause movement, also act as stabilizing structures. Without these external structures, the joint would have excessive instability that would cause additional biomechanical stresses to the joint. Any of the structures in and around the joint can become damaged or inflamed, which can lead to joint pain.

DATA GATHERING

When one approaches a patient with a painful joint, the differential diagnosis needs to be made. The history is extremely important (Tables 11.1 and 11.2). Certain key forces can cause acute or chronic swelling and disability. The following discussion will

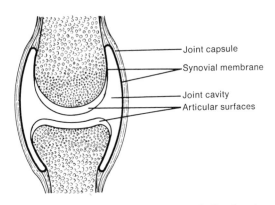

Figure 11.1. Typical structure of diarthrotic joint. (From Hilt NE, Cogburn SB: *Manual of Orthopaedics.* St. Louis, CV Mosby, 1980, p. 22.)

238

Table 11.1

Interview Guidelines for the Clinical History of Patient with Arthritis

Age at onset
Joints involved
Morning stiffness
Pattern of pain: constant, waxing and waning, migratory, or weight bearing
Family history of arthritis
Family history of associated illness, e.g., psoriasis, colitis, iritis, sarcoidosis, gout, hypermobility, osteoporosis
Associated systemic symptoms such as: fever, rash, alopecia, weight loss, fatigue, dyspnea, depression, sleep disturbance, Raynaud's disease, or oral ulcers
Sexual history
Recent changes in activities of daily living
Recent or remote trauma to affected joints
Recent changes in performance at school (children)

Table 11.2

Assessment History and Physical Exam of the Arthritic Patient

	History
Pain	Most frequent complaint
	Subjective sensation
	Location of pain
	Quality, e.g., sharp, radiating, or burning
	Radiation
	Activities that worsen or improve pain
Swelling	Possible anatomic distribution: bursa, joint, or muscle
Stiffness	Duration of stiffness
	Time of day
	Differentiate from neurologic diseases, such as Parkinson's
Weakness	Secondary to painful joint
	Possible disuse atrophy
	Myopathies: inflammatory, endocrine, or other
Fatigue	Often seen with inflammatory rheumatic diseases

	Physical Examination
Swelling	Location, either intra- or extra-articular in the synovial sac, tendon sheaths, or bursae
Heat	Indicates an inflammatory process
Erythema	Usually indicates a traumatic or inflammatory process
Range of motion	Compare with normal and progression over time
Crepitation	Usually indicates loss of smooth gliding cartilaginous surface in joint; sometimes made from tendons slipping
Pain	During active/passive range of motion or with palpation
Instability	Loss of external ligament support or muscle strength
Deformity	Description
Strength	Normal or decreased
Flexibility	Especially important in the lumbar spine exam when considering seronegative spondyloarthropathies

and disability. The following discussion will emphasize the clues to classification of inflammatory (RA) versus noninflammatory (OA) arthritis.

Typically the patient with early inflammatory arthritis will be a young woman who, for the past several weeks or months, has had 1 hour of morning stiffness of the hands, difficulty opening jars, and noted improvement in function during the day. She presents in the office with similar complaints of the forefoot. During the review of systems the patient may complain of recent hair loss, mouth blisters, and fever that suggest a systemic disease. On physical examination swollen, tender joints usually symmetrical of the MCP and PIP joints of the hand are found. Frequently the joints of the knees, elbows, ankles, and small joints of the feet are involved. Evaluate the patient systematically using the rheumatic complaints algorithm (Fig. 11.2).

Continue the assessment with an evaluation of activities of daily living using the Stanford Arthritis Assessment Tool (Figs. 11.3 and 11.4). An accurate assessment leads to a individualized care plan (see Appendix N for a typical nursing care plan for the arthritis patient).

OSTEOARTHRITIS

The most common type of arthritis is osteoarthritis (OA), also known as wear and tear arthritis or degenerative arthritis. Most individuals over 65 years of age will have x-ray evidence of this problem but only about 30% will have significant joint discomfort. The underlying mechanism for osteoarthritis is a gradual thinning of the articular cartilage lining the joint space that leaves exposed bone in contact with bone. The underlying bone becomes thickened and frequently one sees bony spurs adja-

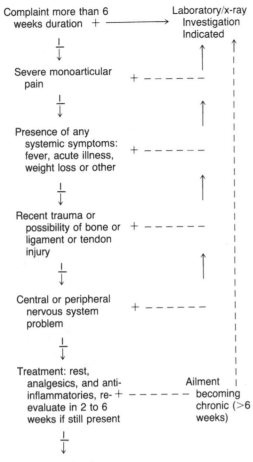

Figure 11.2. Algorithm for evaluation of the patient with rheumatic complaints. (Adapted from Kelley WN, Harris E, Ruddy S, Sledge CB: *Textbook of Rheumatology*, Vol. 1, (ed 2) Philadelphia, WB Saunders, 1985.)

cent to the joint. This type of arthritis is an example of a noninflammatory arthritis that historically has been very different from rheumatoid arthritis. Joint fluids are usually noninflammatory although not uncommonly there may be an associated crystal disease, such as pseudogout. The involved joints are those subjected to the most mechanical stress: cervical spine, distal interphalangeal joints, lumbar spine, hips, knees, and first metacarpophalangeal joints. The pain is described as an aching pain that increases with use and abates with rest. In more advanced stages discomfort

may be present in nonweight bearing positions. The current belief is that there is a family predisposition to OA and there are also several metabolic and endocrinologic disorders that are listed as etiologic. Previous trauma to a joint can often predispose individuals to accelerated degenerative disease because of cartilaginous injury or malalignment of the joint secondary to ligamentous instability.

Therapy or treatment of osteoarthritis is aimed at decreasing the work required of a joint in combination with acetaminophen or a nonsteroidal anti-inflammatory medication and a physical therapy program. Patients should be encouraged to lose weight, especially for painful hips, knees, and feet, wear soft soled shoes to decrease the impact of walking, and avoid high-impact activities such as jogging and aerobics. A structured exercise program is very helpful in maximizing conservative therapy. Thigh strengthening exercises should be encouraged for patients with painful knees; passive and active range of motion exercises are also beneficial for all involved areas. Generally speaking, isometric exercises provide the greatest increase in strength without excessive stress on a joint. Swimming and water exercise therapy should be encouraged.

RHEUMATOID ARTHRITIS

Rheumatoid arthritis is the most common inflammatory arthritis, affecting between 1 to 3% of the general population. As an inflammatory arthritis, rheumatoid arthritis is a good example of the differences in history and physical examination that are crucial to making an accurate working assessment. RA has a predilection for women in their childbearing years. Typically, the disease presents with severe morning stiffness and pain in the small joints of the hands, wrists, and feet. It may continue to involve joints not typically involved in OA such as elbows, shoulders, and ankles as well as the cervical spine, hips, and knees. Frequently the patient feels ill with fatigue, and almost universally has prolonged morning stiffness. Less frequently, rheumatoid arthritis may have systemic involvement of other organ systems such as the lung, heart, skin, eye, or gastrointestinal or urinary tract. Anemia, an elevated sedimentation rate, and a positive rheumatoid factor are commonly associated with RA but alone are not diagnostic of the disease.

Pathologically, the synovial membrane becomes tremendously thickened and inflamed, which leads to red, hot, swollen, and tender joints and surrounding tendons. Many of the rheumatic illnesses affect people during the prime of their lives. Therefore these individuals deserve special attention concerning adjustments in lifestyle, self-care, employment, and family planning. With the current therapies available, many people are able to live normal, productive lives. Others may need to change their life-styles and expectations, and those expectations of a spouse or family.

Treatment is aimed at controlling the inflammation and, in more prolonged cases, attempting to promote an early remission. Initial therapy is aspirin or nonsteroidal anti-inflammatory medications. The physician may then choose to try the antimalarial drugs (hydroxychloroquine, chloroquine), injectable or oral gold, and penicillamine or immunosuppressives such as methotrexate, imuran, or cytoxan. In addition, corticosteroids may be used to improve patient function. The choice of drug therapy is tailored to the individual's pain tolerance and home/work responsibilities. All patients with suspected inflammatory arthritis should be referred to a rheumatoligst (Table 11.3).

THE MANAGEMENT OF COMMON PROBLEMS

Infectious Arthritis

Infectious arthritis commonly presents as an acutely hot, tender, painful, and swollen joint. There are many different pathogens causing the problem, but the diagnosis needs to be made rapidly so appropriate antibiotic therapy can be instituted.

Disseminated Gonorrhea

Disseminated gonorrhea commonly affects women. It often occurs immediately after menses and may be associated with fever, a pustular rash, and tenosynovitis. A sexual history should be obtained from any sexually active individual who has a new onset of an arthritis affecting only a few joints. All patients should have an RPR drawn. As the joint aspirant is rarely positive, it is necessary to do urethra, cervix, rectum, and pharynx cultures for the organism. Patients are treated with intravenous penicillin with improvement noted within 48 hours. Often the diagnosis is confirmed when the patient improves with the treatment. All sexual contacts must be notified and treatment promptly begun.

Pyogenic Arthritis

Pyogenic arthritis usually occurs as a monoarticular arthritis, most commonly with staphylococcus or streptococcus. Inquiry should be made concerning recent skin infections, dental work, surgery, or trauma. Prior to antibiotic therapy, joint aspiration must be performed. This is important for discovering the infectious agent.

Lyme Disease

Carried by a tick, Lyme disease is a spirochetal infection that initially presents as an acute flu-like illness. It may also mimic other systemic diseases, such as pericarditis, meningitis, or Bell's palsy. Approximately 10% of patients may develop a chronic inflammatory arthritis that affects only a few joints. For Lyme disease, the diagnosis is made by a blood test. The arthritis may be responsive to intravenous or oral antibiotics. Care should be taken to ask any patient with a new inflammatory arthritis about exposure to ticks or whether the characteristic rash of erythema chronicum migrans (an annular red rash with central clearing) had been noticed.

Figure 11.3. **A** and **B**, Stanford arthritis assessment tool. (Printed with permission from James Fries, M.D., Stanford Arthritis Center Disability and Discomfort Scales, 1981.)

> In this section we are interested in learning how your illness affects your ability to function in daily life.

Name _____

Date _____

• Please check the one response which best describes your usual abilities OVER THE PAST WEEK:

	Without ANY Difficulty	With SOME Difficulty	With MUCH Difficulty	UNABLE To Do	FOR PHYSICIAN USE ONLY DO NOT WRITE IN THIS COLUMN

DRESSING & GROOMING

Are you able to:

Dress yourself, including tying shoelaces and doing buttons?

Shampoo your hair?

ARISING

Are you able to:

Stand up from an armless straight chair?

Get in and out of bed?

EATING

Are you able to:

Cut your meat?

Lift a full cup or glass to your mouth?

Open a new milk carton?

WALKING

Are you able to:

Walk outdoors on flat ground?

Climb up five steps?

• Please check any AIDS OR DEVICES that you usually use for any of these activities:

_____ Cane

_____ Walker

_____ Crutches

_____ Wheelchair

_____ Devices Used for Dressing (button hook, zipper pull, long-handled shoehorn, etc.)

_____ Built-Up or Special Utensils

_____ Special or Built-Up Chair

_____ Other (Specify: _____)

• Please check any categories for which you usually need HELP FROM ANOTHER PERSON:

_____ Dressing and Grooming

_____ Arising

_____ Eating

_____ Walking

Stanford Arthritis Center Disability and Discomfort Scales, 1981.

• Please check the one response which best describes your usual abilities OVER THE PAST WEEK:

	Without ANY Difficulty	With SOME Difficulty	With MUCH Difficulty	UNABLE To Do	FOR PHYSICIAN USE ONLY DO NOT WRITE IN THIS COLUMN

HYGIENE

Are you able to:

Wash and dry your entire body?

Take a tub bath?

Get on and off the toilet?

REACH

Are you able to:

Reach and get down a 5-pound object (such as a bag of sugar) from just above your head?

Bend down to pick up clothing from the floor?

GRIP

Are you able to:

Open car doors?

Open jars which have been previously opened?

Turn faucets on and off?

ACTIVITIES

Are you able to:

Run errands and shop?

Get in and out of car?

Do chores such as vacuuming or yardwork?

• Please check any AIDS OR DEVICES that you usually use for any of these activities:

_____ Raised Toilet Seat   _____ Long-Handled Appliances for Reach

_____ Bathtub Seat   _____ Long-Handled Appliances in Bathroom

_____ Jar Opener (for jars previously   _____ Other (Specify: _____)
         opened)

_____ Bathtub Bar

• Please check any categories for which you usually need HELP FROM ANOTHER PERSON:

_____ Hygiene   _____ Gripping and Opening Things

_____ Reach   _____ Errands and Chores

Disability Index

We are also interested in learning whether or not you are affected by pain because of your illness.

• How much pain have you had because of your illness IN THE PAST WEEK?

Pain

PLACE A MARK ON THE LINE TO INDICATE THE SEVERITY OF THE PAIN

NO PAIN   VERY SEVERE PAIN

0   100

Stanford Arthritis Center Disability and Discomfort Scales, 1981.

HOW TO ADMINISTER THE ARTHRITIS HEALTH ASSESSMENT QUESTIONNAIRE

Purpose

Recent attitudinal studies revealed that patients frequently judge the success of their therapy by its ability to improve functional status, to complete common everyday tasks and to live a more or less normal daily life. Therefore, functional status is clearly an important goal to be measured. This Health Assessment Questionnaire (HAQ) is designed to provide physicians with a qualitative and quantitative assessment of the functional status of individual arthritis patients.

Administration

The HAQ questionnaire is self-administered. Patients should be given the questionnaire and asked to complete it without additional instructions. When they return the questionnaire to you, use the scoring methods provided here to measure the severity of pain and to calculate a Disability Index.

Specifics

Throughout the questionnaire, patients are asked to record the amount of difficulty they may have in performing different tasks. Do not define terms such as SOME, MUCH, or USUAL, for your patients. It is important that they use their own frame of reference. Likewise, the time frame is OVER THE PAST WEEK…not a particularly good or bad week… just OVER THE PAST WEEK. By repeating the questionnaire at different periods during the course of therapy, you can look at the patient's patterns of functional ability and thereby get a more accurate picture of functional status. If you look at information from only a good or bad week, you will not get as true a picture.

Scoring

Each category (DRESSING AND GROOMING, ARISING, etc.) has two or more component questions.

Possible responses for the component questions are:

Without ANY difficulty	= 0
With SOME difficulty	= 1
With MUCH difficulty	= 2
UNABLE to do	= 3

The highest score for any component question determines the score for that category. If a component question is left blank or the response is too ambiguous to assign a score, then the score for that category is determined by the remaining completed question(s). If all component questions are blank, then the category is left blank.

If the patient's mark is between the response columns, then move it to the closest one. If it's directly between the two, move it to the higher one.

If either devices and/or help from another person is checked for a category, the score = 2. This may determine the score unless the score on any other component question = 3. For example, the response to "Dress yourself…" is with SOME difficulty (score = 1). The patient has checked the use of a device for dressing, thereby increasing the score to 2. The response to "Shampoo your hair…" is UNABLE to do (score = 3). Therefore, the score for the DRESSING category is 3.

Devices associated with each category:

DRESSING & GROOMING	Devices used for dressing (button hook, zipper pull, long-handled shoehorn, etc.)
ARISING	built-up or special chair
EATING	built-up or special utensils
WALKING	cane, walker, crutches
HYGIENE	raised toilet seat bathtub seat bathtub bar long-handled appliances in bathroom
REACH	long-handled appliances for reach
GRIP	jar opener (for jars previously opened)

Devices written in the "Other" sections are considered only if they would be used for any of the stated categories.

Disability Index Calculation:

The index is calculated by adding the scores for each of the categories and dividing by the number of categories answered. This gives a score in the 0 to 3.0 range.

Pain Severity Coding

Pain is measured on a visual analog scale (a horizontal line where each end represents opposite ends of a continuum) 15 cm long, with "no pain" or 0 at one end and "very severe pain" or 100 at the other.

A score from 0 to 3.0 is determined based on the location of the respondent's mark. Some patients put more than one mark on the line. If that is the case, take the midpoint.

Using a metric rule, measure the distance from the left-hand side of the line to the mark (0 to 15.0 cm) and multiply by 0.2 to obtain a value from 0 to 3.0. Round to the even number of cm if the mark falls between two points. For example, if the mark is between 4.2 and 4.3 cm, use 4.2. There is a pain severity coding sheet (which follows) for your use. It converts the number of cm into the appropriate score.

PAIN SEVERITY CODING
(USING THE VISUAL ANALOG SCALE)

MEASUREMENT (CM) = SCORE	MEASUREMENT (CM) = SCORE
0 = 0	7.8 — 8.2 = 1.6
.1 — .7 = .1	8.3 — 8.7 = 1.7
.8 — 1.2 = .2	8.8 — 9.2 = 1.8
1.3 — 1.7 = .3	9.3 — 9.7 = 1.9
1.8 — 2.2 = .4	9.8 — 10.2 = 2.0
2.3 — 2.7 = .5	10.3 — 10.7 = 2.1
2.8 — 3.2 = .6	10.8 — 11.2 = 2.2
3.3 — 3.7 = .7	11.3 — 11.7 = 2.3
3.8 — 4.2 = .8	11.8 — 12.2 = 2.4
4.3 — 4.7 = .9	12.3 — 12.7 = 2.5
4.8 — 5.2 = 1.0	12.8 — 13.2 = 2.6
5.3 — 5.7 = 1.1	13.3 — 13.7 = 2.7
5.8 — 6.2 = 1.2	13.8 — 14.2 = 2.8
6.3 — 6.7 = 1.3	14.3 — 14.7 = 2.9
6.8 — 7.2 = 1.4	14.8 — 15.0 = 3.0
7.3 — 7.7 = 1.5	

Table 11.3
Differential Diagnosis

	Osteoarthritis	Rheumatoid Arthritis
Pathology	Cartilage degeneration bone regeneration (spurs)	Inflammation of synovial membrane Bone destruction Damage to ligaments, tendons, cartilage, joint capsule
Joints affected	Hands, spine, knees, hips, may be asymmetrical	Symmetrical (both sides): wrists, knees, knuckles
Features, symptoms	Localized pain, stiffness Heberden's nodules Usually not much swelling	Swelling, redness, warmth, pain, tenderness, nodules, fatigue, stiffness, muscle aches, fever
Other systems affected	None	Lungs, heart, skin
Prognosis: long-term	Less pain for some, more pain and disability for others Few severely disabled	Less aggressive with time Deformity can often be prevented
Age: onset	Age 45 to 90. Most people have some features with increasing age	Age 25 to 50 Bimodal peaks 3rd to 4th decade to 5th to 6th decade
Sex	Males and females about equal 1:1	Females affected more often 25:1
Heredity	One form is familial	Familial tendency
Tests	X-rays	Rheumatoid factor (80%) Blood test, x-rays, examination of joint fluid, negative Lyme titer
Treatment	Maintain activity level, exercise, joint protection, weight control, relaxation, heat, sometimes medication and/or surgery	Reduce inflammation, balanced exercise program, joint protection, weight control, relaxation, heat, medication and/or surgery

Hypermobility Syndrome (Double Jointed)

Hypermobility syndromes are a common cause of regional rheumatic pain. The features of the benign hypermobility syndrome include: (1) symmetrical joint pain and stiffness, (2) sensation of joint swelling, (3) onset after prolonged inactivity, (4) joint laxity in other family members, and (5) no other contributing illnesses. The diagnosis is made when three of the five following features are found on physical examination: (1) passive apposition of thumb to forearm, (2) passive hyperextension of fingers to 90°, (3) active hyperextension of the elbow greater than 10°, (4) active hyperextension of the knee greater than 10°, and (5) ability to flex spine and place palm on floor with knees straight.

The benign hypermobility syndrome responds well to mild anti-inflammatory drugs and strengthening and conditioning exercises. Young athletes need to be cautioned about avoiding aggravating sports. The condition may predispose the individual to premature osteoarthritis.

Inherited Disease of Cartilage

Certain systemic diseases have joint hyperlaxity and often are associated with internal organ pathology. Some of these diseases include Marfan's, Ehlers-Danlos syndrome, and osteogenesis imperfecta. Patients with extreme hypermobility, a heart murmur, brittle bones, or a family history of brittle bones or sudden death require physician referral.

Figure 11.4. Scoring directions for the arthritis health assessment questionnaire. (Printed with permission from James Fries, M.D., Stanford Arthritis Center.)

Seronegative Spondyloarthropathies

As a group, these arthropathies are characterized by the absence of rheumatoid factor and other autoantibodies and by the predilection for inflammatory disease in the spine, peripheral joint arthritis, tendinitis with new bone formation, extraarticular manifestations in the eyes, heart, skin, and mucous membranes. These arthropathies are found predominantly in young adult males. A strong association with the HLA-B27 antigen has been found.

Ankylosing Spondylitis

Ankylosing spondylitis is a chronic inflammatory axial arthritis with a ratio of 3:1 male/female and an incidence of 0.1 to 0.2% in white men. Clinically, an indolent history of lower back stiffness (usually upon arising in the morning or when a static posture is maintained) is found to improve with activity. Physical examination findings may consist of lumbar spine rigidity in forward flexion, a decreased chest expansion, and pain on side-to-side compression of the pelvis. More than 90% of patients have a positive HLA-B27 marker. Fuzziness of the sacroiliac joints is a classic x-ray finding. Obtain anteroposterior views of the spine and SI joint views at the initial visit. A minority of individuals may get cardiac, eye, or pulmonary diseases. The treatment consists of anti-inflammatories (indomethacin) and hyperextension exercises for the neck and thoracic spine. The treatment goal, in addition to pain relief, is to prevent flexion contractures of the cervical and thoracic spine. Patients are advised to sleep without a pillow.

Reiter's Syndrome

Reiter's syndrome is the presence of the clinical triad of urethritis, conjunctivitis, and an inflammatory arthritis. It may follow genitourinary infections and/or be associated with a diarrheal illness (also known as reactive arthritis). Rashes on the feet, fever, oral ulcers, and penile ulcers may occur. Sacroiliitis tends to be asymmetric. HLA-B27 may be positive in up to 75% of patients. Reiter's syndrome may be the most common cause of inflammatory arthritis in young men.

Psoriatic Arthritis

Psoriatic arthritis may resemble rheumatoid arthritis but has a slightly different joint distribution. Psoriatic arthritis typically involves the distal interphalangeal joints of the hands and feet, giving the appearance of "sausage digits." Psoriatic skin disease often precedes the arthritis. The presence of nail pits occurs in 80% of patients with this arthritis; spondylitis also may develop.

Arthritis Associated with Inflammatory Bowel Disease

Arthritis associated with inflammatory bowel disease, Crohn's disease, and ulcerative colitis may each be associated with either a peripheral arthritis or an axial (spinal) arthritis. Management is a problem because often the nonsteroidal anti-inflammatory drugs may worsen the bowel irritability.

Polymyositis and Dermatomyositis

Polymyositis is an inflammatory disease of striated muscle most commonly affecting the proximal limb girdle, neck, and pharynx, and occasionally involving the heart. The etiology is unknown and it may occur at any age. Women are more commonly affected than men. Patients present with proximal muscle weakness and complain of being unable to comb their hair or ascend stairs. In dermatomyositis there may be a classic violaceous rash around the eyes (heliotrope rash) or on the extensor surface of the extremities. Muscle enzymes (CPK, aldolase) and EMG are commonly abnormal and muscle biopsies will show inflammation.

In the patient over 40 years of age, care should be taken to exclude an underlying neoplasm. Myositis can be seen as part of other rheumatic diseases, most commonly scleroderma and systemic lupus. Other etiologies for proximal weakness should also be sought such as hypothyroidism, steroid myopathy, and electrolyte imbalances. Myositis is treated with high-dose steroids or in steroid resistant cases with methotrexate. As the inflammation subsides, care should be taken to continue passive range of motion and gradually progress to assisted active range of motion. Flexion contractures are not uncommon. Refer all patients with elevated enzymes and muscle weakness to a rheumatologist. The long-term outcome is best for the younger adult patient.

Rheumatic Fever

The prevalence of rheumatic fever has markedly decreased (compared to the preantibiotic era), but at least 100,000 new cases are diagnosed annually in the United States. Recently, there has been a resurgence of new cases of rheumatic fever. The illness follows infection with Group A betahemolytic streptococcal infections and the attack rate can be as high as 3% after epidemic streptococcal outbreaks.

The disease affects both children and adults. A febrile illness associated with a sore throat precedes the symptoms associated with acute rheumatic fever. Migrating, inflammatory arthritis, carditis, subcutaneous nodules, fevers and rashes, fatigue, malaise and a movement disorder (although rare) can all be associated with rheumatic fever. Treatment is directed toward eradication of the streptococcal infection with antibiotics and appropriate anti-inflammatories. After rheumatic fever prophylaxis with antibiotics (penicillin or erythromycin) should be continued for at least 5 years. Antibiotics should be given 48 hours prior to, and following, tooth extraction, root canal, and certain GI and GYN procedures.

Raynaud's Phenomenon

Raynaud's phenomenon is a tri-phasic color change (blue, white, or red) of the extremities, most commonly the fingers. The etiology is unclear and many people have no underlying connective tissue disorder. Cold often provokes the symptoms, which can range from mild discomfort to intense pain in the digits.

Many connective tissue diseases can have an associated Raynaud's phenomenon including scleroderma, lupus, and rheumatoid arthritis. Treatment is aimed at preventing attacks by having the patient wear gloves or mittens. Certain drugs have been used, with varying degrees of success, including nitropaste and nifedipine. The patient needs at least one initial rheumatologic evaluation for the possibility of an underlying disease.

Scleroderma

Scleroderma is a disease of unknown etiology that is characterized by the deposition of abundant collagen in the skin and, less commonly, in internal organs such as the kidney, stomach, heart, and lungs. Patients complain of puffiness and tightening of the skin of the fingers and sometimes the feet. Many people have Raynaud's disease and may have chronic recurring superficial digital ulcers that are prone to infection.

Treatment is aimed at keeping the joints mobilized to prevent flexion contractures and palliative drugs, such as nonsteroidal anti-inflammatories, are used to treat joint pains. Occasionally, additional medications for dilating blood vessels are helpful for severe Raynaud's disease. Reflex esophagitis is often symptomatic and responds well to H_2 blockers. For rapidly progressive skin involvement or in pulmonary disease D-penicillamine is sometimes used. Patients need to be monitored for the development of hypertension that may signal kidney involvement. There is no cure for scleroderma.

Systemic Lupus Erythematosus (SLE)

SLE is an autoimmune disease that most commonly affects women in their childbearing years. Fatigue and fevers are commonly present. Other symptoms are pleuritis, a facial butterfly rash, alopecia, photosensitivity, arthralgias and arthritis, anemia, and oral ulcers. Most patients have a positive ANA (>90%) and surveillance for other organ involvement needs to be done, especially the kidney. Currently the prognosis is generally good for lupus, but the disease creates great psychosocial stress because of the age and stage of the patient and the many symptoms, such as profound fatigue and arthralgias, which are not visible on the exterior of the patient. The individual should be counseled to rest when possible, avoid prolonged sun exposure, and use sunscreens and hats. Steroids are often used for more serious cases of lupus that are not adequately controlled by hydroxychloroquine or NSAIDs.

Polymyalgia Rheumatica (PMR)

Polymyalgia rheumatica is a common disease in persons over 50 years of age; it is predominantly seen in females. The disease is characterized by myalgia and arthralgias and profound morning stiffness in the proximal limb girdle muscles. Very little is found on physical examination except diffusely tender muscles.

The diagnosis is made with the typical symptoms associated with an elevated ESR; the disease responds rapidly to low-dose steroids.

Temporal Arteritis

Temporal arteritis is a vasculitis that is characterized by inflammation in medium sized blood vessels. Patients are usually elderly women with headaches, tender temporal arteries, weight loss, and occasionally fever. Fifty percent of patients with temporal arteritis will have symptoms of polymyalgia rheumatica as well.

Evaluate for jaw claudication, anorexia, and systemic illness. As there is a risk of blindness, tenderness on palpation of the temporal artery requires immediate referral.

Treatment is moderate- to high-dose steroids for several months. The elderly are very sensitive to this high-steroid dose and may have secondary psychosis, insomnia, depression, myopathy, new diabetes, and hypertension.

Fibromyositis

Fibromyositis is a soft tissue rheumatic disease characterized by multiple tender spots known as trigger points, stiffness, and fatigue. Some evidence suggests that a disorder of non-REM sleep may be a contributing factor in this disease. Patients with documented diseases such as rheumatoid arthritis may develop fibromyositis secondarily.

Treatment includes anti-inflammatories, such as aspirin, amitriptyline in very-low doses, and occasional muscle relaxants. Massage, heat, and local injections may give temporary relief.

Before making the diagnosis of fibromyositis care should be given to search for other underlying causes for the complaints such as polymyalgia rheumatica.

Crystal Diseases

Gout

Gout is a common disorder of middle-aged and older males and becomes more common in women after menopause. The characteristic pattern of the arthritis is to develop an acutely painful joint, most often the first metatarsophalangeal joint. The pain is excruciating. Gout is a consequence of hyperuricemia (elevated serum uric acid levels). This may be secondary to overproduction of urate as with psoriasis, a reduced renal excretion of urate, or certain genetic diseases that have defects in purine metabolism.

Uric acid is soluble in serum up to levels of 8.0 mg/dl. In patients with hyperuricemia (uric acid levels greater than 8.0 mg/dl) small crystals of uric acid get deposited in joints, bursa, tendons, and in nodular skin deposits called tophi. Renal calculi are found in 10% of patients with gout. All joints may be affected, though by far the most common joint is the first metatarsophalangeal joint, followed by the hips, knees, and hands.

Chronic hyperuricemia with gout can lead to an erosive destructive arthritis. The diagnosis can only be made by examination of the joint fluid for intracellular monosodium urate crystals.

Treatment is aimed at rapid relief of the acute attack, usually by nonsteroidal anti-inflammatory agents followed by long-term prevention of repetitive episodes. Patients with normal renal function and no history of kidney stones may be placed on probenecid to increase renal clearance of urate. Colchicine has been found useful for both acute treatment (though in high doses it may cause GI side effects) and prophylaxis. Allopurinol, which inhibits purine degradation to uric acid, is often the drug of choice and subsequent attacks can be prevented and the tophi gradually resorbed.

Pseudogout: Calcium Pyrophosphate Deposition Disease (CPPD)

The attack of CPPD arthritis may mimic gout or septic arthritis. The diagnosis is made by examination of joint fluid for the typical crystals. An associated x-ray finding is calcification of the articular cartilage known as chondrocalcinosis. The disease may be associated with other conditions such as hyperparathyroidism, hemochromatosis, hypothyroidism, gout, and osteoarthritis. Treatment with nonsteroidal anti-inflammatories is usually successful.

Juvenile Rheumatoid Arthritis (JRA)

Arthritis is frequently seen in children and JRA affects approximately 60,000 to 200,000 children in the United States. The disease is characterized by synovial inflammation and is divided into subgroups; prognosis is by mode of onset, seropositivity, and related systemic symptoms. The systemic symptoms include fever, rash, splenomegaly, and adenopathy. Certain types of JRA have a predisposition for eye involvement.

Treatment is aimed at relief of painful joints and presenting systemic symptoms. Anti-inflammatories such as aspirin and NSAIDs are the first-line drugs of choice. Adolescents should be monitored closely for drug side effects. These drugs should be withheld if the child gets an acute febrile illness, as the combination of the drugs and the acute illness may predispose the child to Reye's syndrome. Recognition should be made also of possible limb length discrepancy that may occur after a chronic inflammatory process that is adjacent to a growth plate. Family counseling is important (see "Psychosocial Considerations" in this chapter).

Drug-Associated Musculoskeletal Syndromes

Drug reactions or allergies are quite common and can present as acute febrile illness with rash, myalgia and arthritis, oral ulcers, and renal findings. This is also known as serum-sickness. The most common offending agent is an antibiotic but many drugs have a similar effect. There are certain medications (i.e., procaine, pronestyl, hydralazine, beta blockers, aldomet, and hydrochlorothiazide) that are often given for hypertension or cardiac disease, which may induce a picture much like lupus. Any patient with rheumatic complaints needs to have a careful drug history taken.

DRUG THERAPY FOR ARTHRITIS

Prior to initiating either a prescription or nonprescription drug program for a rheumatic disease, the exact diagnosis needs to be established. When this is done, the drug with the fewest side effects for the greatest possible benefit is administered. In conditions such as osteoarthritis, a nonsteroidal anti-inflammatory (NSAID) is often beneficial in conjunction with joint preservation advice. The inflammatory arthropathies often require additional medications known as disease modifying agents or immunosuppressants. All patients need baseline liver and kidney function tests, with periodic testing at 6 weeks, 3 months, and every 3 months thereafter. Changes in normal function warrant discontinuation of the drug and consultation with a physician.

Aspirin and Aspirin Compound Drugs (Over the Counter)

In low doses, aspirin (4 to 6 tablets daily) is an analgesic. A high dose of aspirin (12 to 16 tablets/day) has traditionally been used as the initial anti-inflammatory and analgesic medication for the pain of numerous arthritic conditions. When salicylates are given in high doses, there are certain toxic side effects that may occur. Patients must be closely observed. Individuals, especially the elderly who are more sensitive to side effects and forgetful of doses taken, should be questioned about tinnitus, loss of hearing, dyspepsia, melena, abdominal pain, or an altered mental status. An inadvertent overdose is not uncommon because many over the counter medications for colds, back pain, or indigestion may contain salicylates. A complete review of all medications is indicated in any person suspected of receiving a supratherapeutic dose of salicylates.

Enteric coated aspirin that may have fewer side effects is available. Other prescription forms of salicylates are also available; these are more expensive but are often better tolerated because they need only to be taken twice daily and cause fewer gastrointestinal symptoms.

Acetaminophen

Patients can take acetaminophen in conjunction with other drugs for arthritis. Acetaminophen is a good analgesic for mild to moderate pain but has no anti-inflammatory properties. Patients should take no more than 4000 mg/day. With higher doses (near 7000 mg/day) liver toxicity and kidney failure are possible. In doses under 4000/mg, side effects are negligible.

Ibuprofen

The over the counter strength of ibuprofen is 200 mg. This is the same drug as Motrin or Rufen, which are given by prescription only. Advertising for the over the counter agents has been directed at treatment of minor pain, such as headaches. Ibuprofen is a nonsteroidal anti-inflammatory drug and should not be taken in addition to aspirin or other NSAIDs. Acetaminophen is the mild analgesic of choice.

Antimalarials (Hydroxychloroquine, Chloroquine)

The antimalarials are found to be beneficial in the treatment of rheumatoid arthritis and systemic lupus. These drugs, especially hydroxychloroquine, have relatively low toxicity, but may cause retinal damage. Ophthalmologic examinations are recommended every 6 months.

Gold Therapy (Oral and Injectable)

Gold is one of the "remittive" drugs in rheumatoid arthritis. Side effects are very common and include a decreased leukocyte count and thrombocytopenia, rash, proteinuria, diarrhea (more common with the oral preparation). The mechanism of action is unknown and any beneficial effect does not occur for 3 months. Injections, blood counts, and urinalysis are performed weekly with injectable gold and monthly with oral gold.

D-Penicillamine

This drug is used primarily in rheumatoid arthritis and scleroderma and may work by inhibiting collagen deposition. Many patients respond well to D-penicillamine after 6 months of treatment. Unfortunately, a large number need to discontinue the drug because of the side effects, including loss of taste, leukopenia, rash, proteinuria, and drug-induced lupus.

Corticosteroids

Oral Preparation

The most commonly administered steroid is prednisone, but many other preparations are also available. Topically applied steroid creams, when applied to large areas of the body, can also have the effect of systemic steroids. Steroids are given for refractory inflammatory conditions and severe allergic reactions. If used over a long period of time, they can have severe consequences.

Some of the more common and important side effects include: adrenal insufficiency, diabetes, hypertension, accelerated atherosclerosis, accelerated osteoporosis, truncal obesity, striae, cataracts, gastritis, decreased immunity to infections, edema, myopathy, aseptic necrosis of bone, psychosis, and headaches. Discontinuation of steroids, especially after prolonged use, requires a gradual withdrawal with a tapered dose schedule. Because of the possibility of sudden adrenal insufficiency *steroids should never be withdrawn abruptly.*

Teach patients the dangers of abrupt discontinuation and the necessity of strict adherence to the prescribed dosing schedule.

Steroid Injections

Injections can be made into the joints or the soft tissues (for treatment of carpal tunnel syndrome or bursitis). Intraarticular injections should be used judiciously. The risk of infection is low but repeated injections may soften the cartilage or ligaments.

Immunomodulators (Cytoxan, Imuran, Methotrexate)

Immunomodulators are drugs reserved for advanced refractory diseases where conventional (less toxic) therapy has been inadequate. Gastrointestinal symptoms, mucosal ulcers, and decreased blood counts are the most common side effects. Patients on cytoxan are at an increased risk to develop hemorrhagic cystitis and bladder cancer. Patients need to drink copious amounts of fluids to minimize the concentration in the bladder. All patients on immunosuppressants are at an increased risk for infections so any fever or even superficial skin infection should be reported to a physician.

DIAGNOSTIC TESTS FOR ARTHRITIS PATIENTS

(1) CBC (Complete Blood Count). The CBC is a very helpful test to determine if there are concurrent abnormalities indicating an underlying inflammatory condition. Leukocytosis can be seen with an infectious process or an inflammatory etiology. Leukopenia (WBC < 4000) may suggest a disease such as systemic lupus erythematosus.

Anemia is not found in a normal healthy patient, even in the elderly, and thus can also be a marker of an underlying systemic disease. Screen for anemia after prolonged use of NSAIDs because of associated gastritis and occult gastrointestinal bleeding.

(2) Westergren Erythrocyte Sedimentation Rate. This is a very sensitive but nonspecific test for inflammation. The ESR may be elevated with infections and inflammatory autoimmune diseases. It is usually normal in individuals with noninflammatory conditions, such as osteoarthritis or a traumatic joint injury.

(3) Renal and Liver Functions. Chemistry profiles should be obtained prior to starting older patients on aspirin or nonsteroidal anti-inflammatory agents. The kidney function should also be checked intermittently while the patient is taking these medications, because occasionally they may cause renal insufficiency and elevated blood pressure. These hazards are especially common in a patient with preexisting hypertension or a mild degree of creatinine elevation.

(4) Synovial Fluid Analysis. Joint fluid analysis is used for differentiating inflammatory from noninflammatory processes. The fluid should also be sent for culture to exclude a pyogenic cause and a thorough examination for crystals (urate in gout, calcium pyrophosphate in pseudogout) should be performed.

(5) Rheumatoid Factor. An aggregation of immune complexes that is found in the sera of the majority of people with rheumatoid arthritis. It is not necessary to have a positive RF to be labeled rheumatoid arthritis. Rheumatoid factor can be seen in other diseases such as endocarditis, sarcoid, and systemic lupus and leprosy.

(6) ANA (Antinuclear Antigen). A positive ANA is found in more than 90% of persons who are diagnosed as having systemic lupus erythematosus. ANA may also be present in patients with rheumatoid arthritis, progressive systemic sclerosis, and poorly differentiated connective tissue diseases, polymyositis, and sarcoidosis. Not unusually, low-titer ANA appears in the elderly and may not indicate the presence of an associated connective tissue disease. Several medications have been linked with

the syndrome of drug-induced lupus. Two of the most common ones are procainamide and hydralazine.

(7) Tine or PPD. All patients to be treated with steroids must first be tested for tuberculosis. Patients with a positive result must be treated with isoniazid concomitantly with the steroid therapy.

(8) Lyme Titer. All patients who present with inflammatory arthritis or tick exposure must be tested.

RADIOGRAPHS

Radiographs are very helpful in evaluating a patient with arthritis. Diagnostic changes are seen with certain types of arthritis and the stage and prognosis can also be determined by x-rays. For example, typical changes seen in osteoarthritis include asymmetric loss of the joint space from the narrowing of cartilage with osteophyte or bony spur production and subchondral sclerosis. An inflammatory arthritis will give a picture of symmetrical joint space narrowing and possible juxta-articular erosions. Changes with acute infectious arthritis are swelling of the soft tissues with bony changes seen with chronic infection (osteomyelitis). These changes include osteopenia and loss of the bony cortex. Certain crystal diseases have pathognomonic calcification seen in cartilage. Often after an injury only soft tissue swelling will be visualized, but fractures and foreign bodies need to be excluded, especially if the skin integrity has been broken.

THERAPEUTIC MODALITIES

Physical Therapy

Physical therapy is often recommended to treat the sore, stiff joints and muscles of individuals with arthritis and to teach patients adaptive, appropriate skills for home therapy and prevention of disability.

Treatment consists of various modalities including: hot packs, ultrasound, whirlpool, paraffin wax, and massage. The therapist uses gentle, passive range of motion to stretch tightened muscles and prevent

flexion contractures. "Hot" joints are handled carefully, limiting movement to passive range of motion. As symptoms subside, exercise can continue to include a strengthening exercise program emphasizing isometric techniques and mild resistance exercises using elastic bands and light weights. The daily routine includes use of massage, use of hot/cold therapy for 20 minutes x3/day, and the proper sequencing of anti-inflammatory and mild pain relieving medications prior to showers that are then followed by range of motion exercise and relaxation techniques.

Despite small gains, the physical therapist has the opportunity to soothe and encourage the patient through the use of techniques in touch, helpful modalities, and constant encouragement. Most importantly, the therapist teaches the patient not to overdo or to build too quickly.

Exercise

Patients are instructed to do range of motion exercises 3 to 4 times/day, gradually increasing strengthening exercises daily. Finally, an endurance exercise program can be included after careful evaluation of the patient's major joint dysfunctions and overall conditioning. Again, gradual progression is important from the beginning. Activities such as free style swimming (the water temperature should be at least 82°) or swimming with flotation devices, fast walking (treadmill or street), and bike riding (stationary or mobile) light racquet games (badminton and ping pong), croquet, dancing, and light weight resistance exercises (<20 lbs) are most often recommended.

Patients are advised to avoid the following activities unless suitable adaptation can be made. Activities that impact or jar the joints (jogging, jumping, running, and aerobics), activities that require heavy racquets (tennis), highly competitive team sports and contact sports (Banwell, 1987).

Occupational Therapy

The occupational therapist contributes to the rehabilitation process of the patients by teaching activities of daily living, joint protection, energy conservation techniques, and splinting. The arthritic patient is taught coping skills for everyday living. The patient learns to put on stockings, open jars, and adapt to their chronic illness in a manner that preserves their self-esteem. The occupational therapist uses self-help aides and teaches the importance of balancing rest with work activities to avoid fatigue. Patients usually need special help in alternating their work and rest periods. Teach them to rest when they feel tired or in pain; doing a little each day rather than over-exerting on one day is essential.

The learned techniques in joint protection and energy conservation allow patients to continue with a more normal daily life at home and at work.

Making splints for patients to provide proper alignment of joints and adequate rest of inflamed joints has also become a major responsibility of the occupational therapist. Proper alignment helps prevent joint contractures, tendon ruptures, and deformities. Rest for joints, alternating with gentle range of motion exercise helps to reduce inflammation and pain while maintaining joint function.

Nontraditional Treatments

Nontraditional treatments and/or remedies used for rheumatic diseases are common. A patient who has been told that there is no cure for the chronic, painful condition will naturally try almost anything to obtain relief of pain and (hopefully) a cure. In addition to the feelings of desperation, well meaning friends and relatives continue to bombard the patient with suggestions and recommendations. Some suggestions are as easy as purchasing and wearing of a simple copper bracelet or as strange as drinking a gallon of carrot juice daily. Others include more expensive fare such as mail order high-potency vitamins, or a trip to a Mexican clinic.

The Arthritis Foundation publishes an excellent pamphlet on this subject. Patients often need the reassurance of a health professional that most people do experiment sometimes but that it is good to investigate each possible remedy through the Foundation, nurse, or physician.

Help the patient learn to evaluate non-traditional treatments by asking the following questions:
(1) Does it help or cure all kinds of arthritis?
(2) Was a control group used in the study?
(3) Is it based on a secret formula?
(4) Is it promoted only in the media (books or by mail order)?
(5) Does it use case histories and testimonials in promotion?
(6) Does it eliminate any basic foods or nutrients?

PSYCHOSOCIAL CONSIDERATIONS

Psychosocial aspects must always be addressed when caring for the person who has arthritis. The lack of cure and chronicity of the disease makes adjustment difficult. The patient who deals with pain and disability on a daily basis experiences fears of increasing disability and harmful medications, guilt about being ill or burdensome to the family, and depression from decreased social opportunities.

Most people with arthritis are amazingly resourceful and determined to be independent. Life for people with arthritis is in constant flux. It is through excellent medical care and comprehensive patient education that this roller coaster existence can be modified and normal goals and plans for day-to-day living can be developed.

Education on self-help techniques, involvement in support groups, and interaction with others in the same or similar circumstances seem to be particularly helpful in resolving and promoting a healthy psychological outlook. Counseling for the patient and family may be necessary for overwhelming or chronic depression that results from the loss of health. Once different, but realistic goals, projects, and social interactions can be reinstituted, psychosocial adjustment is usually accomplished more easily. If the patients and their families master appropriate and helpful interventions for depression, situational stress, and flare-ups, these reactions appear less frequently and are more easily controllable. Most important is that the health professionals to whom the person with arthritis is directed are knowledgeable about the diseases, community resources, and chronic illness adjustment methods.

The adolescent with arthritis presents an additional challenge. The adolescent is normally maturing and becoming increasingly independent; the parent must allow the normal growth process to continue despite concerns about health issues, such as getting enough rest and joint protection. The adolescent must be encouraged to develop activities, hobbies, and interests that will not do damage to their joints; overprotection is not helpful. The young person needs to be as active as the disease process will allow. Career planning should take into consideration the physical limitations imposed by the disease. Physical appearance is of special concern to the adolescent. When disability, even slight, does exist the teenager may choose to avoid activities. Teenagers, by nature, want to conform; yet treatment for arthritis often excludes the patient from gym classes. The patient may also experience drug-related cosmetic problems (weight gain and acne). Even the use of a splint can cause loss of self-esteem and make the adolescent feel even further removed from peers. Again, encouragement to participate in activities is important in and out of school so that friendships can be built. Parents should encourage normal activities within the limits set by the physician that promotes normal development. Warm baths and splinting are useful in promoting and maintaining range of motion. Physical or occupational therapy and swimming are additional measures suggested for adolescents with more active inflammation. Counseling may be necessary for both teens and their parents so that the normal process of growing and maturing will not be hindered more than necessary.

ARTHRITIS FOUNDATION

The Arthritis Foundation was established as a national organization in 1947. Originally, it was begun by a group of physicians who wanted to raise funds to support research to find the cause and cure for arthritis.

Presently, the organization has its national headquarters in Atlanta, Georgia and 76 local chapters throughout the United States. The goals of the Foundation are public education and information, patient services, professional education, and research.

The programs of the Arthritis Foundation that are particularly noteworthy include (l) the Arthritis Self-Help Course, (2) the Arthritis Joint Venture Dry Exercise Program and (3) the Arthritis Foundation YMCA Aquatic Program. The national address is: Arthritis Foundation, 1314 Spring Street, N.W., Atlanta, Georgia 30309, (404) 872-7100.

Recommended Reading

Arnett F: Seronegative Spondyloarthropathies, *Bull Rheum Dis*, 37(1):1–12, 1987.

Banwell B F: Exercise and mobility in arthritis. In Hawley D (ed): *The Nursing Clinics of North America*. Philadelphia, Saunders, 1984.

Carr RI: *Lupus Erythematosus, A Handbook*. Washington, DC, Lupus Foundation of America, Inc, ed 2, 1986.

Finsterbush A, Pogrand H: The hypermobility syndrome: musculoskeletal complaints in 100 consecutive cases of generalized joint hypermobility. *Clin Orthop*, 68:124–127, 1982.

Fries JF: *General approach to the rheumatic disease patient*, In Kelley WN, et al., *Textbook of Rheumatology*. Philadelphia, WB Saunders, 1985.

Fues James F: *Arthritis, A Comprehensive Guide*. Reading, MA, Addison-Wesley, 1986.

Hawley D, ed: Symposium on Arthritis and Related Rheumatic Diseases: *Nurs Clin N Am* 19(4), 1984.

Kelley WN, Harris Ed, Ruddy S, Sledge CB: *Textbook of Rheumatology*, Philadelphia, WB Saunders, 1985.

Lorig K, Fries JF: *The Arthritis Helpbook* Reading, MA, Addison-Wesley, 1986.

Pigg JS, Discoll, P: *Rheumatology Nursing, A Problem Oriented Approach*. New York, John Wiley & Sons, 1985.

Phillips, Robert H: *Coping with Lupus*, Wayne, NJ, Avery Publishing Group, Inc., 1984.

Rodnan GP, Schumacker, HR (ed): *Primer on the Rheumatic Diseases*. Atlanta GA, Arthritis Foundation, 1983.

Sheon RP, Kirsner AB, Farber SJ, et al: The hypermobility syndrome. *Post Gradmed*, 71:199–209, 1982.

Drug Therapy for Orthopaedic Conditions

This appendix is a brief overview of the classes of drugs used in orthopaedic drug therapy. The prudent practitioner will consult the pharmacologic references cited at the end of the appendices for more details.

NONSTEROIDAL ANTI-INFLAMMATORY DRUGS (NSAIDs)

General Information

Nonsteroidal anti-inflammatory drugs are indicated most frequently in the orthopaedic patient for mild to moderate pain relief and/or for subduing inflammation. They are often recommended after surgery or injury on an acute basis or for rheumatoid arthritis and degenerative joint disease on a chronic basis. They have analgesic, anti-inflammatory, and antipyretic properties.

NSAIDs are generally classified as salicylates (e.g., aspirin choline salicylate, choline and magnesium trisalicylate), salicylic-acid derivatives (e.g., diflunisal), indoles (e.g., indomethacin, sulindac), oxicam derivatives (piroxicam), propionic acid derivatives (e.g., ibuprofen, naproxen, penopropen, ketopropen), pyrroles (e.g., tolmetin sodium), penamates (e.g., meclofenamate sodium), and rarely indicated pyrazoles (e.g., phenylbutazone, oxyphenbutazone).

NSAIDs work by inhibiting prostaglandin formation. They are rapidly absorbed by the GI tract and are frequently irritating to it. Toxic levels of NSAIDs may cause tinnitus and eighth cranial nerve damage. In addition, they cause sodium and fluid retention, and decrease the ability of platelets to aggregate. Other adverse effects include peptic and duodenal ulcers, gastritis, hemolytic anemia, nephrotoxicity, and elevated liver enzymes. Allergic reactions may occur with any of these drugs and they may induce asthmatic attacks in susceptible individuals.

Nurse and Patient Considerations

The patient should be taught to take NSAIDs with food and/or antacids and at least 8 ounces of fluid to prevent GI irritation or erosions. Hemoccult testing of the stool should be done once a month for those on long-term therapy or without delay if signs of GI bleeding occur. Patients should be taught to observe for bleeding tendencies such as susceptibility to bruises, bleeding gums, smoky-colored urine, and dark tarry stools. It is recommended that renal and hepatic function be tested every 1 to 2 months in patients on long-term NSAIDs, whether or not they display symptoms that are associated with dysfunction. In addition, patients must be questioned about tinnitus. If tinnitus is a complaint the drug dosage should be lowered, and if tinnitus persists the drug should be discontinued. Patients who are taking the drugs for long-term anti-inflammatory effects need to be advised that therapeutic effect may not be noticed for 2 to 4 weeks. A minimum 2 week trial of one drug from each class of NSAIDs is indicated.

Warn patients that many over the counter (OTC) drugs contain NSAIDs and teach the importance of reading the labels. Patients should be encouraged to tell their pharmacist or practitioners about any OTC drugs they may be taking and ask about possible drug interactions or adverse effects.

Because sodium and fluid retention are common side effects of NSAIDs, they should be used cautiously in the elderly and in those with hypertension, cardiac, or renal disease.

Caution is recommended when prescribing NSAIDS in the elderly (see Chapter 4 for Adverse Drug Reactions).

Most NSAID are contraindicated in pregnant women and nursing mothers. The reader is advised to refer to the references listed for specific dosage, considerations, contraindications, adverse reactions and drug interactions.

ACETAMINOPHEN

General Information

Acetaminophen is most useful as a mild analgesic and antipyretic. It is not an anti-inflammatory agent and therefore may not be as effective as a NSAID when inflammation is contributing to pain. However, acetaminophen is less irritating to the GI tract than most oral analgesics.

Nurse and Patient Considerations

Severe liver damage may result if toxic levels are reached. Adult doses should not exceed 4 gm/day or 2.6 gm/day if taken on a long-term basis. Long-term therapy is contraindicated in patients with hepatic or renal disease or in patients with anemia.

CORTICOSTEROIDS

General Information

Corticosteroids are frequently used in rheumatic disorders and collagen diseases for their anti-inflammatory properties. Although the precise mechanisms of action are unknown, corticosteroids nonspecifically inhibit inflammatory effects of many microorganisms, chemical or thermal irritants, allergens, and trauma. These steroids suppress symptoms, but do not treat the underlying cause of the problem.

Continuous daily therapy is usually reserved for acute conditions (for example, trauma or SLE). For chronic disorders enough steroids should be administered to allow function, but usually not enough to provide complete symptomatic relief as this would require much higher doses.

The use of alternate day therapy should be considered in some chronic disease states. Patients receive a 2-day dosage in a single administration every other morning. This mode of administration may reduce side effects, particularly those of adrenal suppression. The theory of this method is that on the "off" days the patient has lower steroid bloods levels. This allows a day of reactivation of the adrenal glands by the normal mechanism of CRF-ACTH and recovery of other tissues from the metabolic effects of exogenous steroids. Steroids that are inactivated in less than 30 to 36 hours must be used to allow the body's own secretory mechanisms to prevail on nontreatment days. The dose should be given in the morning to simulate the normal diurnal rhythm and to achieve maximum benefit with minimum dose (Clayton, 1984).

"When therapeutic dosages of steroids are given for a week or longer, one must assume that endogenous cortisol production has been suppressed. Abrupt withdrawal of the glucocorticoid may result in adrenal insufficiency, so withdrawal of the drug should be gradual" (Clayton, 1984. p. 453).

Nurse and Patient Considerations

Corticoids may increase susceptibility to infection, suppress skin sensitivity tests, and elevate serum amylase and blood glucose. When glucocorticoids are administered over a long period of time, the patient may display sodium and water retention, potassium depletion, and symptoms similar to Cushing's syndrome including hirsutism, a cervicothoracic hump, moon face, edema, amenorrhea, striae and thinning of the skin, hypochloremia, metabolic alkalosis, mental disturbances, and hyperglycemia. In addition increased appetite, weight gain, an improved sense of well-being, peptic ulcer, headache, and dizziness have been reported. Osteoporosis and vertebral compression are well recognized complications of long-term (longer than 2 months) therapy.

Corticosteroid Injections

Local injections can be made into the periarticular sites of inflammation at the tendon insertions, in the bursae or joint capsule. Most physicians recommend no more than 2 to 3 injections into weight bearing joints each year. Injections into the soft tissues can be done more frequently. Concomitant anti-inflammatory drug therapy is essential for effective treatment.

Nursing and Patient Considerations

Following injection patients are advised to rest the joint and apply an ice pack to the injected site for 24 to 48 hours. Patients need to be aware of the potential for increased pain as a result of intra-articular joint injections. Five percent of all injected individuals will experience crystal induced inflammation with a pain intensity that mimics crystal synovitis. Instruct patients to inform the physician of any pain after injection. Although rare, patients need to be aware of the possibility of the following complications following steroid injection: infection, "postinjection flare," localized subcutaneous or cutaneous atrophy (a depigmented, depressed area develops on the skin at the site of injection), and arthropathy. All patients should be contacted in 48 hours to determine the effect of the intra-articular injection.

ANTIMALARIALS— HYDROXYCHLOROQUINE SULPHATE, CHLOROQUINE PHOSPHATE

General Information

These drugs were originally used to treat malaria and were subsequently found to have anti-inflammatory properties, which are useful in the treatment of RA and both systemic and discoid lupus erythematosus. The mechanism of action is unknown.

The most common side effects are GI disturbances, including heartburn. Other adverse reactions include headaches, visual disturbances, tinnitus, vertigo, blood dyscrasias, dermatitis, and neuropathies.

Nurse and Patient Considerations

Retinopathy is a rare side effect, but nevertheless visual acuity and slit lamp ophthalmologic exam should precede administration of these drugs and should be repeated every 3 to 6 months. For this reason the drugs are contraindicated in those with retinal or visual field changes and are not recommended for diabetics. The drugs concentrate in the liver, therefore extreme caution is urged in using these medications in those with hepatic problems or those who are alcoholics. CBC and liver function tests should be obtained routinely in those on long-term therapy.

Overdosage can quickly lead to toxic symptoms; headache, drowsiness, visual disturbances, cardiovascular collapse and convulsions, followed by respiratory and cardiac arrest. Children are extremely susceptible to toxicity; avoid long-term treatment (Hamilton, 1987, p. 37).

Patients should be cautioned to avoid sun exposure as drug-induced dermatosis may result.

GOLD THERAPY (REMITTIVE DRUGS)

General Information

Gold salts have been shown to be effective against rheumatoid arthritis. Seventy-five percent of patients started on the therapy have a favorable response. However, numerous and serious side effects, which are frequently a dose-related problem, may require the discontinuation of the drug. Due to the frequency and severity of these adverse reactions, gold salts are indicated only in patients in which NSAIDs and D-penicillamine were not helpful.

Nurse and Patient Considerations

Gold salts are contraindicated in the presence of many medical conditions (consult references at end of appendices), but show no significant drug interactions. Advise patients that benefits of the therapy may not be observed for 6 to 12 weeks.

Patients may remain on gold therapy for years.

Warn patients to report any adverse reactions promptly to their practitioner, as some reactions are life threatening.

Dermatitis is the most common adverse reaction including rash and/or pruritus. Presence of pruritic skin reactions will often progress to more serious skin problems; therefore it is necessary to discontinue the drug until the reaction clears. Concomitant stomatitis often occurs.

Nephrotoxicity with initial proteinuria and albuminuria may occur; therefore frequent urine dipstick urinalysis is crucial. Blood dyscrasias, most notably thrombocytopenia (with or without purpura), aplastic anemia, agranulocytosis, are well known side effects. A CBC and platelet count must be obtained biweekly. Other adverse reactions include nausea, vomiting, diarrhea, metallic taste, hepatitis, and jaundice.

IM injection should be into large muscles. Patients should lie down for 10 to 20 minutes after injection and then be observed for 30 minutes for acute reactions. Gold sodium thiomalate is a suspension. It requires warming and agitation in order to resuspend and to obtain an accurate dose. It is pale yellow in color and should not be used if the solution has darkened.

As thrombocytopenia, aplastic anemia, agranulocytosis, proteinuria, and nephrotic syndrome are common and potentially life threatening side effects, authorities advise that a urinalysis or dipstick for urine protein and a hematocrit (Hct) precede every gold injection. Dimercaprol is used to treat acute gold toxicity.

D-PENICILLAMINE

General Information

Many patients respond well to D-penicillamine after 6 to 8 weeks of treatment. Unfortunately, a large number need to discontinue the drug due to side effects including renal and hepatotoxicity, leukopenia, thrombocytopenia, rash, drug-induced lupus, and loss of taste.

The mechanism of action is not known.

Nurse and Patient Considerations

Urinalysis, CBC with differential, and platelet count must be obtained every 2 weeks and, if abnormalities are seen, D-penicillamine usually should be discontinued. Proteinuria of more than 2 to 5 gm/day calls for discontinuation to preserve renal function.

It is important to take D-penicillamine on an empty stomach to prevent binding with dietary metals. Binding can cause the loss of essential minerals as well as decrease drug efficacy.

IMMUNOMODULATORS

Azathioprine, (Imuran), Cyclophosphamide (Cytoxan), Methotrexate.

General Information

Immunomodulators are highly effective against arthritis and certain inflammatory diseases. They must be used with caution and are reserved for advance refractory conditions. Adverse reactions may include hepatotoxicity, infections (from viral, bacterial, and/or fungal organisms), parasitic infestation, sterility, and cancer.

Giving immunosuppressives in conjunction with steroids may reduce the dose of steroids needed.

Patient and Nurse Considerations

Response may take up to 6 weeks. Leukopenia, bone marrow depression, hepatotoxicity, and other blood dyscrasias necessitate monitoring of CBC and liver enzymes. Therapy must be stopped to prevent irreversible bone marrow depression, if WBC is less than 3000/mm^3.

Advise patients to observe for opportunistic infections—thrush, herpes zoster, and colds, and to consult their practitioner promptly when even mild fever or symptoms occur.

GI complaints are frequent, including nausea, vomiting, diarrhea, and stomatitis. Taking the drug with meals and an antiemetic may help the nausea and vomiting; scrupulous oral hygiene may help the stomatitis.

Patients on Cytoxan are at risk for hemorrhagic cystitis and bladder cancer; therefore they should drink copious amounts of fluid to minimize the concentration in the bladder. Taking the drug in the early morning helps prevent overnight retention of the metabolites in the bladder.

DRUGS FOR GOUT

Allopurinol

General Information

Allopurinol acts as a hypouricemic agent and is used for long-term treatment of gout. "It is of particular benefit for those who 'overproduce' uric acid, have renal insufficiency, or cannot use uricosuric drugs" (Miller and Greenblatt, 1980). Side effects are generally rare and mild, but side effects indicative of hypersensitivity include rash, hepatotoxicity, and/or blood dyscrasias. These usually occur 1 to 6 weeks into treatment, but may occur at any time during therapy. The drug must be discontinued if these side effects occur.

Allopurinol is contraindicated in those with idiopathic hemochromatosis and should not be given to those on iron therapy.

Nurse and Patient Considerations

Liver function tests and CBC are indicated on a weekly basis during first several months of therapy to screen for hepatic and/or blood problems.

Advise patients that a rash can lead to serious complications (exfoliative dermatitis and toxic epidermal neurolysis) and that their practitioner should be notified promptly so that the drug can be discontinued.

Encourage patients to drink large amounts of fluid. Urine output should be at least 2 liters/day.

Colchicine

General Information

Colchicine or the NSAIDs are the drugs of choice for acute gout. Colchicine can be used as a prophylactic agent on a long-term basis. It has been used for centuries to treat gout. Colchicine is believed to act by inhibiting the migration of granulocytes to an area of inflammation. It has mild anti-inflammatory effects, but no analgesic properties.

Nausea, vomiting, and diarrhea are common side effects and reasons for discontinuing. Infrequently, chronic administration may result in bone marrow depression.

Nurse and Patient Considerations

Baseline CBC should be obtained and monitored as leukopenia, aplastic anemia, and/or agranulocytosis may occur in chronic use. Many special considerations must be observed when the drug is administered IV. Consult one of the references for further information, when administering this drug IV.

Probenecid, Sulfinpyrazone

General Information

These medications are indicated in hyperuricemia and chronic gout. They should not be administered for an acute gouty attack. They work by blocking tubular resorption and thereby cause a marked increase in the excretion of uric acid.

Nurse and Patient Considerations

Treatment should begin with small doses to decrease the probability of renal stones. Instruct patients to drink enough fluid to maintain a urine output of 2 to 3 liters/day (also to prevent renal stones). Alkalinization of the urine increases the solubility of urates and reduces the possibility of renal stone formation. A dietitian can provide information on foods that will help alkalize the urine.

As GI irritation is a frequent complaint, these medications should be given with food to decrease GI irritation. Antacids may also be given with probenecid to decrease GI irritation.

The drug is to be avoided in patients with BUN greater than 40 or creatinine clearance of less than 40ml/minute and in those with blood dyscrasias.

Advise patients that this drug may take up to 6 to 12 months to become effective and gouty attacks may increase the first 6 to 12 months of therapy. Nevertheless, treatment should continue in conjunction with colchicine or other anti-inflammatory agents.

Salicylates inhibit the uricosuric activities of the drug and therefore should be avoided; they also may prolong the half-life of oral hypoglycemics.

appendix b

1988 Prices of Commonly Used Drugs

	Generic Name	Trade Name(s)	How Supplied	1988 Costs
Nonsteroidal Anti-inflammatory Drugs	Aspirin	Generic Bayer	325mg 325mg	$.98/100 $3.49/100[a] $1.89/100~ $4.49/100~
	Ascriptin	ASA/Maalox	325mg	$5.59/100~ $9.00/100*
	Ascriptin A/D	ASA/Maalox	500mg	$5.39/100 + $12.96/100*
	Enteric coated Ecotrin	Easprin	975mg 325mg 325mg 500mg	$27.43/100 + $7.89/100 + $6.34/100* $8.45/100 +
	ASA zero order release	Zorprin	800mg	$25.29/100 +
	Choline Magnesium Salicylate	Trilisate	500mg 750mg	$32.79/100 + $45.56/100* $39.89/100 + $51.98/100*
	Diflunisal	Dolobid	250mg 500mg	$63.79/100 + $72.79/100* $73.79/100 + $85.24/100*
	Magnesium Salicylate	Magan	545mg	$32.39/100 +
	Salsalate	Disalcid	750mg 500mg	$39.69/100 + $51.60/100* $35.69/100 + $47.50/100*
Nonsalicylates	Fenoprofen	Naflon	200mg	$38.99/100 + $51.47/100*
	Calcium		300mg 600mg	$42.99/100 + 56.50/100* $58.49/100 + $70.40/100*
	Ibuprofen	Motrin Generic Motrin Motrin Motrin Generic Advil	400mg 400mg 600mg 600mg 800mg 800mg 200mg	$16.49/100 + $12.00/100 + $31.49/100 + $36.27/100* $27.79/100 + $20.79/100 + $3.15/100~ $7.50/100~
	Indomethacin	Indocin	25mg 50mg 75mg SR	$37.53/100 + $51.70/100* $67.73/100 + $71.73/100* $96.43/100 +
	Ketoprofen	Orudis	50mg	$49.99/100 + $54.95/100*

1988 Prices of Commonly Used Drugs—*Continued*

	Generic Name	Trade Name(s)	How Supplied	1988 Costs
			75mg	$54.99/100 + $63.56/100*
	Meclofenamate sodium	Meclomen Generic	50mg 50mg	$47.69/100 + $33.99/100 + $51.91/100*
		Meclomen Generic	100mg 100mg	$63.59/100 + $44.99/100 +
	Naproxen	Naprosyn	250mg 375mg 500mg	$73.38/100* $87.98/100* $103.35/100*
	Piroxicam	Feldene	10mg	$102.43/100 + $96.15/100*
			20mg	$176.93/100 + $150.51/100*
	Phenylbutazone	Butazolidin	100mg	$54.19/100 + $63.32/100*
	Sulindac	Clinoril	150mg	$73.93/100 + $75.53/100*
			200mg	$90.93/100 + $88.24/100*
	Tolmetin sodium	Tolectin	200mg	$44.29/100 + $54.88/100*
			400mg	$66.69/100 + $77.34/100*
Analgesics (non-NSAIDs)	Acetaminophen	Tylenol	500mg	$3.39/100~ $4.79/100~
		Generic	500mg	$1.39/100~ $3.29/100~
Disease Modifying Agents for Rheumatoid Arthritis	Auranofin	Radaura	3mg	$83.56/100 + $91.59/100*
	Aurothioglucose	Solganal	50mg/ml 10ml (multidose vial)	$68.25/vial*
	D-penicillamine	Depen	250mg	$61.73/100 + $71.77/100*
	Gold sodium thiomalate	Myochrysine	50mg/ml (multidose vial)	$62.50/vial*
	Hydroxychloroquine sulfate	Plaquenil	200mg	$67.79/100 + $80.67/100*
	Allopurinol	Zyloprim	100mg 300mg	$24.90/100 + $30.75/100* $49.90/100 + $41.89/100 +
		Lupurin	100mg 300mg	$24.49/100 + $40.49/100 +
	Colchicine		1mg	$28.53/100* $24.25/100 +
	Anturane	Sulfinpyrazone	200mg	$56.66/100* $50.73/100 +
	Probenecid	Benemid	250mg 500mg	$24.63/100 + $37.32/100*
		Generic	500mg	$27.34/100 +
	Colbenemid (colchicine 0.5mg, benemid 500mg)			$40.17/100* $35.12/100 +
	Azathioprine	Imuran	50mg	$85.66/100*
	Chlorambucil	Luekeran	2mg	$74.36/100*

1988 Prices of Commonly Used Drugs—*Continued*

	Generic Name	Trade Name(s)	How Supplied	1988 Costs
	Cyclophosphamide	Cytoxan	25mg	$87.38/100*
			50mg	$153.68/100*
	Cyclosporine	Sandimmune	100mg/ml	$208.64/50ml*
	Methotrexate		2.5mg	$208.24/100*

[a]~, there was a great variation in price (a range is given); +, the price listed is an average of two or more large pharmacy chains in the Philadelphia area; *, the price listed is that at a Philadelphia hospital outpatient pharmacy.

All drug prices with great variation are from the pharmacy chains. Many pharmacies have a 10% discount for senior citizens.

appendix c

Laboratory Tests

SERUM ANALYSIS

Complete Blood Count

Explanation of the Test

Included in the CBC are white blood cell count (WBC) and differential, red blood cell count (RBC), erythrocyte indices, hematocrit, and hemoglobin. Aspects of the CBC that are useful to the orthopaedic nurse are discussed below.

Red Blood Count (RBC)

Normal Values: Men 4.7 to 6.1ml/mm^3; Women 4.2 to 5.4ml/mm^3

Explanation of the Test

The RBC determines the number of red blood cells in a microliter of capillary or venous blood. It is part of the diagnostic workup for anemia and polycythemia.

Clinical Implications

An RBC that is 10% or more below the normal value indicates anemia. Normal values decrease with age and normal values for men are greater than for women. RBC count is decreased in patients with SLE, RA, rheumatic fever, and chronic inflammation.

White Blood Count (WBC)

Normal Values: 4,500 to 11,500/mm^3 (may be less in black individuals)

Explanation of the Test

This test measures the total number of WBCs in a cubic millimeter of venous blood. The WBC is the body's first defense against infection. The WBC fights infection and defends against microorganisms by phagocytosis.

Clinical Implications

The WBC is a method of evaluating for toxicity from medication (gold, indocin, penicillamine) or presence of infection. The WBC increases with infection and decreases with the previously mentioned drugs. The drugs may mask signs of infection by lowering the WBC. Leukopenia may occur with SLE, Felty's syndrome, and RA.

Differential

Normal Values: Adult

Cell Type	Mean %	Range of Absolute Counts
Segmented neutrophils	56	2500 to 7000/microliter
Bands	3	0 to 700/microliter
Lymphocytes	21 to 35	1000 to 4800/microliter
Monocytes	4	0 to 800/microliter
Eosinophils	2.7	0 to 450/microliter
Basophils	0.3	0 to 150/microliter

Explanation of the Test

Visual examination of a stained slide permits an estimation of alteration in size, shape, number, and structure of different WBCs. The different WBCs are then reported as a percent of the total WBCs, with additional notes about abnormalities.

Interfering Factors

Corticosteroid will decrease the eosinophil count and the lymphocyte count, which in turn will increase the neutrophil count.

Clinical Implications

Neutrophilia, the most common form of leukocytosis is usually caused by bacterial infections, inflammatory disorders, tumors, stresses, and drugs. Rheumatoid arthritis causes neutropenia.

Hematocrit (Hct)

Normal Values: Men 42 to 52%; Women 37 to 47%

Explanation of the Test

The hematocrit is expressed as a percentage, is indicative of the volume of red blood cells in 100ml of blood, and is another diagnostic test for anemia.

Clinical Implications

Normal values vary with age and gender. Hematocrit is frequently decreased due to chronic inflammation and blood loss through the bowel due to medication.

Hemoglobin (Hb)

Normal Values: Men 13 to 18g/100ml; Women 12 to 16g/100ml

Explanation of the Test

Hemoglobin is the iron containing pigment of the red blood cells that carries oxygen to the cells and removes carbon dioxide. It is reported in gm/100ml of blood. Hemoglobin levels usually parallel the HCT and RBC.

Clinical Implications

Hemoglobin is decreased in chronic inflammation. Levels lower than normal indicate anemia.

Erythrocyte Sedimentation Rate (ESR)

Normal Values: Men up to 15mm/hr; Women up to 20mm/hr (higher in the elderly)

Explanation of the Test

The ESR is the speed at which red blood cells settle in well mixed venous blood.

Clinical Implications

ESR is valuable for tracking malignant or inflammatory disease and as a diagnostic test for detecting occult disease. The ESR is elevated in individuals with rheumatoid arthritis, chronic inflammation, and neoplasms.

Platelet Count

Normal Values: 150,00 to 400,000

Explanation of the Test

The test measures the number of platelets (thrombocytes). Platelets are disk-shaped nonnucleated cells that help form the hemostatic plug and are visible on stained blood smears. Decrease in platelets prolongs the clotting process and reflects bone marrow response to various diseases and to physiologic or chemical stimuli.

Clinical Implications

A decreased platelet count occurs in rheumatic fever and SLE or from toxic effect of drugs, especially gold therapy drugs. Platelet aggregation is often impeded in those taking aspirin.

Uric Acid

Normal Values: Men 2.1 to 7.5mg/100ml; Women 2.0 to 6.6mg/100ml

Explanation of the Test

Uric acid is the nitrogen containing end product of purine metabolism in the serum. It is cleared from the plasma by glomerular filtration and perhaps by tubular secretion.

It is a screening test for kidney disease and an indicator of disorders of nucleic acid metabolism.

Clinical Implications

Elevated uric acid levels may occur with arthritis, gout, psoriasis, acute infections, and other conditions, including low-dose aspirin therapy.

C-Reactive Protein

Normal Values: Less than 6 mcg/ml

Explanation of the Test

The C-reactive protein test measures for an abnormal plasma protein (glycoprotein)

that appears as a nonspecific response to a variety of inflammatory stimuli, both infectious and noninfectious. It is a nonspecific diagnostic tool used to reflect the extent and severity of a disease process.

Clinical Implications

An elevated C-reactive protein level indicates an acute inflammatory response, especially in RA, rheumatic fever, disseminated lupus erythematosus, and bacterial and viral infections.

Serum Total Protein and Protein Electrophoresis

Normal Values: Total protein 6 to 8.4 g/dl, Albumin 3.5 to 5.0 g/dl, globulin 2.3 to 3.5 g/dl.

Explanation of the Test

Electrical current is used to separate the globulins in the serum which assume characteristic patterns. The patterns are then analyzed and specific patterns show varying amounts and proportions of six distinct protein fractions. The different patterns assumed by the globulins are characteristic of various disease states. (See References.)

Patient Instruction

Instruct the patient to fast, except for water, for 8 hours prior to the test.

Serum Salicylate Level

Normal Values: No salicylate in the blood
Therapeutic and Toxic Levels:

Up to 50mg/dl,	therapeutic, no ill effects
50 to 80mg/dl,	mild intoxication
80 to 100mg/dl,	moderate intoxication
100 to 160mg/dl,	severe toxicity
Over 160mg/dl,	lethal toxicity

Explanation of the Test

This test measures salicylate levels in the serum.

Clinical Implications

This test allows the clinician to assess for toxicity and therapeutic salicylate levels.

Total Calcium

Normal Values: 8.5 to 10.5 mg/dl adult

Explanation of the Test

The test measures the amount of calcium in milligrams/deciliter of blood. It is primarily used to detect bone disease, parathyroid disorders, and nonspecific hypercalcemic states.

Clinical Implications

Hypercalcemia may occur with noncutaneous neoplasms including myeloma, acute leukemia, cancers that have metastasized to the bone, and neoplasm secretion of parathyroid hormone (PTH). Other conditions associated with hypercalcemia include:

Primary hyperparathyroidism
Sarcoidosis
Thiazide diuretics (always evaluate for occult hyperparathyroidism)
Idiopathic bone fractures, especially during bedrest
Acromegaly
Estrogen therapy

Conditions associated with hypocalcemia:

Primary hypoparathyroidism
Pseudohypoparathyroidism
Malabsorption
Renal failure
Magnesium deficiency
Vitamin D deficiency
Tumor
Cortisone therapy

Calcium levels must frequently be examined in the context of other lab values, especially serum albumin, in order to make accurate assumptions and diagnoses.

Interfering Factors

Radiopaque materials (delay the test until 24 hours, after injection of radiopaque contrast media)
Large amounts of milk products
Alkaline antacids
Calcium salts
Estrogen preparations
Vitamin D
Cortisone

Gentamicin
Methicillin
Antacids
Heparin
Insulin
Dilantin
Diamox
Mithramycin

SELECTIVE SERUM IMMUNOLOGY ANALYSIS

Antistreptolysin O Titer (ASO Titer)

Normal Values: Less than or equal to 85 Todd Units/m

Explanation of the Test

This test measures the relative serum concentrations of the antibody streptolysin O, an oxygen-labile enzyme produced by a group A beta hemolytic streptococci.

Clinical Implications

The test results can verify a recent ongoing infection with beta-hemolytic streptococcal infections when used in conjunction with other tests. A change of two or more units is a clue to recent streptococcal infection but would not, by itself, establish the diagnosis of rheumatic fever (Schoen, 1988, p. 36). When joint pain is present, it is used to help distinguish between RA and rheumatic fever.

Antinuclear Antibodies (ANA, FANA, FNA)

Normal Values: A titer of less than or equal to 1:32

Explanation of the Test

Titer measurement of ANA (single stranded DNA), which includes fluorescent pattern (F in FAN and FANA), detects the presence of antinucleoprotein factors associated with some autoimmune diseases. ANA are gammaglobulins that react to specific antigens when mixed in the laboratory. Antibodies are produced in response to the nuclear part of white blood cells.

Clinical Implications

ANA levels seem to increase with age even in people without immune disease. High titer increases the chance of connective tissue diseases (e.g., SLE, RA, PSS, Sjögren's syndrome).

Anti-DNA, DNA Binding Farr's Test

Normal Values: Considered negative at a 1:10 dilution of serum

Explanation of the Test

Detects antibodies against native double stranded DNA. Used to diagnose and monitor the progress of SLE.

Clinical Implications

High titers are seen in patients with SLE and the titers may increase with increased disease activity. The test may be useful in monitoring some patients' response to therapy.

Rheumatoid Factor (RF)

Normal Values: Latex fixation greater than or equal to 1:160 is considered significant. Agglutination titer greater than or equal to 1:16 is considered significant.

Explanation of the Test

The test provides titer measurement of the rheumatoid factor, which is an antibody directed against the gamma globulin IgG. The most commonly used tests are latex fixation and sheep red cell agglutinations.

Clinical Implications

Clinical significance of elevated RF needs to be interpreted cautiously. People without disease may have positive RF, and RF may be positive in other connective tissue diseases, especially viral infections, SLE, scleroderma, sarcoidosis, and immune complex glomerulonephritis. A negative test for RF can be found in 10 to 30% of patients clinically diagnosed as having rheumatoid arthritis.

SYNOVIAL FLUID ANALYSIS (SEE CHAPTER 9)

Mucin Clot Test

The addition of 5% acetic acid to normal joint fluid results in a thick, ropy clot that will not fragment when shaken. Fluid from an acutely inflamed joint results in a stringy, loose clot.

Viscosity

After taking normal synovial fluid between the thumb and the index finger a string of fluid 1 to 2 inches will develop as the thumb and index finger are separated. Inflamed joints produce a less viscous and more watery synovial fluid. This test is rarely performed.

Color, Clarity, Amount

Normal joint fluid varies in color from yellow to straw, is clear, and is present in the joint in minute quantities only. Inflamed joints produce increased fluid that is turbid.

White Blood Cells

Normal synovial fluid has a low concentration of white blood cells and has predominantly mononuclear cells. WBC less than 2000/mm^3 occurs in osteoarthritis, WBC is greater than 10,000 with sepsis and inflammatory arthritis. Gram stain and culture should be done on all samples with inflammatory fluid.

Crystal Studies

Crystal arthritis is diagnosed only by visualization of the causative crystal. The two most common crystal diseases are gout and pseudogout. Monosodium urate crystals are found in the synovial WBCs when gout is present.

Rheumatoid Factor

Rheumatoid factor may be found in synovial fluid before becoming evident in the blood.

URINALYSIS

Explanation of the Test

A complete urinalysis includes analysis of specific gravity, color/appearance, odor, pH, protein/albumin, glucose, ketones, and hemoglobin; microscopic findings include RBCs, WBCs, casts, crystals, and squamous epithelial cells.

Clinical Implications

Many of these tests can be done quickly with multiple reagent strips and are useful in screening for many pathologies such as diabetes and renal disease. Those aspects of the urinalysis more pertinent to the orthopaedic practitioner are elaborated further.

Specific Gravity

Normal Values: 1.003 to 1.035

Explanation of the Test

The weight of urine is compared to the equal weight of an equal volume of distilled water.

Clinical Implications

Specific gravity is used as an initial screening tool, and any abnormal value warrants further investigation for possible pathology. Numerous conditions can change the specific gravity of the urine; some of the more pertinent and typical ones are discussed further. Urine with a low specific gravity is a clue to the inability of the kidney to concentrate urine and may indicate distal renal tubular disease. In the absence of protein or sugar in the urine, the specific gravity should then be 1.020 or greater. Specific gravity is increased for 1 to 2 days following the administration of radiocontrast material. A more helpful clinical picture is obtained if the patient is able to fast for 16 hours prior to giving the sample, as fasting will more accurately reflect the concentrating ability of the kidneys.

Protein

Normal Value: None present

Explanation of the Test

A dip stick measures the amount of protein in the sample.

Clinical Implications

This test measures the effectiveness of glomerular function.

The presence of protein in the urine is indicative of renal disease. Protein in the urine may also be a result of extreme muscle exertion. Endurance athletes may have some proteinuria following an event.

Crystals

Normal Values: None present
Uric acid 0.3 to 0.5gm/24h in low-purine diet
Uric acid 0.4 to 0.8gm/24h in a normal diet

Explanation of the Test

This test measures crystal formation in the urine.

Clinical Implications

Uric acid and urate crystals may occur with or without clinical gout or renal calculi.

BODY TISSUE ANALYSIS AND TYPING

Synovial Tissue Analysis

A histologic examination of synovial tissue can detect pigmented villonodular synovitis. However, a synovial biopsy may not differentiate among rheumatoid arthritis, ankylosing spondylitis, juvenile polyarthroses, or psoriatic arthritis.

Renal Tissue Analysis

A renal biopsy is performed to discover the pathological type of renal disease that is usually associated with significant renal insufficiency.

Temporal Artery

A biopsy of the temporal artery may indicate the presence of inflammatory cells; with polymyalgia rheumatica the test may detect giant cell arteritis (even without symptoms).

Skin

A punch biopsy of skin examined by light microscopy or by immune fluorescence microscopy assists in diagnosing SLE, progressive systemic scleroderma, psoriasis, or any poorly characterized or suspicious skin lesion.

Muscle

A muscle biopsy is sometimes done with a skin biopsy. It is used to evaluate muscle weakness, especially in patients with polymyositis or dermatomyositis. It is useful for establishing an inflammatory, noninflammatory, or infectious etiology for myopathy.

HLA-B27 Tissue Type

One of the major histocompatibility antigens important to tissue recognition, HLA-B27 is found commonly in patients with ankylosing spondylitis, Reiter's syndrome, and other connective tissue disorders. Presence does not mean disease; HLA-B27 is found in 5 to 7% of normal patients, but 80–90% of patients with ankylosing spondylitis syndrome have it.

Much of the information for this appendix was obtained from "Assessment for Arthritis" by Delores C. Schoen. Published in the March/April 1988 issue of *Orthopaedic Nursing* (Vol. 7, No. 2, pp. 31–39).

appendix d

Prices of Commonly Used Laboratory Tests[a]

Complete Blood Count (CBC)	With differential	$8.50
	Without differential	$7.00
Hematocrit		$7.00
Hemoglobin		$7.00
Serum calcium		$20.00
Total calcium		$9.00
Ionized calcium		$43.00
Serum phosphorous		$9.00
Acid phosphatase		$22.00
Alkaline phosphatase		$9.00
HLA B 27 antigen		$61.00
Synovial fluid analysis		$71.50
Synovial fluid analysis of rheumatoid factor		$24.00

[a]Prices are the average of prices from a hospital laboratory, and a large nonhospital lab in the spring of 1988 in the Philadelphia area.

appendix e

Diagnostic Procedures

General Information for Patient Preparation for Orthopaedic Procedures

RADIOLOGY

Plain Film X-ray

Explanation

The plain film x-ray produces a shadow made on a sensitized film or plate by roentgen rays, without the use of enhancement dyes.

Patient Teaching, Preparation, and Nursing Implications

Explain to the patient that an x-ray is similar to taking a photograph. Therefore, in order to obtain a clear view, it is crucial that the patient remain motionless when the film is taken. Usually there is no special preparation for plain film x-rays. However, to ensure optimum visualization of bone and surrounding soft tissue, proper positioning of the patient is essential. Special positioning can enhance the picture and assure accurate diagnosis. Viewing an injury or abnormality requires centering the film on this area; with orthopaedic problems it is often important to view the joints above and below the problem.

Spinal films especially may require views from several positions and angles. X-rays may be performed standing, in flexion, in extension, bending, in traction, or in compression. For example, a patient may be x-rayed with a heavy pack on the back to demonstrate compression.

Bone Scan

Explanation

Radioactive isotopes are injected intravenously. These isotopes go preferentially to the bone and concentrate in areas that have an increased rate of bone mineral turnover or are hypervascular. These areas appear darker on the x-ray film. The entire skeleton or any part of it may be viewed. The scan may reveal tumors, infection, and trauma, but it is not possible to distinguish one from the other without further diagnostic tests and exams.

Patient Teaching, Preparation, and Nursing Implications

Instruct the patient that the injection feels like any intravenous stick. The isotope material does not cause pain when it is infused. After the isotopes have moved to the bone the films are taken. When the films are taken, as with any x-ray, the patient needs to remain still and may be asked to move or change position for improved viewing. Following the scan the isotope is excreted in the urine. To aid isotope excretion advise the patient to drink several glasses of water following the examination. No precautions are necessary when disposing of the urine.

Tomogram

Explanation

This is an x-ray designed to show detailed images of structures in a selected plane of tissue by manipulating the focal length of the exposure and blurring the images of structures in all other planes.

Patient Teaching, Preparation, and Nursing Implications

No preparation is required; this is similar to having a regular x-ray.

ELECTRODIAGNOSIS

Electromyography (EMG)

Explanation

Electromyography is most useful for diagnosis and documentation of neuromuscular diseases. It evaluates the physiology of the nerve roots for lower motor neuron dysfunction. It does not evaluate sensory or upper motor neuron abnormalities. A small needle with an electrode is inserted into the muscle that is to be evaluated, then electrical activity is recorded at rest and with stimulation. Duration, amplitude, and number of phases of the voluntary motor unit are recorded.

Patient Teaching, Preparation, and Nursing Implications

Explain the procedure to the patient. Many patients complain of pain at the needle insertions site as well as when the muscle is stimulated.

Nerve Conduction Studies

Explanation

Nerve conduction studies measure the speed at which nerve impulses travel. They can differentiate peripheral neuropathy from a central problem.

Patient Teaching, Preparation, and Nursing Implications

Explain to the patient that a recording electrode will be placed over the muscle supplied by the nerve being studied or at a measured distance along the nerve from the point of stimulation. The time it takes from stimulation to response is recorded. Velocities are generally low in persons with poorly controlled diabetes, in long-term dialysis patients, and in patients who have polyneuritis resulting from any of a variety of other causes. Focal slowing of median nerve velocity across the wrist or of the ulnar velocity across the elbow is good evidence of entrapment neuropathy at those locations (Tilkian, 1987, p. 476).

Somatosensory Evoked Potentials (SSEPs)

Explanation

SSEP measures the sensory component of the nerve and is useful in the diagnosis of spinal stenosis. It is most frequently used intraoperatively on patients with scoliosis and major spine reconstructive surgery. It insures that the sensory nerve component is not being adversely effected by the surgery.

Evoked potentials are defined as electrical responses to sensory stimulation. The spinal evoked potential is transmitted through the dorsal column and is mediated by large myelinated fibers which are sensitive to both mechanical compression and ischemia. For testing with somatosensory evoked potentials the technique involves stimulation of a peripheral nerve, e.g., posterior tibial or median, with the signal being picked up by scalp electrodes in preset locations on the sensory cortex and recorded by microprocessor (Herkowitz, 1988 p. 14).

Computerized Tomography (CT)

Explanation

CT scan provides computerized analysis of the variance in absorption of a radiologic beam, and therefore provides visualization of a plane of soft and dense tissue. Sagittal, transverse, and coronal planes can be visualized. The procedure is noninvasive and is usually done on an outpatient basis. Sometimes contrast media is employed to improve visualization.

Patient Teaching, Preparation, and Nursing Implications

Explain the procedure to the patient and explain that the patient will lie on an x-ray table that will move in the middle of a circular piece of x-ray equipment. The patient should be instructed to lie still and breathe normally (Tilkian, 1987). Patients are sometimes given tranquilizers prior to the procedure to allay anxiety and to help the patient remain still during the procedure. All jewelry and metal should be removed to avoid obscuring the image. Additional preparation depends on whether or not a contrast media is employed. Instructions for each media should be available from the hospital radiology department.

Magnetic Resonance Imaging (MRI)

Explanation

With MRI, images are created by radio waves absorbed and remitted from protons rotating about their axis in a magnetic field. It is a very sensitive indicator of water content and is especially useful in diagnosing tumors. The test is usually noninvasive, but a contrast media (gadolinum) may be used to evaluate certain conditions.

Patient Teaching, Preparation, and Nursing Implications

No metal materials may be present; all jewelry must be removed. Patients with metal clips and/or implants may not be suitable for MRI and may need to be evaluated on an individual basis. The reasons for the procedure and a description of the MRI cylinder should be given. Tranquilizers may be given to allay anxiety and help the patient remain still. It should be noted that some patients become claustrophobic during the scan and patient teaching may need to include relaxation or other techniques to help the patient.

Myelography

Explanation

Myelography is the radiologic viewing of the spinal cord through the injection of a radiopaque medium into the intrathecal space. Although newer noninvasive studies have replaced the myelogram, it remains the gold standard for diagnosing spinal stenosis and herniated disc. Metrizamide, a water soluble nonionic contrast agent, is the most commonly used contrast media, although the newer contrast mediums, Iohexol (Omnipaque) or Iopamidol (Isovue), may replace it. Pantopaque, which is oil based, may be used when a pathological condition in the cervical or upper dorsal spine is suspected as it is easier to prevent this material from

going up into the cerebral subarachnoid space (Tilkian, 1987).

Patient Teaching, Preparation, and Nursing Implications

Explain the reasons for the test and how the contrast medium is injected. The physician should have explained the myelogram prior to obtaining consent; therefore this should be a review. The contrast material is most easily injected if space between vertebrae is maximized. This is most commonly done by having the patient lie on the side and hold the knees to the chest until the injecting catheter is in place in the lumbar subarachnoid space. Patients who are unable to assume this position may sit with legs extended on the table and the chest leaning over a bedside table, or the technician may need to improvise a position that maximizes the vertebral space, yet minimizes patient discomfort. Drapes are avoided as the physician must view landmarks in order to locate the correct space.

The patient should fast for 4 hours prior to the myelogram. The nurse must also be sure that no phenothiazine is administered for 24 hours before and 24 hours after the metrizamide myelogram.

Patients with previous anaphylactic reactions to iodine must be screened and referred instead for MRI. To prevent allergic reaction patients who are allergic to iodine, but have not had anaphylactic reactions, may be given steroids prior to the metrizamide iodine myelogram (Herkowitz, 1988, p. 10).

Following a water soluble contrast myelogram the patient should rest in a semi-Fowlers position (the head must be kept above 40°) for 8 to 12 hours. This is done to prevent the dye from traveling up to the cerebral subarachnoid space. Patients should be instructed to force fluids for 24 hours following myelography. This may decrease the chance of developing a post-myelogram headache.

Fifty percent of patients undergoing water soluble myelography have untoward side effects. The most common side effect is headache, followed by nausea and vomiting, and (very rarely) hallucinations and/or seizures.

When oil based dyes are employed (Pantopaque), the patient should remain flat for 4 hours. If a headache develops the patient must remain flat for another 12 to 24 hours.

Arthrogram

Explanation

This is an x-ray of a joint in multiple positions after air or contrast media is injected. This allows soft tissues to be more easily visualized.

Patient Teaching, Preparation, and Nursing Implications

The patient is given local anesthesia for the procedure and should not feel pain, though some patients complain of pain and/or stiffness following the exam. Question the patient about allergies; patients with allergies to local anesthetic, iodine, seafood, or dyes used for diagnostic tests are not candidates for arthrogram.

appendix f

Prices of Commonly Used Orthopaedic Radiologic Studies[a]

X-rays (plain films)		
Spine series	Entire spine	$229.00
	Cervical spine	$ 59.00
	Cervical spine 4 views	$ 86.00
	Trauma cervical spine	$122.00
	Cervical flexion	$108.00
	Thoracic spine	$ 59.00
	Thoracic spine 3 views	$ 70.00
	Spine scoliosis	$114.00
	Spine scoliosis 4 views	$142.00
	Lumbar sacral spine	$ 59.00
	Lumbar sacral 4 views	$116.00
	Lumbar sacral bending	$ 79.00
	Lumbar spine plus pelvis	$171.00
	Sacroiliac joints	$ 59.00
	Sacroiliac joints	$ 79.00
	Sacrum-cocci	$ 59.00
Chest	1 view	$ 59.00
	2 views	$ 63.00
	3 views	$ 77.00
	4 views	$ 79.00
		$ 79.00
Pelvis	Multiple views	$115.00
Hip		$ 79.00
Femur		$ 59.00
Lower leg		$ 59.00
Knee	1 to 2 views	$ 43.00
	3 views	$ 65.00
Ankle	1 to 2 views	$ 51.00
	3 views	$ 65.00
Foot	1 view	$ 43.00
	3 views	$ 65.00
Toe		$ 43.00
Clavicle		$ 43.00
Scapula		$ 59.00
Shoulder	1 view	$ 43.00
	3 views	$ 63.00
Forearm		$ 43.00
Humerus		$ 59.00
Elbow	1 to 2 views	$ 43.00
	3 to 4 views	$ 59.00
	5 views	$ 68.00
Wrist	1 to 2 views	$ 43.00
	3 views	$ 59.00
	5 views	$ 68.00
Hand	1 view	$ 43.00
	3 views	$ 59.00
Fingers		$ 43.00
Tomogram		$181.00

Prices of Commonly Used Orthopaedic Radiologic Studies—*Continued*

Enhanced films		
Bone scan		$196.00
Bone scan (multiple)		$282.00
Bone scan (total body)		$362.00
Joint image (limited)		$149.00
Joint image (multiple)		$282.00
Limited bone absorption		$ 76.00
Scan limited body		$190.00
Scan whole body		$355.00
Bone marrow		$284.00
Myelography	Lumbar	$234.00
	Dorsal cervical	$234.00
	Entire spine	$656.00
Discography		$179.00
Computerized Tomography		
Body enhanced		$569.00
Body unenhanced		$546.00
Body combined		$605.00
Head enhanced		$427.00
Head unenhanced		$384.00
Head combined		$547.00
Arthrography		
Arthrogram of elbow, wrist, hip,		$ 64.00
knee, knee, or ankle		
Magnetic Resonance Imaging (MRI)		
Upper extremity		$649.00
Lower extremity		$644.00
Chest		$677.00
Pelvis		$655.00
Spine		$683.00
Spinal cord cervical		$694.00
Spinal canal thoracic		$694.00
Brain and brain stem		$655.00
Electromyography (EMG)		$ 46.00
Thermography		
Lumbar		$178.00
Cervical		$178.00

[a]Prices listed are prices from a medium size Philadelphia teaching hospital and do not include the radiologist's fee for examining the images.

appendix g

Transcutaneous Nerve Stimulation (TENS)

General Description

TENS units are small, battery operated electrical pulse generators used to help control pain. An electrical current is applied to the skin via electrodes attached to the generator. This current stimulates peripheral nerves, thereby modulating pain sensation. The generator controls electrical output, frequency, and duration. Although TENS units are used for many different chronic pain problems and occasionally for acute pain, the most common use is for controlling chronic low back pain.

There are two methods of delivering the stimulation: conventional high frequency with continuous stimulation or low frequency with the TENS delivered in bursts. The burst mode uses a frequency of 2 to 4 cycles/second with a train of impulses, usually 7 per burst (McQuarrine, 1988).

Many units can be switched from one mode to the other. The mode used is determined by which mode works more successfully for the patient. The conventional mode is tried first. Pain relief may be immediate or may occur after a few weeks of use. The relief may last only when the unit is turned on or it may last for hours and even days after using the unit.

Applying the Unit

With the unit turned off the electrodes are placed over or proximal to the painful area. If pregelled pads are not used, gel must be applied to the pads prior to utilization. The pads may be taped in place if necessary. Once applied the current is slowly adjusted so that maximum pain relief with minimum discomfort is achieved.

appendix h
Cast Care

SYNTHETIC (FIBERGLASS AND PLASTIC) CASTS

The fiberglass cast obtains maximum hardness immediately after application, therefore molding (unwanted shaping, dents, or depressions) during the drying process is not a problem. The patient need not avoid resting the cast on hard surfaces after application.

Weight bearing may begin immediately.

The fiberglass cast may be cleaned with mild soap and a damp cloth. Water on the outside of the cast will not harm it. However, water on the inside of the cast may lead to moldiness and/or skin irritation. To avert any possible skin irritation or infection, advise the patient that the cast should stay dry. If the cast becomes wet a blow dryer set on low may be used to expedite the drying process.

PLASTER CASTS

A plaster cast dries in 24 to 72 hours. Smaller casts such as a child's arm cast will dry in 24 hours, larger casts such as an adult body cast may take up to 72 hours. During the drying process the cast must be positioned to prevent unwanted molding or depressions. Weight bearing must be avoided. Warn the patient that the cast will feel warm when "setting." Until the cast is completely dry, avoid placing it on plastic or other waterproof pillows, as these materials trap heat and condensation may occur. The resulting damp cast will not "set" properly.

After the cast is dry the rough edges may be petaled to prevent skin irritation. To petal a cast, cut 4 inch lengths of 2 inch wide moleskin, adhesive, or silk tape, rounding the cut edges. Place one-half of the strip under the cast, firmly sticking it to the inside of the cast. Bring the remaining end over the edge to the outside of the cast (keeping the tape smooth and taut to avoid wrinkles). Continue to apply petals around the edge of the cast overlapping each piece over the previous one.

The cast may be "cleaned" by using a large eraser to remove marks; white shoe polish may be used to cover marks. Avoid covering the entire cast with polish as it needs to "breathe."

GENERAL CAST CARE AND PATIENT TEACHING

Prior to cast application, baseline neurovascular status and skin integrity should be assessed and documented. Following application of the cast neurovascular status is reassessed. The patient should be instructed how to assess the neurovascular status. Instruct the patient to report any adverse change in this status and to report if the cast is rubbing or otherwise uncomfortable. Following cast application, an x-ray is required to verify proper positioning.

Additional patient instructions include:

(1) Elevate the injured extremity whenever possible (ideally above the heart).
(2) Call the practitioner if the cast is damaged and needs repair, if it has become too loose or rubs, if the cast develops an odor, if a fever develops, or if there is an increase in pain.
(3) Avoid inserting *anything* into the cast, including lotion, powders, backscratchers, or liquids.
(4) Maintain the integrity of the cast. Do not chip, break, crush, or otherwise mutilate the cast.

(5) Keep the skin near the plaster cast's edges clean by using rubbing alcohol.
(6) Immediately report any sign of new bleeding inside the cast or seepage to the outside.

The patient should be provided with a written record of exercises, weight bearing limits, instructions for cleaning the cast, a list of cast dos and don'ts, and the phone number of a resource person to call with questions or problems (see Appendix K).

Ambulatory Assistive Devices

AMBULATORY ASSISTIVE DEVICES

Most people whose mobility is restricted because of lower extremity impairment require some type of ambulatory assistive device. The selection of the appropriate device depends primarily on the injury, the patient's physical strengths and limitations, the degree of weight bearing allowed, and the patient's coordination.

Outpatient education and instruction are necessary to prevent both real and potential patient mobility problems associated with the use of ambulatory assistive devices. This section will:

(1) Describe the methods used to ensure proper measurement of axillary crutches, walkers, and canes.
(2) Describe and demonstrate the proper techniques used to arise from a seated position using axillary crutches and walkers.
(3) Describe and demonstrate the proper techniques used to sit down using axillary crutches and walkers.
(4) Describe and demonstrate the swing-to and swing-through three point gaits using axillary crutches.
(5) Describe and demonstrate the proper ambulatory technique using a walker.
(6) Describe and demonstrate the proper ambulatory technique using a cane.
(7) Describe and demonstrate the proper techniques used to ascend stairs using axillary crutches, walkers, and canes.
(8) Describe and demonstrate the proper techniques used to descend stairs using axillary crutches, walkers, and canes.
(9) Identify safety concerns and tips nec-

essary to promote optimal mobility using ambulatory assistive devices.

Throughout this section on ambulatory assistive devices, references will be made to the partial weight bearing and non-weight bearing patient. A partial weight bearing patient may place *some* weight on the affected limb when ambulating. The non-weight bearing patient uses only his *unaffected* limb and assistive device to ambulate. No weight is placed on the affected limb.

AXILLARY CRUTCHES

Proper Measurement

When checking a pair of crutches for proper fit, it is crucial that there be a hands-breadth between the top pad on the crutch and the patient's axilla. Encourage patients to avoid leaning or placing their body weight on the top of the crutches. Sustained pressure on the radial, ulnar, and median nerves can lead to crutch paralysis.

The patient should be able to flex the elbows comfortably at approximately 20° while bearing weight on the padded hand bars of the crutches. Adjustment of the hand bars should allow for this flexion.

Arising from a Seated Position

Seemingly simple tasks such as sitting and standing can become monumental tasks for the person using an ambulatory assistive device. To rise from a seated position using axillary crutches, have the patient slide forward in the chair. The leg on the unaffected side should be placed firmly on the floor slightly underneath the chair. Holding onto the chair's armrest on the unaffected side and the hand bars of both crutches with the other hand, encourage the patient to push the body upward into a standing position. Once erect, one crutch may be shifted to the other arm.

Sitting Down

Have the patient stand with the back to the chair in which the patient would like to sit (preferably a chair with two armrests). The patient should be close enough to the chair so that the back of the *unaffected* leg touches the chair. Both crutches are then placed under the arm on the *unaffected* side. Holding onto the hand bars of the crutches with one hand, have the patient reach back and grasp the armrest on the affected side and slowly lower the body into a sitting position.

Ambulating

When ambulating with crutches, two types of gaits necessitate consideration: the swing-to and the swing-through. For the non-weight bearing patient, the swing-to gait is the gait of choice, at least initially until the patient is able to master balancing.

Swing-to Gait

The patient who is able to bear weight should be instructed to place both crutches securely on the floor approximately 1 foot in front of the body. With the elbows slightly bent, and bearing weight on the hand bars (not the axilla) have the patient propel or swing both feet up to but not beyond the location of the crutches. The cycle then repeats; both crutches are placed approximately 1 foot ahead, then both feet are propelled to a point up to, but not beyond, the placement of the crutches. The non-weight bearing patient should place weight on the unaffected limb only.

Swing-Through

Once adept at the swing-to gait, the patient may progress to the swing-through gait. The swing-through gait is the most vigorous gait in terms of energy expendi-

ture, but it also provides the most rapid means of ambulation.

The swing-through gait is similar to the swing-to gait, but as the name implies, the swing-through gait requires that the patient propel the feet *beyond* the placement of the crutches. Have the patient (non-weight bearer) move both crutches approximately 1 foot forward. While bearing weight on the hand bars of the crutch (not the axilla), have the patient step through or swing-through with the legs to a point approximately 8 to 12 inches beyond the previously positioned crutches. The non-weight bearer should place weight only on the *unaffected* limb.

Negotiating Stairs

Negotiating stairs may seem an impossible task for an individual with axillary crutches. However, going up and down stairs may be accomplished easily and safely when using the proper technique. A good rule to remember is *up* with the *good* and *down* with the *bad*.

Ascending Stairs

To ascend stairs with hand railings, have the patient position both crutches on the *unaffected* side opposite the railing. With the hand on the affected side, have the patient grasp the railing. Using the crutches on the *unaffected* side and the hand railing for support, the patient should swing the *unaffected* leg up to the next stair, followed by the affected leg and crutches. For stairs without hand railings, both crutches are used for support, the good leg is brought up to the next stair, followed by the affected leg and crutches. The patient who is able to partially bear weight should follow the same sequence.

Descending Stairs

When descending stairs remember *up* with the *good* and *down* with the *bad*. Have the patient place both crutches into position on the *unaffected* side opposite the railing on the stairs. Grasping the railing on the affected side, have the patient lower the crutches and the affected leg to the stair below, followed by the *unaffected* leg. For stairs without railings, both crutches are used for support, one on each side. The sequence is the same for the patient who is able to partially bear weight.

WALKERS

A walker may be used for either the full or partial weight bearer. It is considered a stable walking device. To ensure optimal efficiency of the device with the least amount of strain on the patient, it is necessary to assess proper fit.

Proper Measurement

To adjust the walker size for each patient, have the patient stand "inside" the walker. The hand grips should be at the level of the greater trochanter of the hip allowing for a 15 to 20° flexion at the elbow. If the height is not accurate, adjust the walker accordingly. Once assured of proper walker height for the patient, it is time to help the patient gain independence in mobility.

Standing from a Seated Position

To rise from a seated position, place the walker directly in front of the seated patient and have the patient slide to the chair's edge. The *unaffected* leg should be flexed slightly under the chair. Have the patient rise by grasping both armrests on the chair, pushing up by using the strength of the arms and the *unaffected* leg. With the hand on the *unaffected* side first, have the patient grasp the walker. Next, instruct the patient to release the grip on the chair's armrest with the other hand, and grasp the walker with this hand as well. The patient should shift this body weight forward to the strong or *unaffected* limb and into an erect position. Do not allow the patients to use the walker to pull themselves up.

Sitting Down

To assist the client into a sitting position, encourage the use of chairs of average height, preferably with armrests. Have the patient stand with the back to the chair, making sure the *unaffected* leg touches the chair before the patient begins lowering the body into the chair. The patient should then reach back for the chair's armrest with the hand on the affected side. Releasing the other hand from the walker, the patient should grasp the chair's remaining armrest and, leaning forward, slowly lower the body into the chair.

Ambulating

To begin ambulation, instruct the patient to advance the walker approximately 8 to 10 inches. The patient places the weight on the hands, steps into the walker with the affected leg, and then follows through with the *unaffected* leg. The cycle continues as the patient advances the walker, bears weight using the hands and *unaffected* extremity, steps into the walker with his affected leg, and then with the *unaffected* leg.

Negotiating Stairs

Negotiating stairs with a walker is more complex than with axillary crutches. Walkers are larger and more awkward. As with all ambulatory assistive devices, a thorough assessment of the patient and the home environment is necessary. Assess the patient's home environment for the presence of stair railings. Walkers are available for use in homes without railings but they are rarely used because of their awkward size in relation to most steps. In homes where railings exist, or a relative or friend is able to carry the walker to the destination (up or down stairs), it is recommended that the patient use the stair railing rather than the walker.

Descending Stairs

To descend the stairs, have the patient grasp the railing with one or both hands. Have the patient descend one stair at a time beginning with the affected limb, then the *unaffected* limb. If the patient must carry the walker while descending the stairs, have the patient grasp the stair railing with one hand and place the folded walker on the next stair down. Grasping the top of the walker, the patient should then descend the stairs slowly, the affected foot first, followed by the *unaffected* foot.

Ascending Stairs

To ascend the stairs, the patient should first grasp the railing with one or both hands. Using the railing for leverage, the patient should ascend the stairs, the *unaffected* leg first, followed by the affected leg. If the patient must carry the walker while ascending the stairs, have the patient fold the walker according to the directions. Grasping the hand railing with one hand, and placing the folded walker on the next stair up, have the patient grasp the top of the walker with the free hand and advance to the next stair, the *unaffected* foot first, followed by the affected foot. The sequence is then repeated.

CANES

Canes are another ambulatory assistive device often used in ambulation for balance, security, and support. Additionally, canes function to help absorb the body weight for those who are partial weight bearers. Canes may be used unilaterally or bilaterally depending on the patient's needs. Canes may be triangular or quadrangular based to provide greater support.

Proper Measurement

Metallic canes are adjustable; wood canes may be cut to size. The proper length should allow the patient approximately 20 to 30° flexion at the elbow.

Ambulating

The cane is held in the hand on the *unaffected* side. When ambulating, the patient should move the cane in conjunction with the affected leg. The *unaffected* leg is then brought forward. The patient's body weight and level of balance are maintained with the cane.

Negotiating Stairs

Negotiating stairs using a cane is accomplished by reapplying the *up* with the *good*, *down* with the *bad* rule.

Descending Stairs

To descend stairs, the cane is placed in the hand on the *unaffected* or uninvolved side. Grasping the stair railing on the affected side, the patient should move the cane down one stair. The patient then steps down with the affected limb followed by the *unaffected* limb. Remember *up* with the *good*, *down* with the *bad*.

Ascending Stairs

To ascend stairs, the cane is placed in the hand on the *unaffected* side. Grasping the stair railing on the affected side, the patient should move the *unaffected* leg up the stair, followed by the affected leg.

SAFETY TIPS

Shoes

Have the patient wear flat shoes, with approximately a one-half inch heel. The sole of the shoes should be a nonskid surface. Shoes that strap on are safer than loafers or slip-ons, which are apt to "slip-off."

Device

The rubber suction tip(s) on the bottom of the ambulatory assistive devices, as well as the hand grips, should be checked for secure fit, cracks, or uneven wear.

Environment

All potential obstructions should be removed from the floor to ensure safe passage. Throw rugs, electrical cords, and telephone cords are especially hazardous. Optimal lighting (without excessive glare) should be provided. The room should be arranged so items that are used frequently should be placed in close proximity to the patient.

Stairs

Have someone stand behind the patient when the patient is first learning to ascend stairs, and beside or in front of the patient as the stairs are descended for the first time.

The editors would like to acknowledge Joyce Lichtenstein, M.S.N., for preparation of this Appendix.

appendix j
Anabolic Steroids

The use of anabolic steroids by athletes has become increasingly prevalent. These steroids cause an increase in muscle mass and strength, an increase in body weight, and heightened aggression resulting in improved athletic performance. However, these benefits are balanced by many adverse side effects. Possible long-term side effects include hypertension, liver dysfunction, atherosclerosis, changes in cholesterol, cysts of the spleen, premature aging, and sexual and reproductive disorders. Short-term effects include shrunken testicles, enlarged prostate, reproductive and sexual disorders, and hair loss. In addition, the anabolic steroids are associated with psychotic symptoms (Pope and Katz, 1988). The strong possibility of adverse effects and the strong potential for abuse determine that the use of anabolic steroids in athletes is not sanctioned by the pharmaceutical manufacturers or the FDA. In order to protect athletes, athletic committees, such as the International Olympic Committee, have rules clearly stating that their use is illegal.

Despite the sanctions against anabolic steroids and the potential harm that they may cause, many athletes are willing to gamble for the (possible) lucrative careers, fame, and glory of a great athletic performance. Coaches, trainers, and medical practitioners have also been known to encourage the use of steroids.

Anabolic steroids, such as Stanozolol, are legally prescribed by physicians for medical conditions such as angioedema, but are often prescribed for nonmedical purposes. Anabolic steroids are also readily available to athletes from mail order companies.

Nurses working with athletes need to be aware of the signs and symptoms of anabolic steroid abuse. The most evident sign is a gain in muscle mass and weight. Comparing how the patient appeared a year previously to the present appearance may give some clues. An athlete can gain 15 to 25 pounds of muscle in a 12-week cycle of steroids and training. Another clue is the athlete's performance, especially if there have been drastic improvements in an unexpectedly short period of time. The nurse can look for some of the adverse side effects listed; in addition the athlete can be asked about steroid use and the urine may be tested if the patient consents. (The reference by D.R. Lamb, 1984, is highly recommended.)

appendix k[a]

Patient Information Checklist: Name   Date

1. Rehabilitation: Ice _____, Heat _____, 3 sets of Ten _____, Elevation _____
2. General Exercises: Swimming _____, Walking _____
   Exercise Bike Riding: Easy to Pedal _____/Outdoor Bike-Level Ground _____
3. Ankle Exercises: Towel _____, Table Leg _____, Alphabet _____, Toe & Heel Walking _____,
   Up and Down _____
4. Knee Exercises: Straight Leg Raises _____, Quad Sets _____, Straight Leg Raises With Weights _____,
   Active, Assisted Range of Motion _____, Leg Extensions _____, Leg Curls _____, Lateral Step Ups _____
5. Back Exercise: Pelvic Tilts _____, Knee to Chest _____, Other _____
6. Wrist Exercises: Up & Down _____, In & Out _____, Over & Under _____
7. Shoulder Exercise: Circles _____, Broomstick (Cane) _____, Rotator Cuff _____, Wall Climb _____/
   Neck Exercises: Range of Motion _____, Isometrics _____
8. Iliotibial Band Stretch _____, Heel Cord Stretch _____
9. Hamstring Stretch _____, Quadriceps Stretch _____
10. Crutch Instruction: _____, Cane or 1 Crutch (Opposite Hand) _____, 2 Crutch, 1 Crutch or Cane
    (Opposite Hand), No Crutch _____
11. Medication: _____, Number Given _____
    Number Refills _____, Side Effects Sheet _____, Samples Given _____
12. Instructional Pamphlets: _____, With Exercises _____
13. Cast Care Booklet _____, Instructions: _____
14. Infection Information _____
15. Physical Therapy _____
    Occupational Therapy _____, IUP _____, Other _____
16. No Work _____, No School _____, No Gym _____, Modified Gym Class _____
17. Date to Return to Work: Full Duty _____, Light Duty _____, Disabled _____
18. Date to Return to Gym _____, Sports _____, School _____
19. Date to Return to Physician's Office: _____

20. Miscellaneous: _____
_____
_____
_____
_____

21. Signature of Office Personnel: _____
22. I the undersigned have read the above instructions and understand them as
    given to me by: _____

    Patient Signature: _____

    Telephone (_____)

[a]Adapted from Clifford W. Smith, BSED, RN, ONC, Patient Information Checklist 1988.

appendix 1

Ideal Body Weight (in Pounds)[a]

Nonmetric Height		Men: Acceptable Weight Range		Women: Acceptable Weight Range	
		Low	High	Low	High
ft	*in*				
4	10			92	119
4	11			94	122
5	0			96	125
5	1			99	128
5	2	112	141	102	131
5	3	115	144	105	134
5	4	118	148	108	138
5	5	121	152	111	142
5	6	124	156	114	146
5	7	128	161	118	150
5	8	132	166	122	154
5	9	136	170	126	158
5	10	140	174	130	163
5	11	144	179	134	168
6	0	148	184	138	173
6	1	152	189		
6	2	156	194		
6	3	160	199		
6	4	164	204		

[a] Adapted from Wyngaarden JB, Smith LH: *Cecil's Textbook of Medicine*, Philadelphia, WB Saunders, 1985.

appendix m

Recommended Dietary Intake

Basic Four Guidelines and Values

Basic Four Category	Servings	Foods	Nutrients
Fruits and vegetables	4		Carbohydrate
		Citrus fruits Berries Melons Tomatoes	Vitamin C Fiber

		Dark Green Vegetables
		  Broccoli
		  Peas
		  Kale
			Vitamin A
			Calcium
			Fiber

		Deep Yellow Fruits and
		Vegetables
		  Apricots
		  Carrots
		  Winter squash
		  Peaches
		  Cantaloupe
			Vitamin A
			Fiber

		Cruciferous Vegetables
		  Cabbage
		  Broccoli
		  Cauliflower
		  Brussel sprouts
		  Rutabaga
			Vitamin C
			Fiber

Grains and cereals	4		Carbohydrate

		Breads
		  Especially whole wheat
		  products as increase
		  nutrient density and fiber
		Breakfast cereals
		Macaroni
			Vitamin B
			  Thiamin
			  Riboflavin
			  Niacin
			Fiber

Milk and Dairy	2 to 4		Protein Fat

		Milk
		  Skim and low-fat preferred
		  Cheese
		  Yogurt
		  Custards
			Calcium
			Vitamin D

Protein	2		Protein Fat

		Legumes
		  Economic source
		Peanut butter
		  Economic source
		Fish
		Poultry
		Lean Meats
			Iron
			Zinc
			Riboflavin

Basic Four Food Groups

Group	Daily Serving	One Serving (at 1200 cal/day)
Dairy	2	1 c milk 1 c yogurt 1½ oz cheese 2 c cottage cheese 1 c pudding
Meats	2	2 oz cooked lean meat, fish, or poultry 2 eggs 2 oz hard cheese ½ c cottage cheese 1 c cooked dried beans or peas 4 tbsp peanut butter
Fruit and Vegetables	4	½ c juice ½ c cooked fruit or vegetable 1 medium size fruit
Grains	4	1 slice bread 1 c cold cereal ½ c cooked cereal ½ c pasta, grits, or rice

Calcium and Caloric Content of Foods[a]

Food	Measure	Calories	Calcium mg
Cheese			
Cheddar	1 oz	115	204
Mozarella (skim)	1 oz	80	207
American (process)	1 oz	105	174
Swiss	1 oz	105	272
Cottage Cheese			
Lowfat (2%)	1 cup	205	155
Creamed	1 cup	235	135
Milk			
Skim	1 cup	85	302
1% fat	1 cup	100	300
2% fat	1 cup	120	297
Whole dry, nonfat, instant	1 cup	150	291
	¼ cup	61	209
Yogurt			
Plain, lowfat	8 oz	145	415
Fruit flavored	8 oz	230	345
Seafood			
Shrimp	3 oz	100	98
Salmon, canned	3 oz	120	167
Oysters	1 cup	160	226
Sardines	3 oz	175	371
Vegetables			
Bok choy	1 cup	9	74
Broccoli	1 spear	40	72
Collards	1 cup	60	357
Turnip greens	1 cup	50	249
Soy beans	1 cup	235	131

[a]Adapted from NIH guidelines. Osteoporosis: Cause, Treatment, Prevention, *Orthop Nurs* 5(6), 36–37.

appendix n

Nursing Care Plan for Patients with Rheumatoid Arthritis and Osteoarthritis[a]

Alteration in comfort related to joint stiffness and swelling

Goal:

Patient will experience partial or total relief of pain and decrease in inflammation.

Nursing interventions:

Teach methods for pain control. Teach patient and family members in the proper administration of pain and NSAID medication. Instruct in the application of cold packs 20 minutes $\times$ 3/day or warm moist compresses 20 minutes $\times$ 3/day.

Evaluate patient's understanding of the instructed material by reviewing medication dosing and side effects at each office visit. Have the patient demonstrate application of pain reduction modalities.

Impaired physical mobility related to pain of swollen joints

Goal:

Patient will maintain functional positions and optimum joint mobility with no further joint injury or deformity.

Nursing interventions:

Teach methods to maintain functional status. Warm baths or showers, ROM $3 \times$/day, application of splints, strengthening and endurance exercises as tolerated, frequent change of position, use of assistive devices and equipment for ambulation as necessary, arrange living areas to insure safety.

Evaluate mobility at each office visit.

Self-Care deficit

Feeding, bathing, dressing, toileting as related to impaired physical movement.

Goal:

Patients will demonstrate increased ability to perform independent activities of daily living.

Nursing interventions:

Assess level of function. Refer to occupational therapist, PRN, encourage increased ADL as tolerated. Assist patient in purchase and use of adaptive equipment as necessary. Arrange for home assistance (i.e., housekeeper, home health aid) as needed.

Evaluate functional level at each office visit. Modify the environment as indicated.

Disturbance in self-concept

Body image related to increased dependence secondary to physical limitation resulting from loss of joint function.

Goal:

Patient will adjust to chronic disease limitation and develop new means of enhancing a positive self-concept.

Nursing interventions:

Encourage patient to talk about the loss of health and self-esteem. Identify positive coping skills and accomplishments, encourage patient to participate in positive self-help behaviors (i.e., stress management), encourage patient to consider new activities and future goals, and refer to counselor PRN.

Evaluate at each office visit.

Health maintenance alteration

Goal:

Patient will have sufficient information to understand disease, indication for medication, exercise regimen, rest, joint protection, and community resources.

Nursing interventions:

Assess patient's present level of knowledge and receptiveness, provide information on disease process, exercise, medications, use of hot/cold, joint protection techniques, and community resources. Refer patient to local arthritis foundation.

Evaluate at each office visit and alter the regimen as necessary.

---

[a]The authors wish to acknowledge Wendy McBrain, B.S.N., for developing this nursing care plan.

Appendices References

Brassell M: Pharmacologic management of rheumatic diseases. *Orthop Nurs*, 7(2), 43–51, 1988.

Boothe R: Spinal stenosis. *Instructional Course Lectures*, Vol 35. St. Louis, CV Mosby, 1986, pp 420–435.

Clayton B: *Pharmacology in Nursing* 3rd ed. St. Louis, CV Mosby, 1984. Corrigan B, Maitland GD: *Practical Orthopaedic Medicine*. Boston, Butterworth, 1983.

Hamilton H, ed: *Nursing 87 Drug Handbook*. Springhouse, PA, Springhouse, 1987.

Hamilton H, ed: *Diagnostics*. Springhouse, PA, Springhouse, 1984.

Hamilton H, ed: *Procedures*. Springhouse, PA, Springhouse, 1983.

Herkowitz H: The radiologic and electrodiagnostic evaluation of spinal stenosis. In *Spinal Stenosis*. Philadelphia, Continental Press, 1988, pp 5–20.

McQuarrine A: Physical therapy. In Kiraldy-Willis WH (ed): *Managing Low Back Pain*. New York, Churchill Livingstone, 1988, pp 25–33.

Lamb DR: Anabolic steroids in athletics: how well do they work and how dangerous are they? *Am J Sports Med* 12(1), 31–38, 1984.

Miller R, Greenblatt D: *Handbook of Drug Therapy*. New York, Elsevier Inc, 1980.

Pope HG Jr, Katz DL: Affective and psychotic symptoms associated with anabolic steroid use. *Am J Psychiatry*, 145(4), 487–490, 1988.

Schoen D: Assessment for arthritis. *Orthop Nursing* 7(2), 31–39, 1988.

Stewart JD, Hallet JP: *Traction and Orthopedic Appliances*. New York, Churchill Livingstone, 1983.

Stedman TL: *Stedman's Medical Dictionary*. Baltimore, Williams & Wilkins, 1978.

Tilkian S, Conover M, Tilkian A: *Clinical Implications of Laboratory Tests* 4th ed. St. Louis, CV Mosby, 1987.

INDEX

Page numbers in *italics* denote figures; those followed by "t" denote tables.